Living with HIV and ARVs

Living with HIV and ARVs

Three-letter Lives

Corinne Squire
School of Law and Social Sciences, University of East London, UK

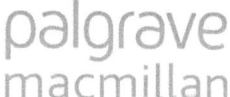

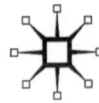

First published 2013 by
PALGRAVE MACMILLAN

Palgrave Macmillan in the UK is an imprint of Macmillan Publishers Limited, registered in England, company number 785998, of Houndmills, Basingstoke, Hampshire RG21 6XS.

Palgrave Macmillan in the US is a division of St Martin's Press LLC, 175 Fifth Avenue, New York, NY 10010.

Palgrave Macmillan is the global academic imprint of the above companies and has companies and representatives throughout the world.

Palgrave® and Macmillan® are registered trademarks in the United States, the United Kingdom, Europe and other countries.

ISBN: 978–0–230–28423–4

This book is printed on paper suitable for recycling and made from fully managed and sustained forest sources. Logging, pulping and manufacturing processes are expected to conform to the environmental regulations of the country of origin.

A catalogue record for this book is available from the British Library.

A catalog record for this book is available from the Library of Congress.

Contents

Acknowledgements

This book has benefited from discussions with many colleagues at the University of East London and in seminars and conferences in the UK and other European countries, Australia, the US, Canada, and South Africa. Centre for Narrative Research colleagues, especially Molly Andrews, Cigdem Esin, Maria Tamboukou, and our associate at Monash University, Mark Davis, have been unfailingly supportive. I have been able to pursue research and writing thanks to travel and sabbatical grants from the School of Law and Social Sciences, UEL, and from UEL's central sabbatical fund, for which I am very grateful. I was also lucky to conduct and later complete writing and editing with the help of visiting fellowships at the Sociology Department of McMaster University, Hamilton, Ontario, and at the Centre for Innovation in International Governance (CIGI), Waterloo, Ontario. I have gained a great deal of understanding from my discussions with UEL students studying HIV issues, to whom I am extremely grateful. In the UK, Harriet Anyangokolo, Rachel Stovold and Royce Clarke were committed and thoughtful research assistants. In South Africa, I am indebted to the work of Nondumiso Hlwele. My family and other friends, in particular Neil, Ruby, Mary and Simon, have been continuing sources of encouragement and sustenance. Without the research interviewees themselves, and all those others within HIV organisations who made the research possible, the book would, of course, have been impossible; I thank them for their openness, insightfulness and courage. The book is dedicated to the memory of James Hyde and Nomonde Khundayi.

Section 1

Living with HIV and ARVs
in the Treatment Possibility Era

1
Why the Three Letters Matter

This book is about living with the Human Immunodeficiency Virus, or HIV, and with anti-retroviral, or ARV, therapy, the combination of medications that helps HIV positive people to live long and healthy lives. Today, when ARV treatment is more and more available to those who need it, and is in prospect for those who do not yet have access, the two three-letter acronyms, HIV and ARV together, increasingly index people's experiences of the pandemic. The book examines lives lived with HIV and ARVs in different national contexts, primarily the United Kingdom and South Africa, where I have conducted interviews about HIV support with people living with HIV, since 1993 in the United Kingdom (most recently in 2011), and since 2001 in South Africa (most recently in 2012).

There have been dramatic improvements in people's access to treatment, and in their health and life expectancies, across the pandemic. In the United Kingdom, ARVs arrived in 1996. In South Africa, they began to be available in the early 2000s, though rollout has been fastest since 2009. The World Health Organisation (WHO) has made strong moves to encourage earlier treatment, to preserve HIV positive people's health so that illness does not compromise it before they start ARVs. South Africa is likely to join the United Kingdom in following these guidelines (World Health Organisation 2013). Annual HIV counselling and testing (HTC) became a universal expectation in South Africa in 2010, and it is an increasingly general part of primary health practice in the UK. Both countries are working to reduce HIV stigma and discrimination, with some success (UNAIDS 2012a). These hopeful characteristics of the two epidemics are reflected more broadly in suggestions within international HIV policy that the end of the HIV pandemic may be in sight, and in assumptions within some social research that, whatever the practical problems, the pandemic no longer poses important theoretical issues.

The major impetus for the book came from hearing my HIV positive research participants in both the United Kingdom and South Africa talk about the continuing difficulties of living three-letter lives. The interviews indicated that in many ways, despite positive indicators, the pandemic was very far from its end. HIV's naturalisation, that is, its incorporation into the natural order of people's lives, through processes of medicalisation, social normalisation and marketisation, seemed to be stalling, undoing itself, and leaving things out (Squire 2010). The interviews intimated that these difficulties derived partly from the global recession's impact on three-letter lives, and the problems of living with HIV alongside many other illnesses, and with socio-economic constraints. Other common difficulties were narrated around what it was like to be diagnosed, still a problematic moment although no longer a death sentence; telling and not telling people about being HIV positive, and their good and sometimes bad reactions; and the impact of HIV on children and relationships.

Some of the commonalities across the interviews were less obviously about problems, and more about the complex shape of HIV experiences. This complexity was emblematised in the clouds of other acronyms suffusing the interviews. 'HIV' itself, for instance, was a term sometimes used interchangeably with 'AIDS' (as happened frequently, earlier in the epidemic). 'ARVs' were described variously, across different national and socio-historical circumstances, as 'ART' (anti-retroviral therapy), 'HAART' (Highly Active Anti-Retroviral Therapy), or 'combination therapy'. I have used the term 'ARVs' throughout this book because it was deployed by the majority of interviewees across both South African and UK studies. Another three-letter (or more accurately, two-letters-and-a-number) acronym, the CD4 + T cell count, signalling immune activity, was used by interviewees to indicate levels of health before and while taking treatment, together with 'viral load' numbers. The many three-figure acronyms that hide behind or substitute for ARV brand or generic names, such as AZT (generic name, Zidovudine), D4T (generic name, Stavudine) and 3TC (generic name, Lamivudine), were regular currency within the interviews. Three-letter lives now also encompass newer, still-uncertain uses and outcomes of ARVs, similarly acronymised. TasP (Treatment As Prevention), PrEP (Pre-Exposure Prophylaxis) and PEP (Post-Exposure Prophylaxis) emblematise the acronymic optimism about treating away the pandemic expressed by many medical and policy organisations, though these acronyms, especially the first two, were used less often by interviewees themselves. The acronyms 'MTCT' or 'PMTCT', for mother to child transmission, or prevention of mother to child transmission, indicate programmes to prevent vertical transmission that involve giving ARVs to both mother and baby, and that interviewees, women interviewees particularly, often mentioned.

As with 'HIV' and 'ARV', other acronymic descriptions of the epidemic have changed over time. The acronym PWA, 'person with AIDS', developed, as Adam Mars-Jones' (1992) character in a story written early in the UK epidemic, 'Slim', puts it, to remind people that he was indeed a person, has been modified, as treatment has developed and people live with HIV rather than progressing to AIDS, to 'PLWHA' or 'person living with HIV/AIDS'. The call for VCT (voluntary counselling and testing) is now often superseded by emphasis on universal testing. The prevention mantra 'ABC', 'Abstain, Be faithful, Condomise', has given way to emphasis on condoms, circumcision, work to reduce risky sexual encounters, and ARV-based prevention, especially TasP. Treatment and prevention initiatives are now frequently related to another acronym, MDG 6 (Millennium Development Goal 6), which aims to provide universal treatment access and to reverse the spread of HIV by 2015 (United Nations 2013). UNAIDS's 'three zeroes' – the triad of zero deaths from AIDS, zero new HIV infections and zero HIV-related discrimination – have shaped many prevention and treatment campaigns since 2010 (UNAIDS 2010b). HIV citizenship, which takes in the ways that people living with HIV or affected by HIV define themselves, and act and campaign in their social worlds, is related to an acronym, this time of four letters: GIPA, the principle of Greater Involvement of People Living with or Affected By HIV/AIDS in all decisions made about them, which has been integral to international HIV policy since 1994 (UNAIDS 2007). Within specific national contexts, local acronyms play large roles in HIV citizenship, particularly those of service and activist organisations such as THT (Terrence Higgins Trust) in the UK, and the TAC (Treatment Action Campaign) in South Africa.

People do not live among all of these letters, all of the time. Moreover, many problematic elements of HIV experience are not acronymised. People who are HIV positive or otherwise affected by HIV and ARVs, however, do now tend to live with crowds of other acronyms as well. They navigate their way through these swirls of letters extremely effectively, and the letters themselves can be useful. They signify medical, social science and policy knowledge in condensed, appropriated and owned forms, without people having to be HIV clinicians, epidemiologists, virologists, behavioural scientists or policy experts in order to use them.

At the same time, acronyms can set up barriers for people who do not know what they mean. They can also create a sense of uncertainty among those who are HIV positive or HIV-affected themselves, even if they use them, because of doubts about what, exactly, they mean, what precisely is the expertise they impart, and what their own relationship is to that expertise. The perpetual recoinings of HIV acronyms testify to the struggles for the power of definition and knowledge conducted by people living with the condition, as well as by doctors, policymakers and activists.

It is medical, social and political shifts in addressing the pandemic that have made these particular sets of letters into powerful determinants of living with HIV. In 2008, the journalist Jonny Steinberg published a book about the difficulties South Africans were facing in getting tested for HIV and in accessing treatment. These difficulties arose not just from resource shortages, but also from competing belief systems, politically as well as culturally produced; concerns around social stigma and discrimination; and psychic conflicts, themselves the results of political and social as well as personal histories (Steinberg 2008). The book drew on interviews and encounters Steinberg had had in times and places where HIV was highly prevalent, mostly untreated, little talked about and usually fatal. In this book, called *Three Letter Plague* (*Sizwe's Test* in the United States), 'HIV' were the three letters referred to. In *Living with HIV and ARVs*, the arrays of letters framing the epidemic are multiple, ARVs are as important as HIV, treatment access is greatly improved, people have the potential for a long and healthy lifespan and stigma is reduced in high-prevalence situations (Zuch and Lurie 2012). Difficulties, including some of those described by Steinberg, remain (Abrahams and Jewkes 2012; Flowers et al. 2006; Zungu 2012). Nevertheless, *Living with HIV and ARVs* addresses the contemporary realities of the HIV pandemic as the difficulties of particular citizenly lives, rather than, as in Steinberg's book, which appeared just five years ago, the problems of living in the midst of a plague. And *Living with HIV and ARVs* focuses on two sets of letters, not one, on ARVs as well as HIV, since these two three-letter sets, taken together, have increasing salience.

One of the ways in which three letters can act is as a declaration. Just saying 'HIV', let alone saying 'I am living with HIV', makes an impact. But three letters can also be a kind of shorthand that evades the actualities of the condition, leaving behind its complexities and difficulties, especially when 'ARVs' are added to HIV, as if, by themselves, they constitute a solution. On the other hand, 'HIV' itself may be too much to say. There are many codes for HIV to avoid saying it. One is indeed the 'three-letter disease'. Others are expressions like 'this thing', 'this torturing disease', and in high-prevalence contexts, 'our disease'. The character in 'Slim' uses the eponymous term, first used to describe the illness in Africa, instead of 'AIDS', because it describes precisely what is happening to him, and plays ironically on the value attached to thinness in the West. This character also insists on his own terms for other aspects of HIV illness: 'blackcurrants', in place of Kaposi's Sarcoma lesions, for instance (Mars-Jones 1992: 10). His lexical creativity allows him to keep hold of his own bodily reality and at the same time to grasp broader control of a disease process that he cannot much affect, giving it his own meanings. Oscar Moore, describing two years of his 'life as an acronym', also sketches out the 'secret fraternity of sickness' which builds around the acronyms, conveying information, sympathy, rage and hope (1996: 3, 62). These are some of the more empowering functions that the slew of words, abbreviations and rhetorical play around HIV generates.

Different forms of expression appear, of course, around other difficult health conditions like cancer (Sontag 1988), but they have been especially prolific within the HIV pandemic. We learn from them that indirectness can be helpful in allowing people to approach HIV issues obliquely (Squire 2007). However, indirectness can also be problematic. It can allow, through its imprecision, associations between HIV and areas of meaning – such as sexuality, death and foreignness – that make it harder for people to understand HIV as an illness. In addition, with conditions like HIV, often characterised by privatised suffering and public silence, it can be very important for some people to talk openly and publicly, and for everyone to be able to talk openly in certain situations (Plummer 1995, 2001). Also, now that many people live with ARVs as well as HIV, the abjectification of HIV has diminished, so indirect ways of approaching it may be becoming less important (Abrahams and Jewkes 2012; Zuch and Lurie 2012).

At the same time, oblique strategies for approaching HIV continue, for a variety of reasons. People living with HIV and ARVs may have lived through a history of HIV as a 'death sentence' that does not leave them. Even those who became HIV positive more recently have heard about and imagine that history, which is also the present reality for perhaps 16 million people needing and not receiving treatment (World Health Organisation 2013; World Health Organisation/UNAIDS/UNICEF 2013). Such a history is also close to the present for people whose treatment is physically or psychologically difficult, or medically failing. An AIDS-free generation may be in sight, but it is not a reality even for the HIV positive people now also living with ARVs. And so acronyms remain important both as indirect strategies for addressing the difficulties of the pandemic and, paradoxically, as indices of optimism.

The material in this book derives primarily from research participant interviews about experiences, expectations and requirements of HIV support in South Africa and the United Kingdom. In the early chapters especially, the book draws, too, on policy and cultural narratives of HIV in the United Kingdom and South Africa, and at international levels. The book's material also comes from listening to HIV volunteers and paid workers in South Africa and the United Kingdom, who, regardless of their status, are all citizens of an HIV-affected, HIV-defined world to some degree, and who discussed many of the same issues as the research participants. In addition, much of the book draws on insights from students who have participated in my 'HIV in the world' module at the University of East London over the past five years, who themselves came from many different country contexts across the pandemic, particularly from sub-Saharan Africa and the Caribbean, and who raised many similar issues to the research participants.

Often, students on the HIV module will say that the current policy picture cannot be right, and the figures must be wrong. They talk about all the people they know back home who don't have free treatment available locally, who can't get to treatment, who can't afford the fees the clinics charge, who fear someone will see them in the clinic, who have never told anyone their test result or received any medical help after their diagnosis, or who, even now, have never gotten tested but have just accepted their illness and likely death. In all this, they are frequently more pessimistic than workers in the HIV field, who are implementing change and measuring improvements, or indeed than my research participants, who, despite their extensive knowledge and understanding of the difficulties of three-letter lives, are well connected to treatment and education services. My students know, or sometimes are themselves, such people. They also know, or in some instances are themselves, people who do not access HIV services, do not know about services, do not know and will not consider their own HIV status. The continuing and new forms of difficulty around living with HIV and ARVs thus show themselves here too, in the conversations of people with close but often incidental connections to the pandemic.

The many directions from which the difficulties, as well as the hopefulness, of contemporary three-letter lives appeared defined the shape of this book. The book starts from a general consideration of a possible end of HIV 'exceptionalism' and the beginning of a new 'particularity' about the pandemic. It continues by examining the different characteristics of HIV's contemporary naturalisation – its medicalisation, normalisation and marketisation – and how these characteristics at the same time denaturalise HIV. It then proceeds to explicate how HIV's particularities appear via its naturalisation and denaturalisation within two contemporary epidemics, in the United Kingdom and South Africa. In doing so, the book tries to describe and understand the new forms of HIV citizenship that are being articulated and performed within the current context of three-letter lives.

Chapter 2 in the book's first section, 'Living with HIV in the treatment possibility era', is called 'From HIV's exceptionalism to HIV's particularity'. It examines contemporary lives lived with HIV and ARVs in the context of medical, social and political gains within the HIV pandemic which promise to turn it into an everyday, rather than an exceptional, condition. It poses the 'acronym' optimism associated with this move away from exceptionalism against continuing medical, social and political difficulties around HIV, as well as difficulties in the arena of personal beliefs and feelings. All of these difficulties still have powerful effects on the pandemic and contribute to what the chapter calls its particularity. Chapter 2 goes on to describe the narrative approach to living with HIV and ARVs which I take in studying HIV support in the UK and South Africa, which allows for the particularities of lives within the pandemic to be registered. The chapter also describes how such studies, focused on the social, historical and personal particularities of epidemic contexts, may allow for transfer or translation of understandings across contexts.

Section 2, 'Being naturalised, being left behind', examines the ways in which HIV has become part of everyday life, and the extent to which it has not, drawing both on my research studies, from the perspectives of people living with and affected by HIV, and on policy statements, professional position papers, corporate representations and the discourses of HIV-related NGOs.

Chapter 3, 'Being naturalised', discusses ways in which the pandemic is becoming naturalised, made to seem an inherent, regular and inalienable part of the established order of power relations through processes of medicalisation, normalisation, and marketisation. It also examines how these processes undermine themselves internally and at the same time undo HIV's naturalisation, leaving lives lived with HIV to some extent outside or on the borders of naturalisation.

Chapter 4, 'When the drugs do work: The medicalised HIV citizen', explores the power of HIV's naturalisation through medicalisation; the benefits of that medicalisation; the constraints operating through medicalisation, which reduce and simplify ways of thinking about the pandemic; and the effects of some complex personal and cultural HIV narratives which try to redefine HIV citizenship in the biological field.

Chapter 5, 'A long-term condition: HIV's normalisation', focuses on the second major naturalisation process operating around the contemporary pandemic, which I call normalisation. Normalisation has many positive aspects to it, and yet its mainstreaming of HIV concerns can make the particularities of the condition hard to talk about or even to recognise.

Chapter 6, 'Investing in the pandemic: The marketised HIV citizen', examines the third naturalisation process in the contemporary pandemic, that of marketisation. This process increasingly structures arguments around prevention and treatment, and appears within personal as much as policy and popular accounts of the pandemic. It has become particularly prevalent since the financial crisis of 2008.

Medicalisation, normalisation and marketisation are processes of naturalisation that appear in many different contemporary fields. Chapter 7, 'Being left behind', goes on to examine some other denaturalising discontinuities in how the contemporary HIV era is lived, which derive from HIV's specific biological, psychological, cultural and sociopolitical characteristics. These discontinuities leave many people living with and affected by HIV at some distance from the relatively hopeful HIV present. The chapter argues that both naturalisation and its failures lead to HIV being 'left behind', and that this is an important element of HIV experience which requires continued attention.

Section 3 examines the particularities of HIV epidemics as they play out in different modalities of naturalisation in two national contexts, those of the United Kingdom and South Africa, drawing predominantly on interviews conducted largely in 2011 and 2012, respectively. Chapter 8, 'Living on: Three-letter lives in the United Kingdom', develops the analysis of narratives built up in the previous chapters, in relation to the particularities of the UK epidemic. To do so, it draws on the fifth round of my study of support used and wanted for living with HIV in the United Kingdom, in which 47 people, roughly half gay men, and half women and heterosexual men, took part in semi-structured interviews, mostly in 2011. The chapter discusses how narratives of medicalisation and de-medicalisation, narratives of normalisation and non-normalisation, and narratives of marketisation and of living outside markets are enacted within the context of UK HIV citizenship. It is especially interested in how these three common narratives within the interviews, and their accompanying countervailing narratives, are inflected by what is often called neoliberalism. It examines what the narratives can tell us about the adequacy of this term in relation to the multiple, 'paraliberal' ways people are developing of living with HIV and ARVs. It also investigates how the notion of living on a variety of HIV 'borders' of health, social and economic life, knowledge and resources (Derrida 1979) might be adapted to describe people's active engagements with uncertainty and other difficulties.

Chapter 9, 'Living with HIV: Three-letter lives in South Africa', examines how the particularities of the pandemic are lived out in a high-prevalence, medium-income country context. Here, 'living with' HIV increasingly seems to characterise research participant narratives as they trace the relations between different HIV statuses, and between HIV and other conditions, particularly in terms of resources needed, mobilised and developed. The chapter suggests that social resources of 'living with' HIV, or a kind of HIV conviviality, have come to have important effects, not just for people who are HIV positive or affected by HIV. At the same time, people living with HIV in under-resourced contexts face particular difficulties of being left behind in resource terms, as well as those difficulties of HIV knowledge and understanding which people living with HIV in higher-income countries also face.

Chapter 10, the last chapter in Section 3, reviews the particularities of contemporary three-letter lives as they have appeared in this book and points to varieties of action and activism that may currently be available in everyday contexts such as those lived in by the interviewees in the HIV support studies. The chapter also suggests that the complexities and contradictions of living with HIV and ARVs, and their socially and historically particular forms, come into view in the long, involved, reflexive and often creative stories that people living with HIV co-construct in interview situations. They are persuasive accounts of the particularities of HIV and of the processes by which its contemporary socio-political place is being negotiated.

To begin the book, I return now to the debate about current HIV optimism, how far concerns with HIV can be mainstreamed, and how we might be able to avoid separating and reifying the pandemic in an exceptionalist way, while still addressing its exceptional, particular characteristics.

2
From HIV's Exceptionalism to HIV's Particularity

We are at a moment of extraordinary optimism in the response to the human immunodeficiency virus (HIV). A series of scientific breakthroughs, including several trials showing the partial efficacy of oral and topical chemoprophylaxis and the first evidence of efficacy for an HIV vaccine candidate, have the potential to markedly expand the available preventive tools. There is evidence of the first cure of an HIV-infected person. And most important, the finding that early initiation of antiretroviral therapy can both improve individual patient outcomes and reduce the risk of HIV transmission to sexual partners by 96% has led many to assert what had so long seemed impossible: that control of the HIV pandemic may be achievable.

(Havlir and Beyrer 2012: 685)

The most significant impact [of the economic crisis] is that we're seeing more people dying. During the Global Fund grant, we achieved reductions in mortality. But now people are not adhering to their treatment because the social and nutritional support they need to do so is not there.

Joan Didier, Executive Director,
St Lucia AIDS Action Foundation
(quoted in UNAIDS 2012b: 14–5)

Yah, you know, really, the HIV is a complicated issue...it affects your health, economic, (social life), people disclose, sometimes you don't disclose your status. And sometimes your health is up and down, and create many many disease, you have blood pressure, hypertension, diabetes and all those, kidney infection, all organs. Yeah this hard when you start with medication and you have to stick with time of medication and you have to eat some kind of food...whereas because even the medication is not like any (laughs) another pills. Many, many three, four tablet, and sometimes the sideeffect, you know when you take it you feel pain, you feel like nausea, like headache, like rash, that's all those things. And sometimes you feel difficult to take with you, you know, especially when around the community, all the people around you....Or if you miss it that is another problem for you....And I saw this when I started medication, I saw even my memory is not like before. Really I forgot many people, and even some people they start to ask me 'what, your shape is changed, and what happened?' My friend he ask me, 'why you took a lot of tablets?' I say 'no this is because I have got some' – sometime I have to lie – 'no, no! I have got some problem with my kidney or my ulcer and the doctor, prescribed me that all those things.' And secondly, you know family, they don't know {my status}, that is another barrier. And your lifestyle, for to have a partner this is another issue, because you have to stick with someone in the same situation. Otherwise it is affecting the law and how that is. And even when you have sex, and you have caution about that, if you have to use condoms. Also if sometimes the lady, say 'why you use condoms?' also suspect you or something, I say 'no no because it's safe for you and for me'...For me because I didn't marry for wife people started – because I have got HIV before wife, maybe for fifteen years, yes – people asking me many 'why why why's' especially that's in our culture you have to {have a wife}.[1]

Quentin (United Kingdom 2011)

Introduction

This chapter examines convergences and conflicts between contemporary positions that people take in relation to HIV, in policy and in everyday lives. The quotations above present three such positions. The first, an optimistic assessment of the current possibilities for prevention and treatment, particularly those arising from new biomedical developments, suggests that HIV may soon cease to be an emergency in the world. I will call this the 'naturalisation' position. It assumes not that HIV will no longer exist, but rather that AIDS will disappear and that HIV will become a regular, natural part of the biosocial order of things, still difficult, but no longer to be seen in catastrophic terms.[2]

The second quotation, from Joan Didier, suggests that dealing with HIV remains difficult, and is even becoming difficult in new ways. The global financial crisis has led to stable, that is, declining in real terms, international contributions to the pandemic. This means, for instance, reductions in psychosocial support and food security programmes. Moreover, ARVs are still only available to around half of those who need them, and HIV remains a highly stigmatised condition. Do these characteristics still render HIV 'exceptional', as was once often claimed: both an emergency and one that is different from other health and social emergencies (Piot 2006; UNAIDS 2012a; World Health Organisation 2006: 2ff)? At times, such claims could be said to move from exceptionality to exceptionalism, that is, to a description of HIV's exceptional characteristics as invariant, or at least relatively stable, across social and historical contexts, and as therefore requiring stable exceptional responses at international, national and local levels. Such HIV exceptionalism has been the subject of extensive criticism and commentary. Some suggest that clinical progress, financial crisis, and moves away from discourses of aid and dependency, towards an emphasis on trade and investment, mean that HIV cannot or should no longer be considered exceptional. Other writers predict, like Didier, that elements of HIV's exceptionality, if not its exceptionalism, will continue, and will need to be kept in mind. Some suggest that aspects of HIV 'exceptionality' thinking, such as its internationalism, open-endedness, commitment and integration, might fruitfully and sustainably be extended to broader health and other requirements in low- and middle-income countries (for instance, Bayer 1999; Ooms et al. 2010; Smith and Whiteside 2010). Perhaps we need another characterisation of the pandemic, one that does not separate it off and associate it with top-down Western decision-making, as exceptionalism often does, but that at the same time pays appropriate attention to the distinct features of HIV, and of existing responses to it.

The third quotation at the start of this chapter is from a 2011 interview I conducted with Quentin (all the names of research participants that I am using here are pseudonyms, chosen by participants themselves if they wanted to do so), a man in his 40's, of African origin, living with HIV in the UK. Quentin suggests that living with HIV, while easier than it used to be, is still 'complicated'. Medicines do not work perfectly, health is uncertain, disclosure is difficult. Living with HIV may indeed now be a matter of living with a long-term illness which has commonalities with other, similar illnesses. At the same time, HIV has many particularities which are also specific to people's social and historical positions within the pandemic. I will argue that a recognition of HIV's *particularity*, rather than a position that endorses naturalisation or exceptionalism, is the most helpful way to approach the condition currently.

I want to follow up Quentin's description of his 'complicated' life with two anecdotes from the different national contexts where I have recently researched people's stories of support for living with HIV. These two anecdotes express something of the continuing particularities of encounters with HIV, in quite different situations, for people who are HIV-affected and unaffected, as well as for people living with HIV.

In summer 2012, in a township outside Cape Town, I was trying to find an NGO I had not visited before. It is a small organisation, rooted in the neighbourhood. In South African terms, it is a CBO, a community-based organisation. I was met at the taxi stand by a young man, whom I'll call Nathaniel, who volunteers for the organisation. He did not talk about his own HIV status, but as we walked towards the office, he told me that he used to work with a larger HIV-oriented CBO nearby. Two million of South Africa's 5.6 million people living with HIV now take ARVs, 80% of those who need them, and people talk about the condition more openly in the country (Irin News 2012; Zungu 2012). And so Nathaniel felt that HIV was now a less urgent area of activity. Instead, he wanted to make a difference by working on local issues that affect everybody. He reeled off a list of them: policing, gender-based violence, sanitation, roads, and other infrastructural problems. It was time, he thought, to adopt a wider perspective.

Nathaniel's approach to the epidemic recognised its wider environment, but still also acknowledged its particularity. He acknowledged that many HIV-specific problems remained to be dealt with, such as lack of food and cash support for people taking ARVs. However, HIV's particularity had, for him, a new context. The no-treatment emergency had passed. Now, he thought, he himself could best address the epidemic by focusing on broader socioeconomic issues. And so it was no longer HIV that drove his own actions.

A few months later, I was in a class I teach to third-year undergraduates, 'HIV in the world'. Students at my university come mainly from the local, East London area, where rates of HIV are high for the United Kingdom, and diagnoses often late (Health Protection Agency 2012). The class contained students from white British, Asian British, Caribbean British and African British backgrounds. As always, some students were relatively recent migrants from countries with high HIV prevalence, several had close family members or friends who were HIV positive, and a few were HIV positive themselves. This year, like every year, students did not talk about their own status. However, some openly discussed relatives who were HIV positive, or who had died from HIV-related illnesses. In this session, we had a speaker from the London-based HIV organisation, Positively UK. After his initial presentation about the organisation, he said, casually and clearly, that he himself was HIV positive. A quiet gasp went round the room. Several students complimented him on how well he looked, his positive attitude, his openness. There were questions about medical treatment and keeping well, but also about traditional treatments and HIV's origins. A couple of students seemed to be suggesting that HIV positive people had an obligation to accept themselves and be self-affirming, like this young man, in order to be healthy and accepted by others. During the class, one young woman wrote the speaker a poem about the impact of his calm announcement. An older man declared that this event would make him more accepting towards a friend whose recent diagnosis had strongly disturbed him; the class turned and applauded this student.

As this incident demonstrates, the specific characteristics of people's responses to HIV still need to be taken into account, even in a national situation like the UK where resources for HIV treatment, care, prevention and education are relatively good. In this case, the particularity of HIV made itself felt in people's accounts of ongoing difficulties with disclosure, distancing and rejection, as well as in ideas about how people living with HIV and ARVs 'should' conduct themselves.

At times, the HIV pandemic may seem, even to people embedded in it, such as Nathaniel, like yesterday's news. HIV is now a treatable condition. Antiretroviral (ARV) treatment restores and preserves HIV positive people's health; people who take ARVs can live for many years. This treatment has been rolled out to nearly 10 million people, 20 times more than in 2003, and 56% of those eligible to receive ARVs are now taking them. Death rates and new infections are falling. Prevalence, the rate of HIV infection in a population, is levelling off in many countries majorly affected by HIV (UNAIDS 2012a; World Health Organisation 2013). Progress is being made on effective vaccines, new forms of medication, and functional cures by earlier or at-infection ARV treatment and by stem cell transplants (for instance, Bacchus 2012; Cohen et al. 2011; Haynes et al. 2012; Henrich et al. 2012; Hutter et al. 2009; Kitahata et al. 2009; Persaud et al. 2013; Rerks-Ngarm et al. 2012). International NGOs such as UNAIDS, the United Nations institution dedicated to HIV work, and the World Health Organisation (WHO), as well as governments, are committed to providing long-term medical treatment, care and prevention services. Many people living with the virus are doing well in medical terms. They are accepted by families and friends. They pursue their education or are successfully employed. They are in supportive partnerships or marriages. They are loving parents of healthy children.

Some suggest that today the HIV pandemic is well enough managed and understood to be treated as simply one target among many others in national and international health programmes. For many politicians and policymakers, the pandemic is less of a priority than it used to be, especially given the current recession. People living within high-prevalence epidemics often express 'AIDS fatigue', sometimes even when they are HIV positive themselves. A number of social and health researchers argue that HIV now requires only applied research on the best way to deliver ARVs and the most effective prevention initiatives. HIV appears in such accounts as an emblematic but not exceptional case of successful medical treatment and of psychosocial and, increasingly, medical control of infection transmission. Sometimes, more critically but no more exceptionally, the pandemic is viewed as one among many illustrations of medicalisation and the power of Big Pharma, of dependency-based development practice, and of the skewing of the global south's priorities by the interests of the global north.

So is the pandemic itself a problem solved – for the world, if not for every individual living with the virus or affected by it? Once, it was a fatal condition about which nothing was known. Later, it manifested itself as a crisis: a pandemic with major effects, particularly in sub-Saharan Africa, on health and social welfare systems, and on people's lives and lifespans. Now, some say, the 'beginning of the end of AIDS' is in sight. Is HIV still a critical condition, if not an exceptional one?

I shall argue that popular and policy downgradings of the pandemic erase or deny some important realities. We are living in an era which we can call, not the treatment era, since nearly half of those who need ARVs are still not getting them (UNAIDS 2012a), but the treatment possibility era (Davis and Squire 2010). In this era, however, HIV's still – powerful impact in high HIV-prevalence areas; its continuing invisibility in many low-prevalence or low-resourced contexts; ongoing stigma and discrimination; new issues that have arisen within the treatment possibility era; the virus's continuing high incidence, or rate of new cases; other, competing resource demands; and the need to sustain and increase HIV funding at a time when the global financial crisis is impacting it: all this means that the pandemic continues to pose significant conceptual as well as practical problems, some of which are shared across different national contexts (Sidibé et al. 2012).

Ten million people are now living three-letter lives in a double sense. Those lives are shaped by the benefits and difficulties of lifetime ARV use, as well as of HIV itself. At the same time, the other 26 million people thought to be HIV positive are living with the possibility of such treatment, when they reach a state of health where it is appropriate, when they take the step of accessing ARVs, or when ARVs become accessible to them. The World Health Organisation's new (2013) guidelines, indeed, call for immediate expansion to another 10 million of those people, to safeguard their health. All these people are living three-letter lives. For, even in the many countries where national and international organisations have not yet raised treatment possibility beyond low levels (UNAIDS 2011a: 22), those organisations are explicitly committed to 'universal' coverage, that is, ARVs for at least 80% of those who need them. And the year-on-year increases are large: 2.3 million more people in sub-Saharan Africa accessed ARVs during 2010 and 2011 (UNAIDS 2012a). Even people living with low levels of treatment access are thus still living with a significant level of treatment possibility, that is, with the possibility of living with ARVs as well as with HIV.

This book draws on studies and representations of HIV epidemics across the world. However, it focuses in particular on people living with HIV in the United Kingdom, a high-income country, with relatively good resources for people living with HIV; and in South Africa, a middle-income country with very high HIV prevalence and only partially adequate medical and other resources, despite ARV treatment's wide availability. The book draws on my own research in these national contexts over the past 20 years in the United Kingdom, and 12 years in South Africa.

In examining these two research contexts, the book aims to avoid simplistic divisions between the pandemic's global-north 'haves' and global-south 'have-nots'. South Africa, like the United Kingdom, is a significant international power. Both countries have high Gini indices (a measure of internal inequalities), and high levels of migration. These common factors impact their HIV epidemics. Nevertheless, South Africa is a medium-income and the United Kingdom a high-income country. Unemployment in the former is around 24%, around 8% in the latter. People living with HIV in high-prevalence, medium-income countries such as South Africa are still less likely to have ARVs than HIV positive people in high-income nations, and they experience severe constraints on other resources such as other health services, social services, infrastructure, and education. In South Africa, people living with HIV live with the aftermath of what is often called 'AIDS denialism', that is, sustained popular and political scepticism about the existence and causes of HIV illness, as well as successful mass activism for treatment and a powerful recent history of political struggle (Mbali 2005; Nattrass 2012; Robins 2008). Such particular conditions of HIV epidemics, tied into local, national and regional contexts, cannot be treated fully here, but they must be recognised (Davis and Squire 2010). For, while the pandemic's naturalisation, and the limits of that naturalisation, appear in many contexts, it is important to acknowledge unevenness across those contexts. This is especially the case because ARV access, and the naturalisation processes associated with successful treatment availability and uptake, happened over a decade later and are still less general in low- and middle-income than in high-income countries.

The differences between UK and South African contexts of HIV are important, but so is what we can learn from what they share. HIV is a pandemic with a major, global impact. It was the first epidemic to be associated with late twentieth-century globalisation (Barnett and Whiteside 2006). It is also a variable, changing and uncertain pandemic. We are all 'living with' these characteristics of HIV, but the pandemic affects us in different ways, depending on its diverse political, economic and social contexts; its different national and local histories; changing and unevenly available medical technologies; and our own HIV statuses. Given these divergences, how can people usefully address HIV in ways that mobilise common understandings across the pandemic, while still recognising the most particularities in how HIV is lived? *Living with HIV and ARVs* tries to address that question, within the necessarily limited framework of a focus primarily on the UK and South African epidemics.

Although the book also refers to HIV epidemics in other, lower-resourced contexts, and in contexts where treatment is less available, it does not describe those contexts in detail. Of course, there are some points of comparison between living with HIV and taking ARVs in low-income country circumstances, and in middle- and high-income contexts such as the South African and UK epidemics. But there is also a great gulf between a country where people still have little access to ARVs, especially outside cities; where there are minimal health services, no social welfare grants, little paid employment and food shortages, and a middle-income country such as South Africa which, despite problems with ARV supply and access, large-scale unemployment and food insecurity, provides pensions, disability grants, child support grants and 80% ARV coverage. The gap is even greater if we consider a high-income country like the United Kingdom, where unemployment benefits are also available, where most people living with HIV are able to travel to specialist clinics relatively easily even if they live in rural areas, where the most recent and effective treatments are still usually offered to all who need them and where minimal resources for food and shelter are provided by the state. The divide is especially stark if we consider sub-Saharan African countries, where epidemics are largest. However, even in many middle-income countries with relatively small HIV epidemics, ARV coverage remains below 40% (UNAIDS 2011a: 22). This situation makes them 'low-resourced' in relation to HIV, even if not in general economic terms.

This book does not give an account of epidemics in low-income countries, or in middle-income countries with very limited resources for HIV treatment, care, and prevention. There are other research projects to be done, other books to be written about the difficult and different circumstances of HIV epidemics and ARV treatment in such countries. Vinh-Kim Nguyen's *The republic of therapy* (2011), an insightful account of the exigencies, triages and possibilities operating around the HIV epidemic in Côte D'Ivoire, is an inspiring example. Sarah Bernays's research on the small, dispersed, almost invisible communities of people living with HIV in Serbia and Montenegro (Bernays and Rhodes 2009) is another. Leslie and Len Doyal (2013) have written a thoughtful and integrative review of social research on the pandemic, *Living with HIV and dying with AIDS*. Anthony Barnett and Alan Whiteside's (2006) *AIDS in the twenty-first century* provides a comprehensive and prescient overview of development and economic accounts of the pandemic.

By contrast, this book has a fine-grained and specific aim: to examine how people are living with HIV in the treatment possibility era, particularly in two countries with very different HIV prevalence and resources, and with distinct economies, infrastructures, social structures, and histories. In these contexts, how are people's three-letter lives, living with HIV and living with the actuality or possibility of ARVs, affected by those letters? How heavily do the letters inscribe themselves across their everyday health, work and relationships? How far do the letters reach across their lives? And as ARV treatment becomes more general across the world, what can these different conditions tell us about possible futures for the increasing numbers of people who will be living three-letter lives?

In this chapter, I discuss recent arguments around the significance of lives lived with HIV and ARVs, in the context of recent medical, social and political advances around HIV treatment, prevention and care. I examine contemporary optimism about the pandemic's future, alongside the ongoing impact of medical, economic and psychosocial difficulties. I also outline the narrative approach to people's accounts of living with HIV and ARVs that my own research takes, and how this approach allows attention to the particularities of three-letter lives.

First, I want to spend a little time describing the positive aspects of the contemporary situation. These aspects are much more encouraging than people living with HIV, affected by HIV, or simply observing the path of the pandemic, might have expected, even five years ago.

The beginning of the end of AIDS?

In 1995, the British journalist Oscar Moore, writing his regular column in a major UK newspaper, reported the positive results from the first ARV 'combination therapy' drug trial, as 'a major battle won against one of the smartest guerrilla insurgents around' (1996: 129). Moore also acknowledged that for him, what had been won was 'the fight for time'. Moore had been seriously ill for a couple of years and had tried other, less helpful ARVs before, both factors that can make combination therapy less successful. The new 'combination' ARV treatment did not work for him. He died in 1996, the year that combinations of ARVs were rolled out as a standard HIV treatment in high-income countries, with notable success. By the end of 2010, ARV combination therapy was thought to have prevented around 2.5 million deaths (UNAIDS 2011a).

Today, the WHO defines HIV as a chronic illness, like any other. The ARV coverage that makes such a definition feasible in a high-income country like the United Kingdom is 88% (Health Protection Agency 2012). In the United Kingdom, people who are classified as 'stable' patients, with good health, effective medication and high levels of adherence to that medication, can choose to receive their ARVs by post and may attend a clinic just twice a year. The United Kingdom's Health Protection Agency (HPA, now Public Health England) presents HIV as a manageable condition and emphasises that early treatment makes for long life (Health Protection Agency 2011a). In pursuit of this goal, the HPA urges people in groups with high prevalence, such as men who have sex with men, people from high-prevalence countries, intravenous drug users, and their sexual partners, to test at least yearly. It suggests tests be offered to everyone at hospitals and doctors' surgeries in high-prevalence areas, and in sexually transmitted infection clinics, drug treatment centres, and antenatally. This expansion of testing is calculated to be economic as well as life-saving, avoiding the costs of late-diagnosed HIV illness, and also enabling lower levels of untreated, transmissible HIV in the population (Health Protection Agency 2011b).

HIV is also increasingly framed as a treatable, manageable condition, worldwide. In at least eleven middle- and low-income countries, including South Africa, as well as in high-income countries, such as the United Kingdom, ARVs are now available 'universally', which is defined to mean for at least 80% of those who need them (UNAIDS 2012a). Almost every country is now trying to implement the World Health Organisation's 2010 guidelines for starting ARV treatment earlier, at a stage when HIV positive people's immune systems are less compromised and can be better protected. The new guidelines for even earlier treatment (World Health Organisation 2013) will be similarly implemented. South Africa, on what might seem like the other side of the HIV world from the UK's small but heavily-treated and well-supported HIV epidemic, with 5.6 million people living with HIV, has been able to meet the 2010 guidelines (UNAIDS 2012a) and is now applying the latest ones. Its large-scale HIV Testing and Counselling programme has expanded from clinics, via mobile units working in public spaces such as shopping centres, taxi termini, even churches and schools. As in the United Kingdom, government advice is for those at risk, which in South Africa includes everyone potentially sexually active, to get tested yearly. In South Africa as well, most people on ARVs are regarded as healthy. If blood tests show good levels of immune functioning and low levels of HIV, they no longer get disability grants.

Across the pandemic, too, newer treatment and prevention options are coming onstream. Post-exposure prophylaxis, or PEP, involving immediate ARV treatment after high-transmission-risk activities such as unprotected sex with an HIV positive person or needle-stick injuries, has proved extremely effective in preventing new HIV infections. Functional cures, resulting in no active, replicating virus, although small amounts of virus can still be detected in the body, have been achieved by ARV treatment immediately after infection or in the first ten weeks – a regime that builds on PEP procedures – and by stem cell transplant in cases of HIV combined with leukaemia (Henrich et al. 2013; Hutter et al. 2009; Persaud et al. 2013; Saez-Cirion et al. 2013). Less dramatic perhaps, but of lasting and worldwide significance, is the highly effective ARV treatment for PMTCT, the prevention of mother-to-child transmission. This treatment, involving voluntary HIV testing and counselling for all pregnant women, the provision of ARVs for HIV positive pregnant women, and ARV medication for newborn infants, has grown alongside the expansion of ARV treatment. 57% of HIV positive pregnant women in low- and middle-income countries now receive it. During 2010 and 2011, it is estimated to have saved 490,000 infants from becoming HIV positive (UNAIDS 2012a).

Across the pandemic, ARV treatment is much simpler and less prone to producing side effects than it used to be. ARV treatment also now starts much earlier than before, allowing people to safeguard their immune systems before they are too compromised. Such treatment, by lowering HIV levels in a population, can in addition help to reduce transmission, a process known as 'treatment as prevention' or TasP, supported by the HPTN 052 study across eight countries and three continents (Cohen et al. 2011, 2012; Donnell et al. 2010; Fang et al. 2004). Researchers have in addition trialled the prophylactic or preventive use of ARVs, or PrEP, to prevent infection among some vulnerable people. In summer 2012, indeed, the US Food and Drug Administration approved the Gilead-made drug Truvada, an antiretroviral medication, to be taken as a preventive by HIV negative people unable to guarantee they can avoid unsafe sex, such as people who have unprotected sex with unknown – status partners, have sex for money or commodities, or are in sero-discordant partnerships with HIV positive partners (Food and Drug Administration 2012). PrEP means that HIV's medical prevention is now within everyone's knowledge and, potentially, reach. Botswana, Kenya, and Uganda are among the sub-Saharan African contexts where PrEP has been trialled with heterosexual populations, cutting HIV transmission by around 50%, if used consistently (Van Damme et al. 2012). PrEP has been used with similar success by men who have sex with men in a variety of national contexts, and by drug users in Thailand (Baeten and Celum 2011; Centers for Disease Control 2013; Grant et al. 2010; Thigpen et al. 2011). Circumcision and vaginally-applied microbicides are showing promise in lowering transmission risk (UNAIDS 2012). Publicly-funded adult men's circumcision is part of the WHO's HIV/AIDS strategy for high-prevalence countries (World Health Organisation 2011) such as South Africa. Microbicides are themselves PrEP mechanisms, and South Africa is trialling a gel containing tenofovir (a component of Truvada), which may be rolled out for women nationally (Abdool Karim et al. 2010). Behavioural strategies such as condom use and later-starting and fewer sexual partnerships have and will continue to play a major role in reducing transmission (UNAIDS 2011a, 2012a). As mentioned earlier, vaccine development is showing promising signs (Haynes et al. 2012; Rerks-Ngarm et al. 2009)

Taking into account these new options, particularly those made possible by treatment advances and TasP, the 17,000-strong International Association of Providers of AIDS Care (IAPAC) thinks there is a possibility 'of welcoming an AIDS-free generation within our lifetimes' (International Association of Providers of AIDS Care 2012: 2). Diane Havlir and Chris Beyrer (2012), a clinician and a researcher respectively with longstanding HIV expertise in the United States and internationally, in their article, 'The beginning of the end of AIDS?', quoted at the beginning of this chapter, also raise the possibility of such a generation, mooted first in 2011 by the then-US Secretary of State, Hillary Clinton. Havlir and Beyrer (2012: 685) suggest that we are living in a 'moment of extraordinary optimism' within the pandemic.

At the beginning of this chapter, I described a young South African man, Nathaniel, deeply involved with HIV issues but now framing his community work within a broader context. HIV is now often less of an issue in people's lives than many other circumstances, such as other illnesses, getting an education, finding a job, having a relationship, caring for others and poverty, with which they live. Extending this argument about the importance of other aspects of people's lives, it is frequently argued, as I indicated earlier, that 'HIV exceptionalism', that is, treating HIV as a special case because of its nature or extent, must now be ditched. Added to contemporary optimism about the HIV pandemic in this argument are a large array of other criticisms. The pandemic is said to be overfunded and ring-fenced at the expense of other health fields. HIV funding is claimed to intensify aid dependency. Some suggest that the ongoing policy focus on HIV stigma strengthens rather than erodes it. Poor governance is alleged in the administration of HIV funds. Programmes beyond ARV and other medication provision, particularly outside the health sector, in the psychosocial field, are declared of limited or no effectiveness. Economies and social structures, once the subject of dire warnings about their imminent HIV-related collapse, are asserted to be much more resilient to the pandemic's effects than previously thought. Some maintain the redundancy of HIV-dedicated organisations, including UNAIDS itself, which, they think, could be rolled into the WHO. Roger England, chair of a policy group focused on middle- and low-income countries, Health Systems Workshop, made this case strongly and controversially in 2008, before the large curtailments of HIV spending demanded by the financial crisis. He wrote,

> Although HIV can tip households into poverty and constrain national development, so can all serious diseases and disasters. HIV is a major disease in southern Africa, but it is not a global catastrophe...multi- sectoral programmes were misguided and have got nowhere slowly and expensively....Vast sums have been wasted through national

commissions and in funding esoteric disciplines and projects instead of beefing up public health capacity that could have controlled transmission.... It is no longer heresy to point out that far too much is spent on HIV relative to other needs and that this is damaging health systems ... HIV exceptionalism is dead – and the writing is on the wall for UNAIDS. Why a UN agency for HIV and not for pneumonia or diabetes, which both kill more people? (England 2008: 1072)

England's perspective is not widely endorsed (see, for example, Poku et al. 2007; Sidibe et al. 2012). His criticisms of the international HIV sector and its partners echo criticisms made of 'development' initiatives in many arenas, without being specific to HIV. His calls for funding to shift away from HIV and towards health systems generally recall many similar pleas made by stakeholders with interests other than those currently being funded. At the same time, the argument that HIV does not now, if it ever did, require the amount of resources given to it, and that this overprovision skews health and social service sectors in many countries, is one commonly heard within government policy organisations and NGOs at all levels. Funding applicants are often of interest to external donors, or think they will be, if they include HIV among their priorities. At present, many HIV organisations are struggling to preserve or increase funds within a new climate of HIV optimism underpinned by global recession. Frequently, they reframe their activities for the current context as requiring financial and social 'investment', not aid. Is this reframing enough to convey a picture of the contemporary HIV epidemic that describes its difficult realities, without the simplification and reductiveness that exceptionalism has sometimes involved?

HIV's psychosocial realities

England's argument is one, somewhat extreme, manifestation of the many varieties of 'endgame' optimism suffusing contemporary accounts of the HIV pandemic. What of the other, less optimistic side, the continuing difficulties of living with, treating and preventing HIV, as told from within the pandemic? Fifteen years after Moore's *PWA* appeared, HIV trainer Elaine Maane, of Zambian origin but living in South Africa, wrote her account of living with HIV, titled *Umzala* (2009), after the viral 'cousin' who accompanies her everywhere and whom she accommodates without giving in to. The book is the story of how she lives with the virus, brings up her child, takes the drugs that keep her looking and feeling healthy, and encourages her HIV positive friends. Adopting one of those friends' advice, she thinks of taking ARVs as an everyday, routine matter, like taking vitamins. Living positively with her HIV positive status, she says,

> I have hope that one day there will not be any more HIV infections. I have faith that young mothers will enjoy their husbands longer, rather than losing them to premature deaths. All this is possible if we stand as one to encourage one another to take our medicines and take them correctly. Children will have their parents around much longer too and health workers will be less overworked. I have faith and hope that it will be better someday. (Maane 2009: 190)

But *Umzala* is also, as perhaps the subtext of this quotation might suggest, the story of the medications' distressing side effects, many sad bereavements, ongoing difficulties in relationships, and how Maane mourns or feels frustrated about those friends who could not get ARVs or who, even now, will not take them.

These difficulties are not just South African or developing-world issues. The extract from Quentin's interview at the beginning of this chapter describes the many troubles that accompany three-letter lives even in contexts where HIV resources are relatively abundant. Quentin started treatment late; his health, unsurprisingly, is still not good. However, in my UK interviews, some recently diagnosed people, who began treatment promptly, also reported considerable medical problems. Moreover, for those research participants, as for Quentin, a large number of their difficulties with living with HIV were not medical, but could be called psychosocial in nature, and they resemble those that Maane reports.

The most common policy application of the term 'psychosocial' is to integrative initiatives. It is used, for example, to describe initiatives within the WHO that pay attention to subjectively experienced difficulties which larger social programmes around occupational health may be ignoring; that provide socially-sensitive mental health services during emergencies or post-conflict; or that supplement medical HIV testing and treatment with psychological, social and community care (World Health Organisation 2010a, 2008, not dated). However, the term 'psychosocial' also applies academically to a critical interplay between psychological, sociological, cultural-studies and political approaches alongside an array of uses of psychoanalysis. Researchers view a 'psychosocial' approach as a way of critically questioning all of these fields, and of focusing on psychological subjects as emerging at their intersections. This is the way I will use the term in this book (for examples, see Frosh and Baraitzer

2008; Stenner and Taylor 2008; Walkerdine and Jiminez 2012). More specifically, I will be deploying the term to capture, as Judith Butler (2005) does, the way in which the 'self' is called into being, socially and ethically, and is politically formed at its most fundamental levels. Within this approach, subjectivity also comes to operate as a force in its own right, with intimate and unalienable, though ambiguous, histories and associations running across it.

Quentin's account provides many examples of this 'psychosocial' complexity. As Quentin makes clear, ARVs are not always easy physically. Many people stop taking them or do not even start because of the side effects, which can make the high level of adherence that ARVs require in order to work well (usually cited as at least 95%), difficult in itself. As Quentin says, missing doses is a real problem, quickly reducing ARVs' effectiveness. Moreover, taking ARVs can make you feel more ill than not taking them.

At the same time, for some, ARVs also carry the psychological difficulty of reminding those who take them of their condition daily, and the stigma associated or feared to be associated with going to the clinic, taking the medications, and ARV side effects like the shape change which Quentin mentions. Side effects may develop which themselves need difficult treatment. Some HIV-related conditions may persist. These too may require challenging forms of treatment, in Quentin's case, for kidney failure. Long-term effects of living with HIV, similar to those often experienced in late middle age, but exacerbated by HIV, such as cardiovascular problems, are also increasingly likely to arise as people such as Quentin and Maane enter their 50s and 60s, demanding further adjustments in their lives. All these issues are socially shaped. They are harder to deal with in situations of poverty and resource constraint, faced by Maane especially, and of social exclusion, particularly relevant for Quentin.

Another psychosocial area of commonality between Maane's South African-based and Quentin's UK-based accounts appears around secrecy and disclosure. Maane is unusually open about her life with HIV. She is, indeed, an HIV activist. Nevertheless, there are many discussions within her autobiography of deliberations about when and to whom to disclose, and the mixed results of disclosing: sometimes unexpectedly positive, as with her sister-in-law, sometimes negative or ambivalent, as with male relationship partners. Quentin is involved in similar deliberations, though his conclusions are usually more negative. But we can also read in Quentin's account a strong and distinct emphasis on secrecy, fear of criminalisation if he does not disclose to partners, and isolation, something that leads to severe restrictions in his social and relationship life, and indeed, to depression. This constellation of psychosocial difficulties does not seem to be touched by the relative richness of HIV and other resources with which Quentin lives. Such troubles may be more intense within the largely invisible, low-prevalence HIV epidemics of high-income countries. For people living with HIV in low-resourced, high-prevalence situations, HIV is at least part of the life of every family, even if, as for Elaine Maane, it is not talked about much there. HIV positive people's isolation in the developed world is also particularly likely if, like Quentin, they are migrants with reduced family networks, living in countries like the United Kingdom which seek legal redress for non-disclosure.

Many social and psychological researchers (Davis 2009; Kippax 2012; Nguyen et al. 2011) suggest that psychosocial troubles of the kind discussed here need a lot more attention than they are currently getting. Without such attention, they may have effects that severely counterbalance current optimistic takes on the pandemic. TasP, PrEP and circumcision, for instance, may lead to 'disinhibition', to the attitude that transmission risk is sufficiently low to make condoms unnecessary. ARVs may not be taken consistently, may be given up, or may not be accessed, because of their difficulties and stigmatisation (Rao et al. 2009; Roura et al. 2009). People may find condoms hard to use because of how they and others see them. People who are HIV positive may not be able to disclose and get support. There are high levels of depression among HIV positive people in many national contexts, which affect their ability to access testing and treatment take-up, ARV use, and life expectancy (Wada et al. 2013).

Medical, service and other resource constraints

The psychosocial difficulties within the contemporary pandemic do not just exist by themselves. They are linked to and are sometimes indeed direct results of a wider set of problems that the HIV pandemic continues to present. For instance, treatment possibility is itself just that: possibility. Even the newest ARVs, taken promptly, may not work, or work well. As Quentin's account suggests, many medical problems can attend living with HIV and ARVs. People's physiological reactions to them differ unpredictably. Viral load fluctuates. Resistance, side effects such as diarrhoea, and the long-term physical effects of both HIV and ARVs, can be problematic to manage medically, especially with older, less-tolerated, more complex and cheaper medications. The point at which treatment should optimally start is debated; it is particularly difficult to start it during the early, highly infective period, when people do not test positive. It is not clear that TasP, or still less, PrEP, will work physiologically in all situations. People's responses to the medications also vary with time, again not entirely predictably (see, for example, Bertagnolio et al. 2012; Jain and Deeks 2010; Kitahata et al. 2009; MacArthur and DuPont 2012).

Universal early treatment, treatment as prevention and prophylactic ARVs are, therefore, like non-pharmacological initiatives such as male circumcision, microbicides and condoms, not fail-safe. They may be particularly faulty if they come to operate as substitutes for psychosocial prevention technologies. At the same time, existing psychosocial technologies, as they are currently implemented, seem now not to be lowering rates of new infections, or HIV incidence, much beyond what they have already achieved. However, the future balance between these two types of prevention technology remains uncertain and is strongly debated (England 2008; Granich et al. 2009; Kippax 2012; Rosengarten and Michaels 2010).

Havlir and Beyrer (2012: 685), while suggesting that the new treatment and treatment-as-prevention strategies may portend the 'end of AIDS', also emphasise that medically, this will require more dramatic progress: 'A combination approach to prevention that includes HIV treatment {as well as behaviour change initiatives} can generate tremendous gains in the short term by curtailing new HIV infections, but ending the AIDS epidemic will probably require a vaccine, a cure, or both'.

Treatment possibility is also just 'possibility' for many in a more obvious sense: they know about treatment, but it does not reach them. HIV-related deaths remain at high levels, around 1.7 million a year. Death rates from HIV-related causes remain stable in many countries with long-established epidemics, including the United Kingdom and Uganda. Only about 54% of people who, according to WHO guidelines, need ARVs in low- and middle-income countries, currently get them, and the figure is consistently lower for men than for women. Worldwide, around 50% of HIV positive people do not know their status. A falling but still large number of people, around 2.5 million, become HIV positive each year. All of those people will need ARVs, and medical opinion is moving to provide them sooner, rather than later. Prevention, regular testing and prompt treatment thus remain urgent priorities (UNAIDS 2012a).

Millennium Development Goal 6 is to 'Have halted by 2015 and begun to reverse the spread of HIV/AIDS', and to provide universal treatment and care, defined as reaching 80% of those who need them (United Nations 2013). This is a laudable but currently still unlikely aim for many high-prevalence countries. In these countries, HIV has generated illnesses and deaths that affect every family, every workplace, every group of friends. The consequent crises in health, the economy and social structure across large geographical regions are unprecedented in recent times, however well individuals, neighbourhoods and countries manage to deal with them (Poku et al. 2007; De Waal 2006). By contrast, in high-income countries with low HIV prevalence, ARV treatment has been available since 1996. Here, HIV is often seen as a problem for other people in other, less fortunate places. These countries' own HIV epidemics are frequently rendered invisible.

The pandemic must not, though, be read as a tale of two separate, developing- and developed-world epidemics. In high-income countries, those most affected, such as gay men, sex workers, drug users and African migrants, remain highly socially stigmatised, as are HIV positive women (Carr and Gramling 2004). Treatment has, as we have seen, its own difficulties and stigmatising side effects. In high-income just as in middle- and low-income countries, many HIV positive people do not access treatment and are unaware of their status (Health Protection Agency 2012). Rates of new infections are growing among young heterosexuals, young gay men, and people of colour in many high-income countries, generating severe local epidemics. Moreover, developing- and developed-world epidemics are increasingly geographically connected. Many of us move between these epidemic worlds: tourists move predominantly in one direction, migrants and refugees in the other; migrant workers move both ways.

Nevertheless, many of the difficulties that qualify recent optimism about the HIV pandemic and ARV treatment remain heavily stratified: shaped by economic and social differences. ARVs' availability and effectiveness in low- and middle-income countries, for instance, are particularly curtailed by economic constraints. The most recent medications, those with fewest side effects, and second- and third-line ARV regimes for people for whom ARVs of first resort are not working, are often not available within the low-cost, largely generic ARV provision of these epidemics. There are severe cost implications of WHO guidelines advising that treatment should start when people are less severely ill than previously recommended. Not all countries are yet following these guidelines. In low- and middle-income contexts, treatment for side effects and HIV-related infections may be limited. There may be lapses in supply and failures in human and physical infrastructure, for instance, problematic pharmaceutical management, too few doctors, or no afford-able transport. The nutritious food required by people who are HIV posi-tive, in order for ARVs to have their best effects, makes severe financial demands that many in low-income situations cannot meet, as my South African interviewees repeatedly emphasised (Abdullah and Squire 2010; Geffen 2013; Ivers et al. 2009; Jain and Deeks 2010; Lodi et al. 2011). As Didier notes at the beginning of the chapter, this problem has been exacerbated by financial crisis-driven cuts in nutritional programmes.

In low- and middle-income countries, wherever ARVs are not accessed free, they often cost more than a middle-class wage. If medicine is paid for, if ARVs are at distant clinics, or if, as is often the case, clinics or doctors charge visit fees, people must devote enormous proportions of their resources to buying the medications or simply to keeping their appointments. Social networks may determine who gets ARV access. Free ARVs may 'leak' from the system and get sold. Shortly after Truvada was registered for PrEP use in the United States, reports appeared in Ugandan media suggesting that pharmacists were selling ARVs for PrEP to men keen to stop using condoms, a thought-provoking meeting of economic need with new HIV knowledge (Uganda Radio Network 2012).

Living with HIV imposes other severe resource costs: losses of economic, social and cultural productivity, educational attainment, and income for people who are ill, people who are caring for them, and their relatives. All these have short-term effects on people's ability to pay for food and rent; services like electricity, travel, other medical needs, and school fees, as well as for important social events such as marriages and funerals. These costs are having longer-term effects, too, on countries' economic, social and cultural potential, and also on the psychosocial fabric of people's lives, for instance, hindering some people's precarious efforts at staving off poverty (Poku et al. 2007), narrowing young people's views of possi-bilities within their lives (Lana 2012) and entrenching some men's views of their sexualities and relationships in fatalism (Zungu 2012).

The costs of the treatment era are not just difficult for middle- and low-income countries. In the United States, for example, low-end health insurers have always made access to more expensive and unusual medi-cations difficult. Now too, earlier treatments – especially in the USA, which has opted for immediate treatment for everyone testing HIV posi-tive – as well as TasP and PrEP are increasing the expense of HIV treat-ment for high-income countries. The new WHO guidelines may save costs from later illnesses and transmission by untreated HIV positive people, but they will raise the treatment budget by 10% and the number needing ARVs by perhaps 10 million (World Health Organisation 2013).

Since the advent of effective treatment in the mid-1990s, psychosocial services around the epidemic, including prevention services, have been cut in many high-income countries and their measurability and effectiveness put in question, not just by commentators such as England (2008) but also by larger bodies (World Bank 2010; see also Padian et al. 2010). My UK research participants have been noting these 'soft' service cuts since the 1990s, as well as their currently increasing impact. Yet from their qualitative accounts, the importance and effectiveness of such services is very clear.

The financial crisis has severely exacerbated difficulties in providing HIV services, though these have again been more acute in low- and middle-income countries. Not just ARVs but also the support services around them, food supplementation for instance, are under threat. As Joan Didier indicates at the beginning of the chapter, this is something that threatens many recent health gains. High-income countries are encouraging people living with HIV to start with cheaper drugs, and are intensifying social welfare cuts (for instance, see Dangerfield 2011). In low-income countries, donor countries' failures to deliver on budgetary promises have led to service curtailments, for instance, Uganda ceasing enrolment of people onto ARVs for a period (Bogere 2009). Income-generation projects with internal and external markets have faltered or closed. The crisis has also led to a heightened emphasis on value for money among the public and private financial supporters of HIV organisations, and within the organisations (World Bank/UNAIDS 2009) And it has cast new and serious international doubt on the long-term sustainability, let alone expansion, of many HIV programmes.

The resource requirements of HIV now make themselves felt globally, giving a transnational economic character to all our national HIV epidemics. Developing-world countries with high-prevalence epidemics face internal debate about devoting ever-larger proportions of their budgets to HIV as well as increasing demands from international NGOs to do exactly this (UNAIDS 2011a). Developed-world countries try to avoid the costs of treating HIV positive migrants within their own borders. Citing the global financial crisis, they may renege on promised contributions towards developing-world HIV costs. The costs of the pandemic will inevitably increase, since almost all HIV positive people will at some time require ARVs, governments and international NGOs are committed to providing them, and prevention initiatives will not soon reduce new infections to zero. For international drug companies, the cost of providing free or cheap drugs to the developing world must be weighed against the high public relations cost of not doing so.

And for all governments, the bill for providing aid for HIV treatment, support and education must be assessed against the possibility that the pandemic, under-resourced, will contribute to countries', indeed whole regions', failure to develop, and in some cases, will foster destabilisation and insecurity.

Social and cultural contexts

Variability in social and cultural situatings of HIV, as well as economically constrained resources, also qualify any general optimism about the treatment possibility era. There are pronounced differences in the comprehensiveness and success of HIV programmes even between countries at similar income and prevalence levels which relate to their histories of engagement with the pandemic and to their structures of medical and social provision. In the United States, for instance, where engagement with the epidemic was tardy in the 1980s and has been inhibited by social conservatism, particularly in relation to intravenous drug users, 58% of people known to be positive are in good touch with HIV services, whereas the rate is 90% in the UK (UNAIDS 2012; Health Protection Agency 2012). The US epidemic's intransigence has indeed recently spurred the resurgence of one of the earliest and most effective HIV activist organisations, ACT UP, the AIDS Coalition to Unleash Power, now active in many of the cities where it began in the 1980s. Public psychosocial services, welfare benefits, publicly available infrastructure and the range of HIV medications available to those on low incomes remain at a better level in the United Kingdom. However, difficulties in the UK epidemic have not disappeared. A number of HIV positive people died in 2011 after rejecting ARVs for faith healing. HIV stigma remains high and stops people testing, disclosing, and accessing treatment. It affects people at work, in their families and in relationships (Dangerfield 2012; Health Protection Agency 2012).

In middle- and low-income countries, similarly, there is great unevenness in provision, even at comparable levels of prevalence. In South Africa and Botswana, almost every family has lost members to HIV, but the epidemics' histories are different. Botswana has a history of strong engagement at the government and NGO levels; South Africa's national-level engagement came later. Thai and Brazilian governments committed early to treatment and prevention programmes, compared to neighbouring countries. Malawi has recently made similar commitments, much stronger than those of many other low-income, high-prevalence countries; Uganda was well known for making such commitments earlier in the pandemic (Epstein 2006). The absence of national-level political commitments and open popular dialogue about HIV makes tackling it more problematic, but such commitments alone do not obviate difficulties. HIV prevalence has been rising in Uganda since 2006, partly due to ARV access, but also to decreased condom use and the stigmatisation of HIV-affected communities such as men who have sex with men (UNAIDS 2012).

There are also large differences in prevalence, and thus in the nature of epidemics, within countries. For instance, in the United States, there are high-prevalence cities like Washington, DC, with epidemic-level rates of 3.2% among people over twelve (Denning and Dinenno 2013; Government of the District of Columbia 2010), as well as epidemics in rural areas of the South and within particular communities, especially African American and Latino communities. In the United Kingdom, HIV appears at higher percentages among gay men and people of African origin. It is a truism that the HIV pandemic is made up of many different national epidemics. It is also the case that these epidemics are themselves jigsaws of smaller, local epidemics, creating gradients of difficulty within a country. Some areas of a country may be untouched, as in the United Kingdom where the overall prevalence is low but where particular boroughs in London, for instance, such as Lambeth, Kensington and Chelsea, Camden, and Newham, where many gay men and people of African origin live, have much higher prevalence, setting up radically different sets of local issues and requirements around HIV (Health Protection Agency 2012).

Within countries, HIV resources may also vary dramatically according to local infrastructure. Particular regions or provinces and rural areas in general are less served, especially but not only in low- and middle-income countries. My empirical work has been done mostly in relatively well-resourced, urban and peri-urban areas in both South Africa and the UK. Even in the UK, research participants in rural areas have to travel for some services, though they are much more able to do this than rural South African participants would typically be.

HIV's difficulties also exist, like HIV identities generally, intersectionally, at the juncture of a whole set of social and cultural identities (Hall 1990), some of which may mitigate or intensify the challenges of HIV lives, and all of which will have different salience in different social and historical contexts (Crenshaw 2003; Yuval-Davis 2006). I have already discussed how differential economic statuses affect living with HIV and ARVs. Sexualities, drug use and sex work, citizenship status, age and gender also make big differences. Men, for instance, are especially likely to access ARVs late or not at all (Zungu 2012). Women tend to use psychosocial services around HIV more; in my South African interviews, for example, respondents accessed through organisations dedicated to both men and women have been overwhelmingly female. The epidemic itself has often been said to be feminised. In high-prevalence regions especially, the pandemic has indeed had a dramatic impact on women. For it is women who are not only more easily infected, but who are rendered vulnerable through violence and poverty and who are the principal carers for HIV-infected family members and orphaned children (see for instance Brandt 2008; Ciambrone 2001; Doyal and Anderson 2005; Higgins et al. 2010; Squire 2003).

In many national epidemics, gay male sexuality (or the less identity-defining term commonly used by HIV NGOs, 'men who have sex with men', or MSM) and sex work remain unspeakable and highly HIV-associated. These conjunctions turn HIV into a similarly silenced condition, especially for gay men or 'MSM' who cannot be open about their sexualities,[3] and for sex workers who are not open about their work, but also for heterosexuals who are not sex workers, and who are concerned about HIV's links with pathologised sexualities. Many of the heterosexual study interviewees in both the United Kingdom and South Africa expressed these concerns, particularly when recounting their own preconceptions about HIV and their concerns after diagnosis.

In what is increasingly going to be a greying pandemic, as HIV positive people taking ARVs survive into old age and rates of new infections slowly fall, a fresh set of issues are arising for this group, particularly around long-term health concerns (Power et al. 2010). Within my longitudinal research in the United Kingdom, half of the interviewees now fall into this category. Moreover, specific issues arise for people who become positive over the age of 50, who are very unlikely to get diagnosed early; these, however, were people I was not that likely to see within the HIV support study.

Citizenship status is an under-recognised but major contributor to ongoing difficulties with living with HIV. People without citizenship status in the United Kingdom, especially if they are illegally in the country, and are not registered as asylum seekers, are probably least likely to get help. Indeed, young women recently diagnosed who became positive outside of the United Kingdom are the most likely not to access services regularly (Health Protection Agency 2011a), and this group's often problematic citizenship status may be related to that irregularity. These were perhaps the least likely people to participate in my UK study, though in fact some participants have belonged to this category in every interview round I have done since the late 1990s. There are also many undocumented migrants from sub-Saharan Africa within South Africa, including at least two million Zimbabweans, some of whom are HIV positive. While HIV services often fail to reach them, other issues are usually more pressing (Doctors Without Borders 2010). I did not talk to them in my HIV support study there.

Finally, HIV may be just one of many issues that trouble people's lives. Much of the time, it may not be the most important one, particularly for women (Brandt 2008; Ciambrone 2001; Doyal and Anderson 2005; Squire 2003). However, there are times and contexts where it can become more salient. To remove its exceptionality, mainstreaming it and hence relegating it to one issue among others, can mean that its salience becomes hard to recognise. Yet the partial, integrated, sometimes almost incidental character of positive HIV status in people's lives is going to become an increasing feature of the pandemic, as more people access improved ARVs. Even today, HIV's social salience is frequently at odds with its low profile within people's lives.

In the 2011–2 interviews about HIV support on which this book draws, many of my interviewees, both in the United Kingdom and in South Africa, especially those who have been diagnosed recently, who received medication early and who are doing well health-wise, with or without ARVs, described HIV as just another health condition or life challenge, and often as not the most important one in their lives. At the same time, many others pointed out that HIV has a very particular stigmatised character, a difficult past, uncertain present, and unknowable future. How, for instance, will the medication work, lifelong, for people taking it? Will high-income countries continue to fund ARVs and HIV services in lower-income countries where HIV occurs at high rates, in perpetuity? Sometimes, the same interviewee said both things. They affirmed that HIV does not define them and is a minor part of their life, while at the same time expressing strong concerns about their present and future health and resources, and the effects of HIV on their lives in general.

From exceptionalism to particularity

Given the psychosocial, socio-cultural, medical, and economic resource constraints that operate in specific patterns around HIV, it seems reasonable at this point in the pandemic to argue, not for HIV exceptionalism of the kind described and criticised above, but rather for a recognition of HIV's *exceptionality,* based on its *particular* characteristics. That is, it is crucial to recognise the always shifting aspects of the epidemic, the exceptions that cannot be understood within current frameworks, but that nevertheless insist on making themselves felt (Derrida 2002[4]). It is important to negotiate these exceptions into social understanding by various partial processes of translation that characterise their particularity in ways we can grasp. But some of this particularity will always be left outside, guaranteeing a continuing, radical openness to what HIV involves and means.

This particularity may then be the continuing grounds, as for Havlir and Beyrer (2012), for requiring the appropriate funding of HIV requirements alongside others, and for the maintenance of HIV as a priority even in conditions of fiscal austerity. Like many others, Havlir and Beyrer (2012: 686) buttress this argument with the deliverable promises of HIV science: 'It would be an extraordinary failure of global will and conscience if financial constraints and false dichotomies truncated our ability to begin to end AIDS just when the science is showing that this goal is achievable.'

Despite all the difficulties of living with HIV, and their diverse manifestations, the improved and longer lives that increasing numbers of HIV positive people are now leading on long-term ARV medication do indeed point to a newly optimistic state of the pandemic, as well as to fresh difficulties. The ways in which people now live these three-letter lives also indicate some areas of the pandemic that are increasingly converging, in high- and middle-income countries especially, in both their improvements and their difficulties. The concept of HIV's particularity enables us to bridge the contradiction between these divergent aspects of living with HIV and ARVs.

In South Africa, and to a lesser extent in the United Kingdom, both the contemporary preoccupations of research participants and the ways in which my longer-term research participants' concerns have shifted over the past decade suggest that the move from figuring HIV exceptionalism to HIV particularity, still being debated by policymakers, has happened already, some time ago, in their lives. In their accounts of their day-to-day experiences, their HIV status remains highly but variably significant. It is broadly integrated into their larger set of life concerns, but its specific manifestations and effects continue to disrupt those lives. The same shift is now happening in the policy arena and in activism. The resurgence of ACT UP in the United States involves collaborations with, for instance, Housing Works, a community-based HIV service organisation that arose from ACT UP in the 1990s, and the Occupy movement. HIV organisations in the United Kingdom such as the Terrence Higgins Trust, and the African Health Policy Network (AHPN), which developed materials for recent London HIV prevention campaigns targeting African-origin communities, operate with wider sexual health and health concerns. In South Africa, many HIV activists from the last two decades, such as Nathaniel, are now working in broader social justice fields. At the same time, the continuing particularities of the epidemic still require attention, even within coalitional organisations. However, these particularities appear with special clarity and emphasis in what people say about their specific life circumstances.

The particularised characteristics of living with HIV and ARVs, especially those that are neglected or not yet recognised in politics and policy, are powerfully registered at psychosocial levels, as Quentin's interview and Maane's account suggest. These characteristics can be understood structurally; they are not necessarily or fully experienced in that way. And it is at the psychosocial level that the experience of HIV, across high-, middle- and low-income contexts, are most generally shared. In this book, I shall be treating experience as Joan Scott (1991) describes it: as a form of making sense and understanding, rather than as unmediated knowledge. As the word's etymology suggests, it is an effort, a way of 'trying'. Sometimes experience is multiple and contradictory. Language and other media, as well as social and historical circumstances, shape it. At the same time, it allows us access to subjective phenomena that other HIV research materials, such as physiological samples, behavioural scales, or personality inventories, do not register (Daniel and Squire 2010). As we have seen, HIV experiences are shaped and lived differently in situations of poverty than in high-income situations. In middle- and low-income countries, treatment is less accessible, social services more restricted. HIV may compete as a policy priority, particularly in the midst of recession, with requirements for other health care, notably basic health care, food security, infrastructural elements such as electricity and clean water supplies, employment and political stability. However, much of what people say in, for instance, South Africa, about the astounding gains but also the difficulties of ARVs – about the potential for healthy, productive lives and reductions in stigma, but also about dealing with the continuing stigma, sadness and uncertainties of the condition, and about living 'positively' with HIV positive status and helping others do likewise – sounds very similar to how people in the developed world talk about HIV (Squire 1999, 2003, 2006, 2007, 2010). Like HIV positive people in the United Kingdom, too, people living with HIV in South Africa often want to forget about the virus and think instead about their children, their boyfriends or girlfriends, their jobs and education. And people in both circumstances insist that the specificities of HIV identities, however mobile and variable, be recognised, and call for understanding of and services for living with HIV, specifically, to continue.

Social researchers, especially in the fields of sociology and psychology, have increasingly been emphasising the need to complexify approaches to what we have been calling 'psychosocial' issues around HIV, which can take account of the particularities described in this chapter. Such researchers are developing perspectives that bring together attention to emotions, thinking, interpersonal relations, smaller and larger-scale social structures, and cultural, political and economic formation. Without such approaches, they suggest, the increasingly specialised and extensive biomedical treatment and prevention strategies currently generating policy optimism in the HIV pandemic will run into insoluble problems, as they have before (Campbell et al. 2007; Flowers and Davis 2012; Kippax 2012; Myklahovskiy and Rosengarten 2010; Nguyen et al. 2012; Rosengarten 2009; Squire 2010). Moreover, many researchers emphasise that approaches to contemporary HIV issues benefit from integrating social with humanities research. Developing a long tradition of attention to the cultural and artistic representations operating around HIV, the secondary 'epidemic of signification' accompanying the medical one, researchers note the indissolubility of the links between how HIV is lived, and how it is talked and written about, seen, and heard (Treichler 1999; Watney 2000).

Researching HIV particularities through narrative

The research on which this book draws takes on these concerns by adopting a narrative approach to HIV research. Studying narratives enables the researcher to bring different modalities of representations together, and to engage with psychosocial complexities as well as the social, cultural and political contexts within which such representations are produced. In the case of HIV, narrative research thus seems an apposite psychosocial research technology. It offers a way to address the particularities of the pandemic at many levels.

Why deploy narrative, specifically, to study the particularities of HIV? After all, many qualitative research approaches offer themselves as possible modes of address to highly specific, heavily contextualised and complex phenomena. Here I will describe how a narrative approach to the research materials drawn on in this book, especially the materials from my UK and South African interview studies, helps keep the particularities of the pandemic in focus. Other aspects of the studies will be described in later chapters as they become relevant, and in the next chapter, I will discuss some common and overarching narrative framings of the pandemic that appear in policy and popular-cultural texts as well as in the interviews.Narrative approaches are especially good at taking account of the uncertainties, multiplicities, gaps and contradictions that play out through people's accounts of their lives with HIV. Narrative research does not view these aspects of stories as 'wrong', as they might seem to participants themselves if they had to say or write contradictory things in answer to questions, or as might appear in a thematic analysis that pits one theme against another, rather than viewing themes as succeeding and building on each other throughout an interview (Squire 2005, 2008; Butler 2005; Hyvarinen et al. 2010; Riessman 2008).

Narratives are sequences of symbols, arrayed on dimensions of temporality, probably their most obvious ordering principle, but also of causality and spatiality. From this perspective, they are enactments of experience, but in a specific sense. Narratives express experience, not as summative and authoritative wholes or internal truths, but as processes of linguistic and social engagement (Scott 1991). They may seem to be 'personal', but they enact personhood as a changing social strategy, rather than as a single, stable formation. Narratives are processes of everyday meaning-making, but that does not imply that their meanings are completely accessible, or accessible to everyone; they are historically and socially specific, and their readings therefore depend on specific, situated language communities (Squire 2012; Squire et al. 2013).

Narrative approaches make it possible to bring different types and levels of stories into dialogue with each other. By addressing the apparently 'personal' stories that people tell in interviews, for example, researchers can pay attention to stories of detailed psychic difficulties, which some researchers might say are even being told at an unconscious level (Brandt 2009; Long 2009), alongside mid-level stories that are about conscious subjective, interpersonal and micro-social strategies for living with HIV: factors like information-sharing, discussion in safe social spaces, the building of individual efficacy and community capacity, and the development of various kinds of social resources or 'capitals', which Campbell and colleagues (2007) summarise as 'HIV competence'. NGOs dealing with HIV issues frequently deploy people's stories in their publicity and education materials in this way, showing the detailed texture of HIV positive or HIV-affected people's lives, at the same time as they delineate the local resources that encourage positive ways of living (an example is the UK National AIDS Trust's 'Real Stories' page: http://www.hivaware.org.uk/be-aware/real-stories.php).

Narrative research can in addition address the interplay of people's individual stories with culturally current HIV narratives, which themselves operate in and derive from different fields. In the United Kingdom, for instance, my research participants' storying of their lives at least partly around legal, policy and media accounts of criminalisation, as in Quentin's account of the legally shaped 'caution' he must exercise in relationships, was not a feature of people's HIV accounts in the early 2000s. However, criminalisation affected interviewees' stories quite strongly in 2011. In South Africa in the 2000s, research participants very often told stories of their own salvation through knowledge and in some cases treatment. These stories asserted their own moral agency, against the many current popular and religious narratives that positioned HIV infection as the wages of sin and people living with HIV as excommunicable transgressors (Squire 2007). As in this case, narrative research makes it possible to relate individual to cultural stories in different media and fields; here, for instance, to biblical as well as media narratives, and to narratives that are expressed in large and small social groups, or that appear in print, audio and visual popular media.

Fictional narratives, especially those produced in television soap operas such as *Eastenders* in the United Kingdom, *Soul City* in South Africa, and in a number of African countries, starting with Kenya, the youth-oriented MTV series *Shuga*, are many people's route into understanding HIV issues. Highly effective visual narratives of people's lives are also in operation across the pandemic. Photographic work, as one of the Through Positive Eyes project participants, Alejandro from Mexico, says, allows one to 'find things through pictures that I haven't realised before' and to express 'things that are very hard for me to say in words' (Mendel 2009). Paintings of the body, HIV and ARVs, like those generated by Cape Town's Bambanani Women's Group, through workshops in South Africa, Zambia, Tanzania and Canada, condense the complexities of HIV lives in ways that would be laborious and insufficient if essayed in linear verbal descriptions (Morgan and the Bambanani Women's Group 2004). Poetry offers a means of narrating aspects of lives with HIV that other genres do not attend to. As mentioned at the beginning of this chapter, my student's emotional encounter with someone living with HIV generated, even as she was living it, a poetic reflection. In my work with Lumka Daniel in South Africa, Daniel deployed poetic form to condense the voices of the research participants and, in so doing, brought into more intense focus the emotional progressions of those 'voices' (Daniel and Squire 2010). Narrative research enables cross-media approaches to such materials (Ryan 2004; Squire 2012).

At a still broader level, a narrative approach makes it possible to understand people's expressions of their lives in relation to political metanarratives. This relation was particularly and newly important in the contemporary UK context in my 2011 UK research, most obviously in participants' frequent references to medical and social service cuts and more broadly, in people's accounts of themselves as socially worthy or unworthy, benefit recipients or workers. Frequently, this round of my UK HIV support research seemed to become, *de facto*, research on recessionary living or 'living with the cuts'. In South Africa in 2012, too, as Nathaniel's story at the beginning of this chapter indicates, for many participants, HIV politics had become rolled into wider political stories. To some extent, this expansion was driven by the exigencies of global financial crisis. But it was also shaped by widened access to effective treatment, coming after a decade of struggle for such access. Addressing people's accounts as stories enables one to see such larger moves, and individual progressions, as interrelated, rather than as fundamentally personal, as a grounded theory approach, for instance, might suggest. We can understand such stories as existing in a matrix of narratives with common themes and structures, articulated at different levels and in different media, or as HIV 'story worlds' (Herman 2013) within which we all live.

For the purposes of this book, I am particularly interested in what I shall call 'counteracting narratives', which operate to criticise or comment on the larger and more dominant narratives of the HIV pandemic, working against the naturalisation processes of medicalisation, normalisation, and marketisation. Such narratives are similar to what are often called counter-narratives or counter-stories (Bamberg and Andrews 2004; Fine and Harris 2001), a much-discussed and complicated category. I am restricting the book's interest, however, to stories that act, or counter-act: that clearly, if subtly, perform different meanings to those hegemonic around the pandemic.

Narrative work is not unique to HIV within the field of health and illness. There is a large body of narrative health research, much debated. It is often argued that such research enables the voices of people living with illnesses to be heard, that it has moved medical understandings away from disease, towards illness and that it understands the effects of serious illness on the disruption and the reconstitution of identities (Bury 2001; Frank 1997; Kleinman 1988; Mishler 1986). A narrative approach to health issues can, though, be over-simplistic, operating as if the stories themselves are curative. It can also ignore the positions of many seriously ill people who have other much higher priorities in their lives than illness, such as keeping a job, looking after children, or people close to them who are themselves ill, or surviving in poverty. HIV is, as we have said, a condition for which this is frequently the case, particularly for women (Ciambrone 2001).

Nevertheless, in the case of an often-silenced, stigmatised, serious and new condition such as HIV, around which political campaigns were fought in the high-income world especially in the 1980s and 1990s, and in low- and medium-income countries in the 1990s and the early 2000s, personal stories can often act, as the sociologist Kenneth Plummer (1995) has described, to bring people together, and to catalyse political actions. The sociology of social movements has been increasingly interested in the emotional loads that stories carry, and how stories can work to precipitate or to shift activism (Tilly 2002). Francesca Polletta's (2006) work on stories of spontaneity and how they worked to potentiate the civil rights movement in the 1960s United States is a good example. Plummer (1995) has written about the powerful effects of sexual stories, of gay and lesbian sexual identities, sexual harassment, gendered disempowerment and HIV itself, moving from 'private' to 'public' notice, undermining that dichotomy, and becoming part of collectivising consciousness and action. Narratives do not always potentiate or support progressive social change; they may work in the other direction, or have no discernible effects on the broader social world at all (Squire 2013). In instances similar to those Plummer describes, however, stories socially suppressed into suffering can have micro- and macro-social significance when they get told and heard.

There is a considerable amount of research specifically on HIV stories. Not all of it, however, is of the kind just described. Some narrative HIV research describes story categories, and tries to measure people's lives against them. It asks, for instance, whether narratives directed at restoring lives work better for people than what read like unorganised 'chaos' narratives or stories that appear to minimise HIV. Such research may also ask whether narratives that move from biographical disruption towards reconstitution in the light of a new HIV positive identity are useful for people, and how such narratives emerge within people's lives (Crossley 2000; Carricaburu and Pierret 1995). Some narrative HIV research, however, addresses narrative complexities that do not lend themselves to such categorisations. Examples in the South African context are Rene Brandt's (2009) case-study work with very poor women living with HIV, Carol Long's (2009) detailed biographical accounts of compromised HIV positive maternity, Thirusha Naidu's (2012) study of HIV home carers storying a micro-politics of care in rural areas and

Nompumelelo Zungu's (2012) multi-levelled analyses of the meanings of HIV, 'our disease', for men. In UK contexts, Paul Flowers' and colleagues' (2006) phenomenological analyses of the stories of continuing stigma told by HIV positive people of African origin, Leslie Doyal and Jane Anderson's (2005) research on women's accounts of the emotional dilemmas through which they live with HIV, and Mark Davis's (2010) tracings of the intricate narrative arguments gay men develop around relationships, sero-sorting and disclosure, are instructive examples.

This book operates at somewhat of a tangent to both these research paths. It is not concerned with how psychological adjustment relates to particular story types, although this is, of course, sometimes a real issue for research participants. The book also does not focus on life narratives and the complexities embedded in them, though such intricacies certainly make themselves felt in the interview material. Rather, the book examines narratives more specifically, for what they offer as strategies within people's three-letter lives, and also, more broadly, for their intersections with the wider worlds of HIV significations, policy, and politics.

What about narrative research's significance for research participants? Qualitative approaches are often popular with participants, especially if they are from well-researched populations used to ticking endless boxes, as is often the case for people living with HIV. Qualitative research can also be favoured if, as a research participant, you think that your opinion and experience have been ignored, your voice unheard. This was especially the case when I first did research in South Africa, in 2001, and people were extremely keen for their words to be heard through the research and perhaps elsewhere. Some research participants, seeing the research process as a potential conduit to a wider and possibly more receptive world, offered to take their stories into broadcast media. Some wanted to use their real names, to be examples to others. In the 2011 research, though, it was much more the UK interviewees who said they felt erased from the social scene as HIV citizens, rendered invisible; and who wanted their and others' voices heard. In South Africa, a decade of increasing awareness and improved treatment of HIV meant that the participants' witnessing to the difficult realities of their lives, though still outward-facing, was less fraught and urgent.

'Voice' is not a simple matter within narrative research. As with Lumka Daniel's 'Voices' poem, it can involve an interested hearing and relay of multiple, overlapping research participants' voices, rather than a direct representation of discrete voices. When working with HIV-dedicated NGOs, international NGOs, and all levels of government policy organisations, stories are told by and often to those organisations in a policy 'voice', bearing in mind the audiences who do and might support the organisations. In this round of the UK research, for example, many interviewees were in a sense talking 'past' me, to the voluntary organisations providing services threatened by the cuts, and to the government departments charged with making those cuts. Similarly, the South African participants were telling their stories to me, but also to the organisations that help them, and perhaps also to international audiences currently trying to cut and reorganise HIV funding. The ethical questions involved with such voicings take on a more intense significance with narrative research than in many other forms of qualitative study. For narratives are always told *to* someone: to audiences, real or imagined, past, present or future, of others and within the self. And so we cannot avoid thinking about transitivity, and the consequent co-constructions of 'voice', when we are involved in narrative research (Esin and Squire 2013; Riessman 2008).

The voice of the narrator is also more complex than it appears. Narrative research does not necessarily require people to tell stories. Indeed, in my research, I never ask people to do this, still less to tell the story of their lives, or their lives with HIV. I try to avoid the more coercive aspects of entraining people into storytelling, or storytelling of a certain type, particularly that of personal disclosure and redemption (McAdams 2006; Plummer 2001). However, UK and South African participants alike frequently declared they were telling 'their story'. Even when they did not do this, they tended to structure many of their responses to questions as narratives, for instance as temporally organised accounts of their progression through HIV-related conditions, as has been found in much other narrative health research (Bury 2001; Carricaburu and Pierret 1995; Kleinman 1997). Alternatively, participants narrated spatially or conceptually organised progressions, for example charting their moves from clinic to clinic or support service to service, or following disclosures made successively to family members. These progressions are also 'narrative' in the sense of progressing through successions of symbols that build meaning (see also Squire 2012).

Such worked on, cultivated meaning structures are given over to researchers with the participants' ownership of them attached. Alessandro Portelli (2010) has described oral historians as needing to be thankful to those who 'lend' their voices to the work. This is a helpful position, but one that needs development when researchers re-present materials (for 'representation' always involves some degree of reframing), or when researchers bring their own meaning structures to bear on the material, as they necessarily do in narrative analysis. Because of the disjunctions between story readings, and between participants, researchers and other audiences, we always need to address the power relations within which narratives and their meanings, as well as the ways in which stories can operate powerfully to change meanings and lives.

Narrative research therefore has to follow narratives themselves in operating dialogically. Narratives work dialogically through the construction of stories in dialogues between researcher and research participant; between the many voices of each of these participants; between research participants and a whole range of expected or imagined audiences such as family and friends, local communities, policymakers and politicians; and between particular and more general and widespread story meanings. Narrative research must address these interactions, but also its own dialogue with narrators and narrative materials. This ubiquitous dialogism helps produce narrative research's multi-levelled sensibility and its ability to position narratives within power relations, as well as to pay attention to their particularity (Esin and Squire 2013; Riessman 2008).

However, none of this potential complexity of narrative analysis obviates the ethical issues that arise when any researcher, using any methodology, summarises, interprets and quotes from research participants. In the case of this book, care has been taken to anonymise and to remove identifying information at many points. The analyses have been made available to the research participants for comment wherever possible. The text has also been read by people working in the HIV sector in the United Kingdom and South Africa, in order to engage in a critical dialogue that positions the narratives within this book in a more thorough and more useful context during its production as well as its later, wider audiencing.

Narrative dialogism and ethics are not simply matters of equitable conversational exchange and emotional care. They have to be understood as operating from positions that are specifically and diversely aligned with power, and as having, themselves, more or less powerful effects. My own position in the studies as a middle-class white British female academic who is HIV negative is germane to what transpires in the research. However, different aspects of this intersectional position are mobilised by different social contexts, at different times, with different participants. In South Africa, for example, when I conducted research with people who were unemployed or who had low incomes, my class, racialised and national positions seemed most salient, though my unmarked HIV negativity may also have been in play in the interviews. Within a UK research context, HIV status, classed and racialised categories, and also gender and citizenship status, are often all more or less explicitly activated.

All research situations configure power relations in highly particular ways that need to be attended to. In the case of these studies, meeting up with research participants who have taken part in the interviews before means drawing on a long, albeit interrupted, history of research exchanges that invest participants with a more powerful place in the research. The many interviewees in the study who are resource-poor often view the power gradient between researcher and participant with especially clear eyes, overruling the complexities of interpersonal dialogue with the larger ethic of a dialogic position structured by economic inequality. In all the interview rounds, participants are paid on a local university research assistant scale for their time. However, this rubric is not always sufficient to address the everyday inequities with which people live. One man I interviewed in a very under-resourced support group in a South African township in the early 2000s told me, 'Next time you come, you have to bring something, because we have no food. For instance, a box of apples.' When I returned to the group to conduct follow-up interviews in 2012, I heeded the spirit if not the letter of this advice. After consulting with the group coordinator and group members, we used the interview fee allowance for food supplies that were much cheaper to buy in bulk, rather than disbursing individual payments which would have bought less.

Power relations are also in play in the language of narratives. Such language always fails to express everything about experience, but at the same time it fixes people in their stories and to some extent forces them to 'be' their stories. There can be considerable violence attached to telling and listening to a story. As Butler (2005) says, a self-narrative is an implicit response to the question, 'what have you done?' And while such questions are, at their broadest, asked of everyone who participates in social and symbolic human life, they are also often asked by highly regulative interrogators: parents, teachers, employers, doctors, the police, the courts. Even when asked by your friends and family, they require answers; you have to respond in order to be part of any sociality. This humanly coercive potential of narratives is important to be aware of.

At the same time, though, narratives, because they are heterogeneous and fluid, can answer such socio-moral demands by refusal or resistance, though such responses may be ignored or co-opted by an undermining 'sly civility' (Bhabha 1994); by shifting existing answers into a new register, though such shifts may also pass unnoticed; or by directing answers to someone else than the interrogators. Such narratives may not be counter-narratives in any recognisable sense, but they may have *counteracting effects* on hegemonic narratives, which are themselves multiple, contradictory, and susceptible to cracks, breaks and change. In my research, for instance, participants often explicitly declare that they are speaking not just to me and my projected research audiences, but to other HIV positive and HIV-affected people, or to policymakers and policy implementers, or sometimes to research and archive audiences which they imagine in ways that differ from my own projections. Such addresses provide another way to understand the problematic authority of 'voice'. For a narration in a particular 'voice' is also a particular form of knowledge, about experiences of a specific contemporary HIV epidemic. The Latin etymological roots of 'narrative' itself, in words for both knowing and telling, suggest this might be the case. Knowledge is dependent upon lived as well as spoken material practices. The acted and language practices of three-letter lives work together in narratives, to constitute knowledge of those lives. The research participants have more of such knowledge, and they can impart some of it to their diverse audiences through their stories.

It has become apparent in this chapter that 'particularity' is not a straightforward counterpoint to exceptionality in the HIV field. It is, rather, a term that describes well a methodological approach within much qualitative research, centred on what Geerz (1973) has called thick description. Such an approach involves detailed, fine-grained, particularistic accounts of research materials and their relations to their wider contexts and histories, as well as attention to the non-comprehensible, exceptional aspects of empirical materials that call attention to what needs to and cannot yet be explained (Squire 2012). Narrative research, I have suggested, offers special sensitivities to such particularism because of its built-in complexities, dialogism, and negotiation between language, experience and power relations. The challenge for much narrative research is to move beyond the careful and illuminating accounts of specific research contexts, towards what Lincoln and Guba (1985) have called transferable qualitative knowledge: knowledge gained in one particular context that can be applied, usually in part, and with careful attention to similarities and differences, to others.

In the case of HIV, it is clearly valuable if qualitative research can make moves toward transferability. Such moves would enable the narrative strategies mobilised in the United Kingdom and South Africa, now and in the recent past, and analysed in this book, for example, to be considered in relation to the pandemic's broader contexts. Religiously inflected 'conversion' narratives about HIV, of the kind I mentioned earlier, have been reported in many contexts outside of South Africa. Their potential socio-moral effectiveness could make them important to consider in policymaking within those other contexts. HIV's criminalisation has been investigated in many national contexts, usually at the level of variable legal and policy responses. Its difficult psychosocial effects, narrated in my UK study particularly by Quentin and others, and mentioned in many other studies, could helpfully be considered as transferable knowledge germane to criminalisation debates in many national contexts. Such work might, for instance, have had impact on the recent Canadian decision to criminalise non-disclosing HIV positive people who have sex with a 'realistic possibility' of transmission, defined as anything other than penetrative heterosexual vaginal sex with a condom *and* undetectable viral load (Supreme Court of Canada 2012).

As we have seen in Section 1, the HIV pandemic's enormous present and future impact as a 'long wave' event (Barnett and Whiteside 2006) means that it retains ongoing global significance. In addition, developing characteristics of the pandemic require analysis: vastly increased treatment availability; HIV's simultaneous naturalisation and backgrounding among global and national priorities; the difficulties of living with treatment; ongoing resource shortages in many national contexts; the critical global economic situation within which treatment must now be lived; the changing but continuing difficulties of HIV stigmatisation and disclosure; and the shifting character of local and broader activism around HIV. This chapter has argued that such analysis needs to address the particularities of specific HIV epidemics, but also to treat them within a broader context of shared histories and common futures. It has suggested, moreover, that psychosocial commonalities and differences across the pandemic are relevant to all of us, whatever our status, whatever HIV's prevalence in the place where we live and whatever we know or have experienced of HIV.

The rest of this book aims to provide a particular but also transferable analysis of this kind. Its accounts of HIV narratives operating within specific epidemic situations may offer ways to understand similar narratives in different contexts (Squire 2012). This is one way in which we can move from HIV exceptionalism to particularity, while at the same time searching out and recognising the commonalities across different epidemic contexts to which it is also important to pay attention.

Section 2 of *Living with HIV and ARVs* focuses on some commonalities in contemporary narratives of HIV across national contexts, especially those of the United Kingdom and South Africa, that appear across different kinds of narratives, within personal accounts, policy documents and media. The section thus provides examples of transferability in analysis, as well as analysis that defines contemporary HIV particularities. Following on from this, Section 3 excavates more of the particularities of the United Kingdom and South African epidemics, relating them to their 'transferable' contemporary high- and middle-income, recession-enmeshed contexts. The last chapter of Section 3 analyses some wider particularities that appear in the contemporary relations of HIV to other forms of politics and action in first the UK and then the South African context, which may themselves have broader, transferable relevance.

Section 2

Being Naturalised, Being Left Behind

3
Being Naturalised

Nicco: Okay, my name is Nicco surname is (second name), I was diagnosed 2008, I am HIV positive, I am on treatment, ARVs, regime 1, 3TC, D4T, er, nevirapine, mhm, I like my status too much. But once before I was getting challenges through my family but I was able to accept, it was need (ed) to live and to be positive, and also I like to (make) change to my community, because our persons is not open to the status, and also I want to change, to give more information to change the situation of the community.

Nicco (South Africa 2012)

People living with diagnosed HIV in the UK can expect a near-normal life expectancy, particularly if diagnosed promptly... where antiretroviral therapy is available, it has transformed HIV infection from a fatal illness to a chronic manageable condition.

(Health Protection Agency 2011a: 4, 6)

Value for money is best obtained when national AIDS responses make timely investments that are in the right places; utilise the right strategies; increase efficiency, reduce costs and promote innovation.

(UNAIDS 2011a: 31)

Introduction

In the autumn of 2011, I meet Queenie, an HIV positive woman in her 50s who lives in a small flat behind a fast-food restaurant on the North Circular with her children. Queenie came to the United Kingdom as an asylum seeker, discovered her HIV status while waiting for her claim to be decided, and is now doing well on antiretroviral medication. She is hoping to move to a bigger flat soon. She is extremely welcoming, even though I get lost and arrive late. She has two mobile phones and calls me from both to help me find her. In the interview, she describes the network of support of which she is a part, which operates largely through these phones. For instance, she frequently sends encouraging texts to friends of hers whom she has met at support groups, who are more recently diagnosed, less well, still struggling with the asylum process, or all three. While we are doing the interview, the phones are beeping constantly. Sometimes, she breaks off to text back. It turns out that this is a form of support she has developed and is giving out of necessity, not choice. Some local support services have closed; others are too far to reach for those who are not well. She mostly works by texting because texts are cheap, calling costs money, and so does travelling to meeting places. Queenie, despite her optimism and activity, is not well. She finds moving difficult; she has bad neuropathy, that is, damage to peripheral nerves, caused by opportunistic infections, HIV medications, or HIV itself, which causes foot, hand, and limb pain. I see this as she bustles around, but she mentions it only very briefly.

In the summer of 2012, over a decade after I first interviewed Yoliswa in the offices of an NGO dealing with HIV issues in Khayelitsha, near Cape Town, I meet up with her again. Yoliswa has been living openly with HIV since the early 2000s. She is now in her 30s. We have some snacks at a fast-food place in the centre of Cape Town in the middle of her commute homeward, and she brings me up to date. Her health is good, antiretrovirals are working well for her, she has been able to secure a series of short-term contracts despite the low-employment economy, she has even bought a flat. Her son is all grown up and she has had another son since we met, who is also doing well and is now at school. He is HIV negative and she calls him her 'Nevirapine baby', name-checking the medication she took within a PMTCT programme, to reduce the chance of transmitting HIV to him. Yoliswa was open about her status at a time when few were. In earlier years, she appeared in the media, talking about the need for PMTCT. Her middle child, a daughter born when PMTCT was not available, died as a baby. Yoliswa tells me she is very happy with how things are going for her now, except for ongoing job insecurities. As we are getting ready to leave, though, she points out that one thing concerns her, though she does not think about it all the time. What about the global economic situation? All her medications come thanks to international aid programmes. Might these ever be curtailed, or even stopped? The possibility seems remote, but it would be extremely serious, and it is beyond her control. Sometimes, she worries about it.

In a time when it is possible to provide good medical treatment for HIV, that is, the treatment possibility era, what is it like to live with HIV and ARVs? In a pandemic spread across countries of widely different HIV prevalences, with drastically different resources to deal with their epidemics, what are three-letter lives like across these very diverse contexts? Even at a particular income level, among low-income countries, for instance or within any single high-income country, HIV patterns are often very specific. There are HIV epidemics with special characteristics in particular countries, and particular communities within countries. Across this variability, what are the similarities and differences in people's ways of living with HIV and ARVs?

This chapter examines how the particularities of living with HIV are currently expressed, with some commonality, in narratives of a specific kind: stories of HIV's naturalisation and counteracting stories of resistance to that naturalisation.[1] In the treatment possibility era, HIV is increasingly naturalised, that is, constructed as a natural, and therefore general, comprehensible, and relatively stable and manageable (though still difficult to deal with) part of our biological, social and economic worlds. This naturalisation process works against the exceptionalism around HIV that we considered in the previous chapter. Exceptionalism has focused on HIV's serious health consequences, incurability, and stigmatisation, as well as in earlier years on its fatality and untreatability. HIV exceptionalism has also pointed to the condition's high prevalence, depletion of resources, and continuing large resource demands, in national contexts that are already very resource-constrained. The naturalisation of HIV turns such features of the pandemic into problematic, rather than crisis, elements.

The UN foregrounded both medical and social naturalisations of HIV when in 2011 it set up its 2015 goal of three 'zeroes': zero deaths from HIV-related causes, an aim that naturalises early testing and ARV treatment; zero stigma and discrimination, an outcome dependent on the naturalisation of HIV positive status within all communities and countries and zero new infections, an aim that naturalises behavioural change involving low-risk drug use and sex, as well as treatment as prevention (UNAIDS 2012a). The naturalisation of the pandemic is thus written into the broadest of international HIV programmes, as well as being lived out in the everyday conduct of people's lives. Naturalisation is, though, only one aspect of HIV's current particularities. This and subsequent chapters explore how other particularities work within HIV's naturalisation processes, sometimes to further and sometimes to rescind them.

Section 2 of this book begins by describing HIV's contemporary naturalisation within the treatment possibility era, and that naturalisation's limits. In this and the subsequent three chapters, Chapters 4–6, the section details how naturalisation happens, and how it is undermined from within. It examines how HIV's naturalisation relates to the uncertainties of HIV as a biological condition (Chapter 4), to HIV's psychosocial characteristics (Chapter 5), and to HIV-related socioeconomic resources (Chapter 6). Throughout these chapters, Section 2 explores how HIV's naturalisation is put in question, that is to say, *de*naturalised, by many people's physical, economic, political and psychological distance from the apparently hopeful HIV present. The last chapter in Section 2, Chapter 7, examines the HIV particularities of these denaturalisations more closely. This is important to do because such distancing denaturalisations mean that large numbers of people living with or affected by HIV are to some extent 'left behind',[2] living with past difficulties, present uncertainties, and unknowable futures of HIV.

Studying naturalisation and denaturalisation

When describing HIV's naturalisation processes, and the other processes that undo them, it is not a question of ascribing praise or blame for the processes to particular people or organisations. In this chapter and thereafter, I am, rather, treating HIV's naturalisation as a form of governmentality, that is, as a nexus of discourses and practices through which local, national, and international organisations generate and manage their subjects as citizens (Foucault 1991). In this case, I am concerned primarily with the naturalising governmentality operating around citizens living with HIV and ARVs. Many contemporary discussions of HIV citizenship address it along these lines rather than as, more conventionally, a matter of individual or collective rights and responsibilities (though the latter may also be seen as a strategic way of formulating the former; see Mbali 2005; Robins 2009). For in the HIV field, the framing of citizenship as a product of governmentality is supported by the highly socially and politically shaped nature of the pandemic: the socially embedded nature of HIV's transmission, its social stigmatisation, the socioeconomic differentiations across its epidemiology and the strongly politicised histories of national and international approaches to HIV. At the same time, HIV citizenship is, like other forms of citizenship, a complex condition that currently requires further theoretical elaboration (Nguyen 2011; Robins 2009; and more generally, Baubock 2008; Bosniak 2006; Kymlicka 2003; Modood et al. 2006; Pateman 1989; Shachar 2009; Young 1989). Section 2's analyses of naturalising and denaturalising processes build a fuller account of the characteristics of contemporary HIV citizenship. Some of these elaborations may also be relevant to other acute and stigmatised health and social conditions.

To make these analyses, the chapters in Section 2 focus on a range of empirical materials, from interviews and from media and policy documents. This section, as well as those that follow, also draws on my long-term studies of HIV support within the United Kingdom and South Africa. The complex narrative material emerging from these studies demonstrates both the powerful but compromised processes of naturalisation and the subtle yet persistent elements of 'being left behind'. These processes are discernible in other expressions of the pandemic, in policy documents and media accounts, for instance. Such materials are also analysed narratively here, though they originate from a rather different, more abbreviated kind of sampling from key NGO and policy documents, than that deployed in my last two interview rounds. Section 2 spends substantial time considering such materials because the processes of citizenly naturalisation which I am discussing manifest in policy and political contingencies as well as in people's experiences of the pandemic. Such processes become part of matrices of social and cultural as well as personal representations. The personal narratives appearing in interviews, however, often display emergent aspects of HIV citizenship earlier than do other forms of signification. In addition, they exhibit naturalisation alongside denaturalisation processes in highly interlinked and code-termining ways, which display just how complex these processes and interactions are. Personal narratives are thus important in this section, though they acquire a stronger focus in Section 3, which considers the national particularities of the HIV epidemic's naturalisation.

Within narrative research, the selection, extent, and contextualising of story extracts is often debated (Riessman 2008). Here, I use citations from specific interviews to exemplify general narrative patterns in the interview material. For example, if you see a quotation from a UK interviewee living with HIV and taking ARVs in 2011, that means that the narrative discussed in relation to that quotation has features that are also to be found in a large number of the other 2011 UK interviews with participants on treatment. At times, I also quote from less common or even highly exceptional narratives, clarifying the characteristics of such particularity. In addition, in this chapter and in subsequent ones, I have restricted the number of interviews cited, in order to maintain a sense of specific participants' narratives, and the complexities within them. The HIV pandemic is, as mentioned earlier, not a unitary phenomenon. This section tries to pay attention to the divergent contexts of HIV epidemics, especially in the United Kingdom and South Africa, as well as to convergent processes happening at this historically particular moment of the pandemic. I report on material derived from these different national contexts in order to explore common processes of naturalisation and denaturalisation occurring in their distinct high- and middle-income contexts. The national contexts are also distinct in being in the first decade, for South Africa, and the second decade, for the United Kingdom, of treatment possibility. ARVs became generally available in the United Kingdom in 1996; South Africa's ARV rollout began in 2004. However, some of my South African interviewees had ARV access, via drug trials and pilots, in 2001, when I first met them. From 2003, all of the interviewees who needed ARVs had access via international NGOs or the Western Cape Health Department, which operated an early universal ARV policy. And in 2012, as we have seen, South Africa reached the Millennium Development Goal of ARVs for 80% of those who need them.

In the United Kingdom by the late 1990s, and in South Africa by 2003, many interviewees were already dealing with their own projected lifelong ARV use. Only in 2012, however, were interviewees in South Africa as well as the UK living in a context where ARVs were relatively accessible for everyone in the country who needed them, so that living with ARVs lifelong was a general possibility and expectation. Interviewees in both national contexts were therefore living, by 2011–2, with the increasing naturalisation of HIV that accompanies the rollout of effective treatment, and with the continuing uncertainties that undermine that naturalisation. Of course, interviewees were also speaking and living in drastically different social contexts, with distinct HIV and national histories, and sharply divergent resource availability. Nevertheless, some common narrative patterns around HIV's naturalisation, its difficulties, and resistance to it, emerged in the UK and the South African studies. As living long-term with HIV on ARVs becomes regularised, even routine, the common possibilities and challenges of doing so become more apparent, while also varying across social context, time, and treatment 'generations'.

The 'natural order' of the HIV pandemic

Naturalising the 'unnatural'

Even from a cursory look at the progresses in treatment and prevention to which the first two chapters referred, the signs of HIV's naturalisation are numerous. Some of these signs lie in the increasing manageability of HIV prevention, as well as of HIV treatment, by medical means. As one quotation at the beginning of this chapter indicates, the United Kingdom's Health Protection Agency (HPA, now Public Health England), currently presents HIV as a long-term condition, not even an illness, and argues that, with good, early medical treatment, people living with HIV can expect a near-normal lifespan. ARVs, the drugs responsible for this possibility of 'normal' lifespan, are available to all in high-income countries and reach over 50% of those who need them in low- and middle-income countries, a figure that is growing yearly (UNAIDS 2012a; UNAIDS 2011a: 7).

Beginning treatment earlier is preserving the health of people living with HIV. It is also reducing transmission by lowering the viral load of people living with HIV who do not have safe sex. Behaviours which reduce the risk of HIV transmission, especially condom use, have become a more widespread, naturalised part of life, making a large contribution to the shrinking number of new cases worldwide (Cohen et al. 2011; UNAIDS 2011a: 16; World Health Organisation 2013). HIV testing is increasingly a regular part of healthcare in many countries, not just in sexually transmitted infection clinics and antenatal care, but also more generally in hospitals, clinics and pharmacies (Health Protection Agency 2011). Testing is moving out of clinics, into communities. In South Africa, for example, mobile testing units now visit a variety of urban settings such as train stations and malls; in rural areas, team members call on each house individually; home sampling kits can be bought online and in some pharmacies. UK testing has expanded to include community settings such as lesbian and gay community centres, gay bars, and African-oriented NGOs and health centres, as well as home sampling kits obtainable from pharmacies or HIV NGOs.

HIV is also becoming naturalised in some contexts through the lessening, though not the cessation, of stigma, associated in high-income countries with better physical and mental health, and social support, as well as income (Flowers et al. 2006; Logie and Gadalla 2009). Where, as in some areas of South Africa, HIV prevalence is high, people who are not themselves HIV positive almost all intimately know people living with HIV. They have ARV access, they can and increasingly do get HIV tested, and they know about HIV itself. In such circumstances, stigma is decreasing, and HIV is becoming a 'normalised' part of life (Abrahams and Jewkes 2012).

What are the effects of naturalisation on the HIV pandemic? Overall, naturalisation seems to operate, discursively and in practice, to turn a relatively new pandemic, still imperfectly known, and not fully part of established notions of health and illness, into something universal, permanent, and unproblematically incorporated into biological, social, and political relations. At the same time, the HIV pandemic continues to show the traces of otherness that the word 'naturalisation' always carries within its uses around citizenship, and that I will unpack later.

Naturalisation can have very progressive effects. Its constitution of HIV as a condition of general relevance and acceptance can, as UNAIDS clearly plans with its 'zero stigma and discrimination' campaign, reduce pathologising, blaming, and hostility. It can help strengthen HIV-related rights for citizens of all HIV statuses. However, some sociological theories use the term 'naturalisation' to describe processes that turn social and political hierarchies into 'natural', fixed, stable and unchangeable states, assimilated to the biological rather than the sociopolitical field, and made into an unchallengeable part of the rational order, outside of politics (Bourdieu 1977 [1972]; Foucault 1988 [1964]). These theories might suggest that HIV's 'naturalisation' obscures the power relations of the epidemic: the polarities and contests between HIV citizens, between HIV citizenship and other kinds of citizenships, and between the forms of governmentality that constitute these various citizens. Such critical theories of naturalisation indicate the importance of understanding HIV citizenship, like other citizenship, within the frame of multipolar, changeable, agonistic politics (Mouffe 2006), rather than as an achieved state.

Naturalisation, politics, and knowledge

Naturalisation itself needs some explication as a concept. Within Michel Foucault's work, it was developed in relation to European discourses and practices around madness. These, Foucault argued, were always, despite their changeability and contingency, understood as a historical, general, unmarked descriptions of and responses to a natural order. This naturalised order of things could not therefore be resisted or changed. It appeared as existing outside of politics, and it consequently depoliticised all engagements with it (Foucault 1988 [1964]).

Pierre Bourdieu, who wrote later about naturalisation, described it in this way:

> Every established order tends to produce (to very different degrees and with different means) the naturalisation of its own arbitrariness. Of

all the mechanisms tending to produce this effect, the most important and the best concealed is undoubtedly the dialectic of the objective chances and the agents' aspirations, out of which arises the *sense
of limits*, commonly called *the sense of reality*, i.e. the correspondence
between the objective classes and the internalized classes, social structures and mental structures, which is the basis of the most ineradi-
cable adherence to established order. (Bourdieu 1977 [1972]: 164)

Bourdieu was writing here about the naturalisation of concepts such
as class, which are based on socioeconomic realities. The naturalisation
of such concepts imparts to them a rigid certainty which makes itself
felt when 'objective chances' to change socioeconomic realities come
into dialogue with the concepts. Of course, HIV is not exactly the same
kind of concept as class. It does not have the arbitrariness or the potentially fluid relation to change that class has. In the case of HIV, there are
some important biological realities about the virus, and the possibilities
and limits of medical science, with which we have to engage. Moreover,
HIV, and perhaps, in some instances, 'madness' too, the category with
which Foucault was concerned in his account of naturalisation, exists,
in part, within what we often call the 'natural' world, that is, the world
of biological and at a lower level chemical and physical phenomena.
In this sense, HIV is indeed natural, if not naturalised, that is, existing
within the 'reality' of nature. 'Class' is not outside this reality, but it has
a more multiply determined and multidirectional relation to it.

At the same time, what is known scientifically about HIV, as of other
natural phenomena, often suggests a high degree of uncertainty that
policy and popular knowledge tend to erase in favour of more certain,
'naturalised' understandings. 'Objectivity' is difficult in the case of HIV.
Objectivity's implications for the limits of action around HIV are unclear
within debates, for instance, about what the criteria for starting treatment should be, or what constitutes a 'cure'. In dialogue with our aspirations for change, a naturalised concept of HIV with clearer, fixed limits
often comes into play (Latour 2004; Nguyen 2011; Rosengarten 2009).

In addition, the social production of scientific knowledge itself shapes
that knowledge to a large degree, particularly when, as with HIV, the
object of knowledge carries great social urgency and interest. HIV is, like
other illnesses or bodily conditions, disability for example, also a social
condition, an epidemic not just of signification (Treichler 1999) but of
sociality. What constitutes 'successful' treatment or 'effective' prevention programmes, for example, varies socially and historically. Moreover,
what is studied and resourced, and how, the recording and presenting of

findings, and what conclusions are drawn from them, are all inflected by broader political factors. National and international political positions and policy on the phenomenon being investigated; scientific and popular perceptions of the importance of the phenomenon; the power, or lack of it, of people who are affected and scientists who are interested; and levels of local, national. and international resources: all these shape HIV knowledge. South Africa, for instance, has a specific history of some politicians, policymakers and citizens perceiving HIV as not an illness, or as an illness produced simply by poverty, or as an illness best treatable by traditional herbal means. As in many other countries (particularly the United States, where the Tuskegee experiment is perhaps partly responsible for high degrees of doubt about HIV science among African Americans), theories of HIV as punishment for transgression or a deliberately produced weapon against particular countries or racialised groups, have had wide currency in South Africa. This currency is partly, but not entirely, limited by people's familiarity with HIV and the accessibility of treatment (Bogart et al. 2010; Fassin 2007; Kalichman 2009; Niehaus and Jonsson 2005; Rodlach 2006; Steinberg 2008; Thomas and Crause 1991). Religious theories of HIV as a punishment for transgression also continue to be articulated, though much less than before, by spiritual leaders (Squire 2007; Zungu 2012; Prince et al. 2009; Watt et al. 2009). In many epidemics, popular tendencies to 'other' HIV, characterising it as someone else's illness, originating from and belonging elsewhere, continue (Campbell 2003; Joffe 2006; Petros et al. 2006; Winskell et al. 2011). These are all good examples of how the 'epidemic of signification' and the swirl of powerful and less powerful interests around the virus can shape what is known and what knowledge is sought (Robins 2009).

All these patterns of power and signification compete to provide 'objective' HIV knowledges of their own, which then naturalise HIV within these orders of knowledge, setting their own limits on what can and cannot be done about HIV. In some religious accounts, for instance, HIV is naturalised as a condition visited on the body in response to transgression. The sufficiency of your own and others' prayers or other forms of expiation may then be storied in relation to both the degree of spiritual outrage you have provoked, and your own and others' capability to respond with enough humility, enough faith. Even if your prayers fail, cleaving to this route can be narrated as a mark of grace, as submitting to God's will for you.

Where HIV is framed as a developed-world conspiracy, there are diverse possibilities for naturalisation. Science itself may be narrated as, objectively, a thoroughgoing Western conspiracy, in which case HIV is naturalised as an imaginary condition. Alternatively, HIV may be recognised as an illness, with Big Pharma understood as an immense confidence trick played on people experiencing diseases of poverty with their own indigenous solutions ready to hand. HIV treatment is then naturalised within the story as scientific oppression, deliberately and structurally exploitative (Bogart et al. 2010; Zungu 2012). In such a case, both explicit campaigning, and more subaltern, informal kinds of resistance to Big Pharma, like not getting tested, not taking ARVs, or taking them intermittently, might all be naturalised versions of resistant or counteracting narrative responses to the epidemic. The difficulties or failures of ARVs might be explained within stories of the conspiring forces' plans to provide as little and extract as much as possible from the HIV-affected world. Such naturalising conspiracy accounts are less powerful than they were formerly, but they still exist.

Naturalisation's constraints

In the examples so far discussed, naturalisation's effects on forms of knowledge and action are apparent. It depoliticises them, or it politicises them in a singular way which obviates political dialogue.

In philosophy, though, 'naturalisation' refers to something quite different: to an emphasis, within theories of knowledge, on empirical investigations, by ordinary people as well as scientists, about human capacities of, for instance, language and cognition as the route to understanding knowledge, rather than reliance on prior ideas about what knowledge is (Quine 1969).

Of course, prior ideas cannot be erased from knowledge-making, and contemporary naturalist epistemologies acknowledge this; they also do not suggest science is the higher truth. Their naturalism is a pragmatic and heuristic matter (Stich 1993). Such epistemological naturalisation can be applied analogically to HIV knowledge. It suggests that a 'naturalised' knowledge of this new, complex, and changeable field would be the outcome not of assumptions translated from existing personal, religious or even scientific knowledges but rather, of negotiated, limited knowledges, constituted via ongoing academic, professional, and everyday investigations: by investigations, that is, by HIV citizens of all statuses, in every field.

Similarly, many understandings of law heuristically separate out, while accepting their overlap, natural law, governmental law, even divine law, without trying to derive the second from the first or either from the third, or to reduce one to another. Here, the 'natural' indicates a realm of ethical judgement that is not inevitable, unchangeable and foundational, but negotiable. In the case of HIV, this provisionality of the 'natural' is important, especially because HIV is increasingly socially positioned through legal arguments, particularly around the criminalisation of transmission (Monk 2009; Weait 2007). The provisionality of 'natural' law allows us to think about the regimes of HIV knowledge and morality as different from, though overlapping with, the regimes of 'natural' everyday lives, 'governmental' institutional practices, and overarching ethical frameworks. The current 'naturalisation' of HIV frequently involves more absolute oppositions. In its more negative forms, it often involves an elision between the established order of HIV illness and moral pathology. HIV becomes an accepted sign not just of personal but of group, community, even national transgression (Zungu 2012). Sometimes, more positive naturalisations of HIV by people living with HIV seem to involve an opposing canonisation of those previously stigmatised (Steinberg 2008). In this chapter and thereafter, I want to maintain a sense of the disjunctions between and within HIV's physical, psychosocial, politico-legal, and moral naturalisations.

Finally, the meaning of 'naturalisation' within everyday discourse about citizenship provides a further indication of the limits of HIV's naturalisation. In this context, naturalisation indicates both social incorporation and continuing particularity. A 'naturalised' citizen retains this status, always marked out from citizens who did not undergo naturalisation, while being, at the same time, a citizen just like them. This duality characterises HIV's naturalisation, too. For this naturalisation is accompanied by a continuing specificity of the pandemic that limits all naturalised understandings of it, and leaves the status of the 'HIV positive citizen' open to question.

How HIV's naturalisation works

What are the major forms of HIV's contemporary naturalisation? The processes through which it mostly operates are, firstly, medicalisation, that is, the increasing relevance of medicine, especially ARVs, to every aspect of the pandemic, including illness management, care, self-care, and prevention. Second, HIV is normalised, which is to say, constituted as a regular part of health and social relations. This naturalisation process is the one that at first glance appears the most useful and the least problematic. Thirdly, HIV is marketised, or ordered within and through market relations of production and consumption. In the treatment possibility era, given the clear successes of the science and practice of diagnosis and treatment, growing attempts to integrate services within regular forms of provision, and what seem to be an increasingly general marketised model of HIV services and HIV lives, these seem to be the dominant forms of HIV's naturalisation.

In Chapters 4–6, I explore how HIV's naturalisation is played out in people's lives through the processes of medicalisation, normalisation and marketisation, which all operate in inclusive and progressive, but also at times simplifying and limited, ways. I shall examine what narratives of these naturalised, medicalised, normalised, marketised, HIV citizens are like, and what internal contradictions they display. In Chapter 7, I look at processes of denaturalisation which operate particularly around HIV. First though, I turn to the naturalisation process most strongly associated with the current policy and popular optimism around the HIV pandemic: that of medicalisation.

4
When the Drugs Do Work: The Medicalised HIV Citizen

Today we have the tools we need to confront and overcome AIDS and confine it to the history books where it belongs. We are at a crucial point and must seize the opportunity before us. We must take action now.

President Joyce Banda, Lilongwe, Malawi, 28 June 2013

The (International HIV/AIDS) Alliance welcomes the World Health Organisation's (WHO) new guidelines on the use of antiretroviral therapy (ART) for treating and preventing HIV infection...we do not underestimate the challenges. Millions are still not getting the life-saving tools they are entitled to and at the same time, there is a significant withdrawal of international aid from many of the middle-income countries with large HIV epidemics....There is still insufficient linkage between HIV testing and counselling and a high drop-out of people enrolled in HIV care and treatment....This is a programming priority for the Alliance in our global strategy, HIV, health and rights: sustaining community action.

International HIV/AIDS Alliance, 30 June 2013

Introduction: the medical 'end of AIDS' story.

In March 2013, the media celebrated the case of a baby cured of HIV by aggressive ARV treatment shortly after birth. This treatment was provided because her HIV positive mother had not had the usual prophylactic treatment during pregnancy. Despite a later failure to keep taking ARVs, and evidence that HIV remains in her body, the child now shows no sign of active HIV infection, and so demonstrates 'functional cure'

(Persaud et al. 2013). HIV organisations worldwide were notably cautious in their responses. The United Kingdom's first and largest HIV-focused NGO, the Terrence Higgins Trust (THT), commented that the case had little relevance for them since 98–9% of babies born to UK HIV positive mothers were in any case HIV negative at birth because of the UK's thorough vertical transmission prevention programme (Semple 2013). THT spokespeople tried to move the focus away from 'cure', towards the limited applicability of the results (for women diagnosed during labour or babies discovered early to be HIV positive), the uncertainty of later outcomes of this treatment programme, and the importance of better antenatal screening and PMTCT programmes worldwide (Terrence Higgins Trust 2013). Discussing the notion of cure more widely, in the aftermath of a slightly later announcement suggesting 'functional cure' of adults if treated in the first ten weeks after infection, THT similarly emphasised the importance of using condoms, getting tested regularly, and continuing to take ARVs if you are positive (Innes 2013).

However, the 'baby cure' case garnered disproportionately large amounts of media and popular attention, compared to that given to the announcement of adult 'functional cures' (Saez-Cirion et al. 2013). The baby's cure excited a large amount of attention, even compared to the extensive coverage of falling incidence and expanded treatment during the summer 2012 AIDS conference and in the autumn 2012 UNAIDS report. Colleagues and friends who know I work on HIV issues asked me about this case with an intensity and frequency never shown in relation to World AIDS Day announcements, despite those announcements' recent optimistic tone. They took it, very often, as a hopeful portent of a coming 'end of AIDS'.

In this chapter, I will argue that the responses to the baby's functional cure indicate both the power of HIV's naturalisation through medicalised means of addressing the pandemic and some of the limits of that medicalisation. Most obviously, we can see in this example, as the reaction of the THT marks, how HIV's medicalisation may generate poorly grounded optimism not just about 'the end of AIDS' but about a cure. We can also see that narratives of innocence, stigma and blame underpin such medicalised optimism, by the way it fastens onto what seem to be the least agentic of HIV subjects: babies infected by their mothers.

More broadly, as we shall see later, HIV's medicalisation can lead to the glossing over of problems with medical approaches to the condition, and the bracketing out of non-medical, particularly psychosocial issues. These issues can become difficult to fund, to prioritise in policy, even to talk about. THT's response, emphasising the need to continue work on bringing pregnant women into screening and treatment, acting safely, testing regularly, and using ARVs properly, underscores these concerns. So does the quotation from a statement from the International HIV/AIDS Coalition at the beginning of this chapter, which responded to new World Health Organisation (2013) guidelines on earlier ARV treatment by emphasising the role of community interventions in moving towards more HIV testing, from testing to treatment, and from starting to maintaining treatment.

The naturalising medicalisation of HIV involves enormous medical prevention, treatment and care successes; complex patterns of medical knowledge and ownership; and the claiming and practising of medical knowledge by people living with and affected by HIV as well as by medical professionals. Joyce Banda, President of high-HIV-prevalence Malawi, is quoted at the beginning of this chapter supporting WHO's 2013 treatment guidelines. She, like many others who endorse early, expanded treatment, is aware of the complexities of such treatment, as well as the difficulties of attaining it in a low-income, medically under-resourced country, albeit one with high levels of recent government and civil society commitment to universal HIV testing and rapid ARV scaling-up. How can these intricacies of HIV's medication be thought through and addressed?

Below, I sketch some progressive elements of HIV's medicalisation, before considering some illustrations of how medicalisation can solidify and restrict thinking and action within the pandemic, and how personal and broader cultural HIV narratives counteract such reification.

Narratives of HIV as illness

Medical progress in treating and preventing HIV has contributed to popular and political understandings of the epidemic, not, as before, as fatality, punishment, or stigma, but as an illness like others. To a large extent, this progress has been driven by people affected or infected by HIV themselves. This aspect of HIV's medicalisation has turned the story of the condition from a 'disease' story of dysfunction, into a story of illness, voiced by a complex coalition of HIV citizens, including people living with HIV, policymakers, and politicians as well as medical professionals (Kleinman 1997; see also Epstein 1996; Robins 2009).

We have seen in Chapter 2 that medical optimism around the pandemic now encompasses encouraging advances in vaccine and stem cell curative technologies and the prevention technologies of circumcision and microbicide use, as well as the widening range of ARV-related treatment, prevention and 'functional cure' technologies that includes treatment as prevention, early treatment, immediate treatment, post-exposure prophylaxis and pre-exposure prophylaxis. However, the medical technology with the greatest impact has probably been the rollout of ARVs to 54% of those now needing them in low- and middle-income countries, particularly important for sub-Saharan Africa (UNAIDS 2012a). UN Millennium Development Goal 6 includes the specific medical aims of halting and beginning to reverse the spread of HIV/AIDS and achieving universal HIV/AIDS treatment access for those needing it by 2015. The latter goal is more or less met in high-income countries, as well as in more and more low-and middle-income countries, resulting in an estimated ten million people living with ARVs as well as HIV. International HIV organisations are committed to expanding treatment to those without access; treating people earlier, which improves their survival chances and quality of life (Kitahata et al. 2009; World Health Organisation 2013); and using more effective, better-tolerated and simplified drug regimes. UNAIDS's (2011a) 'zero' aim for HIV-related deaths emblematises this policy version of 'treatment optimism'.

ARV treatment expansion thus offers the most general contemporary case of the medicalisation of HIV positive lives. It also displays many of the complexities associated with what might seem a rather straightforward aspect of HIV's naturalisation. At the beginning of Chapter 3, Nicco, a woman in her mid-30s, taking ARVs since 2006, started her account of living with HIV by enumerating her ARV medications. The list led her to the statement that she 'loves' her status 'too much'. Similarly, Yoliswa, also in her 30s, with nearly a decade of ARV experience, acknowledged jokily the medication that enabled her to have a healthy, HIV negative child when she called him her 'Nevirapine baby', crediting the antiretroviral given to mothers and infants in South Africa at the time of his birth to prevent mother-to-child transmission. The effects of medical advances in the HIV field have been dramatic, life-saving and life-enhancing in the three-letter lives of people like Nicco and Yoliswa. Yet people living with HIV and ARVs in this way are not just objects of the medical technology, or grateful patients; they claim ARVs for themselves. They may need to know about HIV and ARVs in medical terms in order to access treatment (Nguyen 2011) and to use it effectively, but they also insert themselves into and take over this regime of knowledge. They are not simply colonised by it (Rose 2007).

For instance, Yoliswa, Nicco, and the large majority of interviewees in both my UK and South African studies, tell stories of themselves being 'expert patients', that is, knowledgeable and proactive about their condition, for and because of themselves and for others like them, as much as 'expert patients' for and because of doctors and other medical professionals. Nicco's knowledge of ARVs came from the speakers who visited her support group, for example, as much as from the local clinic. Her recital of that knowledge performed her ownership of it, and echoed the accounts I have heard she and others give within that support group, to help each other. Often, such medicalised understanding of HIV and ARVs operates in the service of community advocacy or treatment activism, as well as medical efficacy and personal health improvement (Epstein 1996; Kielman and Cataldo 2009; Squire 2007).

In the South African context, and especially in the specific peri-urban area near Cape Town where Nicco lives, HIV prevalence is high and ARVs have only been generally available for a few years. Her statement of her happiness about ARVs was at the same time an activist statement about the importance of treatment provision, and the success of a fight for it which she and her friends in the local support group remembered well. In interviews ten years before, only a handful of people in the group had gained ARV access, through a trial. Longstanding members of the group like Nicco literally embody the success of campaigns for ARV rollout.

More complicatedly, Yoliswa's closing comments about the precariousness of ARV supplies indicate both a personal and political history of medicalisation, and a reminder of the ongoing requirements of treatment activism. A decade before, Yoliswa was one of a few highly visible treatment activists in South Africa. Her campaigning contributed to the medically successful 'three-letter life' she and others now live. In 2012, she was again exceptional in her account, narrating an ARV future of international political, rather than medical and personal, doubt that few other South African or UK interviewees explicitly articulated. In her story, medicalisation was accompanied not so much by physical and psychological uncertainties, but more by economic and political unpredictabilities.

The account of medicalisation that perhaps deals best with such heterogeneity in its nature, effects and resistances, is Nikolas Rose's (2007) Foucauldian formulation of what he calls a new 'politics of life itself' based on biological citizenship. Such citizenship emerges out of biological sciences and the policies and politics around them and works across national citizenship boundaries: it is founded in bio-power, not just biology. In the case of HIV, the transnational demand for medical treatment has given rise to a global apparatus of education, 'safer' behaviour, self-care, 'investment' in the 'three zeroes' and activism around HIV, as well as cutting-edge medical practice. It is thanks to this apparatus that people living with HIV are regulated into being particular kinds of adhering medical subjects in order to have treatment. The apparatus's marketised framework also gives the triaging or rationing of treatment, and early treatment for prevention purposes, an inherent rationale in terms of the cost-effectiveness of such interventions. General rather than HIV-related health, and population rather than individual health, are other current lines of argument and practise within HIV bio-politics.

HIV's bio-political citizenship is, however, lived out very differently in the variously resourced contexts of the ARV era (Nguyen 2011). Even within Nicco's and Yoliswa's stories of their geographically close and generationally similar South African lives with HIV, for example, such citizenship looked different. Both women delineated bio-power as an arena of effective agency, based on their locality's particular history of fighting for treatment access. In Yoliswa's story, though, her ten-year relation to HIV knowledge and practice was marked by its much closer integration with treatment activism. Nicco told a story that ended with medical success and moved on to other local insufficiencies and requirements. Yoliswa, by contrast, qualified her narrative of successful treatment activism with the continuing transnational treatment inequalities of lives lived with HIV and ARVs. She too, though, like Nicco, had moved on to other concerns. She still worked on HIV issues, but she was no longer a treatment activist.

In many situations, the 'politics of life itself' offers the possibility of making claims as biological citizens. People living with HIV may claim the right to treatment, whatever the health resources of the country they live in (Robins 2009). South Africa's Treatment Action Campaign, for example, continues to press local and national government and international organisations for better drugs, additional treatment options to deal with side effects and resistance as people's exposure to ARVs lengthens, and more expeditious treatment delivery. Government and voluntary sector organisations responsible for delivering ARVs frequently pursue issues like those troubling Yoliswa. Are people being denied drugs or given cheaper and less effective ones, they ask. Or will this happen in the future, in order to meet fiscal targets?

The progresses of medical knowledge and practice about HIV, and their accompanying critical appropriations by people living with and affected by HIV, go along with another, less positive aspect of HIV's medicalisation. At times, contemporary narratives of medically treating, preventing and living with HIV return to a medicalised focus on disease that marginalises other aspects of three-letter lives.

Narratives of HIV as disease

Today, the pandemic is more and more being presented in medical and public health terms, even when it is said that other, 'psychosocial' ways of thinking about it are important. There is an accompanying skew of practical and conceptual resources for medical strategies. Such strategies come to be seen as the natural solutions to a condition understood more and more within physiological and pharmacological frameworks. This aspect of medicalisation can lead to HIV being re-narrated as disease, in stories structured around managing and reducing physiological disorder, and performed by medical expertise. These 'disease' stories character-ised earlier years of the pandemic, albeit with much more pessimistic endings (Kleinman 1997; Nguyen et al. 2012). Such re-medicalisation is not unique to HIV. It has been described and criticised in relation to many other socially salient conditions such as activities of children that conflict with educational institutions, states of psychological suffering, and health promotion and education (Sanders et al. 2008; White 2013; Wills and Douglas 2008). It is often accompanied currently by phar-macologisation, a strong emphasis on pharmacological framings of and solutions to medical, psychological and social problems. This move is closely associated with the economic and political clout of international pharmacological companies, and with the current power of biological knowledge in the fields of, for instance, genetics, neuroscience and, particularly relevant in the HIV case, bio-mathematical modelling. Perhaps, too, in the HIV instance, re-medicalisation is being driven intellectually, in policy and to some extent in 'user' communities, by the excitement as well as the hope of large-scale, avowedly somewhat experimental, new treatment directions.

One sign of simplifying medicalisation processes is that even when HIV resources themselves are not all medical, they are increasingly being situated within a medical context. For instance, companies producing ARVs now also offer extensive advice on living with HIV. Merck's 'Healthy Living with HIV' site, charting 'the positive path forwards', focused primarily on medication, though also including other phys-ical, mental and spiritual aspects of health, is an example (http://www.healthywithhiv.com/healthy-with-hiv/healthywithhiv/hiv_support/index.jsp?WT.svl=1).

Another clearer and now often-remarked sign of an over-simple medicalisation of HIV appears in the enthusiasm and optimism that characterise many contemporary discussions of early ARV treatment programmes, with relatively little criticism. Certainly, earlier treatment, alongside expanded testing, can be a medically efficacious shift for HIV positive people's health. It also has positive effects on prevention, for undiagnosed and untreated HIV positive people are the most likely to be infectious (Cohen et al. 2011). However, the programmes have long-term resource impacts at every level as well as implications for how people understand HIV illness and what their long-term treatment paths will be. These complications may get passed over if HIV is understood predominantly as a disease to ameliorate immediately through treatment.

In 2010, the World Health Organisation (2010b) advised starting ARV treatment at the level of 350 CD4+ T cells per cubic millimetre of blood. (This has been the standard measure of poor immune functioning for people who are HIV positive, compared to 600 to $1200/mm^3$ in non-HIV positive, non-immuno compromised people. CD4+ T cells are an important subgroup of lymphocytes, or white blood cells, which HIV infects.) In 2013, WHO moved the advised level up to 500 CD4+ T cells/ mm^3 (World Health Organisation 2013). These advised levels, argued to improve survival rates and reduce transmission (Cohen et al. 2011, 2012; Donnell et al. 2010; Kitahata et al. 2009) were themselves raised from WHO's earlier (2006) 200 CD4+ T cells/mm^3 guideline. They mean that many more people are moving onto ARV treatment, including in high-prevalence low- and middle-income countries, with large resource implications.

President Banda's optimism and enthusiasm about such moves, which started this chapter, are understandable. In Malawi, governments, NGOs and external funders have pushed for measures such as task-shifting from doctors to nurses, decentred ARV distribution, reduced appointments for 'stable patients', better drug supply chains to avoid shortages, expanded funding of medical professionals, and food support, to enable the 2010 guidelines to be met (Médecins sans Frontières 2011; World Health Organisation/UNAIDS/UNICEF 2013). However, many other countries are finding it difficult to provide services that meet the 2010, let alone the 2013 guidelines. It is also hard to get people to initiate treatment before immunity drops below the 350 CD4+ T cells/mm^3 level, when they may feel well. In many epidemics, large numbers of people diagnosed HIV positive do not access medical services regularly. In the United States, where people are advised to start ARVs at diagnosis, one-third of those diagnosed are not in medical care. Late diagnosis figures are also still high across countries in all income groups (UNAIDS 2012a.). ARVs can be hard to tolerate, early treatment is of uncertain general or long-term effectiveness, there are difficult relations between

ARV initiation and people's acceptance of long-term illness, stigma now attaches to ARV use as well as HIV itself, and ARVs require considerable individual resources of transport and food. A policy story of HIV as a disease simply needing better, earlier treatment, tends to drown out these other, complex, less-manageable stories of early treatment.

Treatment-as-prevention or TasP policies, often associated with early treatment programmes, also demonstrate the simplifying aspects of HIV's medicalisation. As well as the prevention benefits of earlier treatment mentioned above, studies have shown the effectiveness of ARV treatment generally for reducing transmission in varying contexts (Cohen et al. 2011; Donnell et al. 2010; Fang et al. 2004). Such studies are leading to the increasing adoption of test-and-treat policies. These polices involve universal, regular, though voluntary, testing, followed by immediate offers of and encouragement for ARV treatment if you are positive, whatever your CD4 count (Granich et al. 2009). There is considerable hope of the policy's good effects, through its positive impact on the health of people living with HIV, on their ability to continue with normal life and work, and on transmission risk, which is driven down by wider diagnosis and ARVs' reduction of viral load in a population.

However, as with the move to treat at higher levels of T cells, treatment as prevention carries with it considerable health problems for people living with HIV and, potentially, for those at risk of becoming HIV positive. For instance, HIV positive people treated mainly for prevention purposes, when they are well, may experience side effects that make them non-adherent, causing later problems of resistance. People taking ARVs and their partners may put aside condoms, overestimating the prevention effectiveness of the medications. People who are fairly newly infected, with high viral loads, are often not diagnosed but feel well, so they will not be affected by the policy. Many HIV positive people also move in and out of care, even when they can access free high-quality health systems (Krentz and Gill 2013), further limiting TasP's benefits. And again, this policy augments the numbers of people taking lifelong ARVs, with many attendant resource and regime problems.

Perhaps more importantly in terms of the simplifying effects of medicalisation, the policy widens the range of ARV uses and blurs those uses' distinctions, eliding the difference between taking ARVs early to protect your own health and taking them early to promote the health of the general population by reducing levels of HIV infectivity or viral load within that population. In policy narratives of TasP, therefore, ARVs become naturalised as agents of freedom from HIV disease, both for HIV positive people whose health they can preserve, and for non-HIV positive people whose status they can protect. This is a shift from ARVs' previous framing as responses to felt as well as measurable symptoms of illness. Again, other health and prevention stories, especially those around behavioural and lower-level, less resource-intensive medical technology, can be edged out. The WHO's (World Health Organisation 2013) stipulation that its early treatment guidelines go along with continued emphasis on condoms, circumcision and education can appear as something of a footnote to medical enthusiasm, as NGOs such as the International HIV/AIDS Coalition, quoted at the beginning of this chapter, warn.

A further set of policies, expanding ARV use to prophylaxis, similarly works well medically while also contributing to medicalised simplifications within discourses and practices around HIV. HIV policymakers advocate ARVs as effective post-exposure prophylaxis, or PEP, after unsafe sex or drug use, or after possible exposure at work or through rape or abuse (World Health Organisation/International Labour Organisation 2007). Many researchers and doctors now also suggest selective use of ARVs for pre-exposure prophylaxis, or PrEP, especially where high prevalence and risky behaviours coexist. This strategy is being trialled in a number of situations (Baeten et al. 2011; Grant et al. 2010; Rosengarten and Michael 2010), once more extending ARVs', rather than condoms', place in the policy story as naturalised resources to preserve people from HIV disease.

Together, PrEP and TasP have generated renewed optimism about UNAIDS's second 'zero' aim, new HIV infections, seeming to promise a medical route to it. The International Association of Providers of AIDS Care (IAPAC), which as we saw in Chapter 1 holds out the possibility of an 'AIDS-free generation', suggests that PrEP alongside early treatment-as-prevention is the paradigm-shifting breakthrough that may make that prospect a reality:

> [T]he time has come to integrate these new prevention approaches into the long established practices of condom use, male medical circumcision, prevention of mother-to-child transmission, and treatment of sexually transmitted infections.…We are convinced that by fully integrating these two biobehavioral interventions into our current armamentarium, we stand a chance of further bending the HIV incidence and AIDS-related mortality curves in a way only imagined years ago and, perhaps – as many have advocated – of welcoming an AIDS-free generation within our lifetimes. (International Association of Providers of AIDS Care 2012: 2)

For IAPAC, these new strategies are the second medical breakthrough in the pandemic, following on from the early use of ARVs. IAPAC seems to view this breakthrough as a reasonably achievable state, although the first breakthrough is still only semi-achieved: around one-half of people needing ARVs according to WHO guidelines have them. The commitment to universal rollout and the rapid progress in extending coverage since the mid-2000s seems to have persuaded IAPAC that HIV policy can now move on to the next medical challenge:

> Early adoption of HAART (antiretrovirals) transformed an HIV diagnosis from 'death sentence' to a manageable chronic condition, saving and enhancing the lives of countless people living with HIV/AIDS. The use of HAART for TasP should move forward so that a similar impact on prevention might occur. (ibid: 7)

The IAPAC is explicitly doubtful about the 'slower progress' of psychosocial prevention efforts compared to medical treatment, and thus they advocate a shift to the 'biobehavioural', biomedical TasP strategies. However, the second possibility depends, even here, upon the first. Without patients' ongoing self-administration and monitoring of their medications, and the avoidance of 'risk compensation behaviours' (such as stopping condom use), TasP and PrEP cannot succeed. To present the first via caveats about behaviour management, alongside some concerns with resources and ethics does, indeed, suggest that a degree of medicalisation is in progress within this type of professional medical discourse (International Association of Providers of AIDS Care 2012: 5, 1). For this story of the epidemic's future de-socialises prevention and presents biobehavioural means of lowering HIV transmission as, increasingly, the taken-for-granted, natural solution.

Another prevention-related ARV treatment extension that has the potential to intensify a simplifying medicalisation is the WHO's revision of its guidelines on infant feeding practices to avoid perinatal HIV transmission, to include an option of breastfeeding alongside ARV treatment for HIV positive women and their children for at least the first sixth months after birth. Formula feeding can be problematic because of, for instance, dirty water, poor sanitation and stigma; breast feeding itself has many benefits (World Health Organisation 2010c). At the same time, this option involves ARV use by babies who are negative, and by HIV positive, healthy women who are only taking the medications to reduce the risk of HIV transmission. Once again, it boosts the numbers of people taking ARVs and the power of these medications in people's lives, piggybacking the naturalisation of pharmacological prevention onto the assumed 'naturalness' of breastfeeding. There are clearly many prevention benefits in this extension of ARV use. And mother-to-child transmission prevention has been under-addressed during ARV treatment rollout, although safeguarding their children's health is key to many people's relations with HIV. However, this new approach to vertical transmission reduction once more extends medicalised explanations and practices within the epidemic, at the expense of the addresses to the psychosocial and environmental factors that were more integrally involved with prior, behaviourally focused policies.

HIV treatment and prevention are embedded in a number of other large fields of medical practice and development. Microbicides, circumcision, and better ARVs remain as research focuses, as do treatments and preventative, prophylactic medication for opportunistic infections. In 2011, for example, the Health Protection Agency advised a new vaccination, safe for the immuno-compromised, against pneumococcal disease, to which people living with HIV are particularly susceptible, for everyone in the United Kingdom who is HIV positive. Large numbers of medications exist and are being developed to combat ARVs' side effects, and aspects of HIV not fully dealt with by ARVs. As we have seen, cures, based at present on results from three HIV positive patients with leukaemia who have had stem cell transplants, retain research and popular interest, though these are less likely to feature in major policy documents since their outcomes are uncertain and relatively distant. Early-treatment regimes are perhaps the nearest and most feasible routes towards functional cure, suggesting expanded forms of ARV use, though for limited periods (Bacchus et al. 2012). There are promising vaccine candidates, only now starting to be trialled (Rerks-Ngarm et al. 2009).

All these areas of treatment expansion look medically productive. The re-medicalised stories of HIV as a now-manageable disease that proliferate around them, though, like the story of an infant's functional cure which started this chapter, mark how such expansions can rigidify, discursively and practically, into simplification.

The limits of HIV's medicalisation

We have seen how the contemporary medicalisation of the HIV pandemic can generate simplifying narratives of HIV as a disease, rather than as a multiply determined and heterogeneously lived illness. This segment of the chapter considers in more detail what re-medicalised disease narratives of HIV, and the medical, social and political apparatuses they describe and support, are leaving out.

As conditions related to living long-term with HIV medications or with HIV itself become more common and complex, the amount of medical management required is increasing. However, research and policy attention even on medical aspects of living with HIV focuses primarily on ARVs' effects and on the most life-threatening of HIV-related conditions. Attention to improving treatment for other HIV- or ARV-related conditions seems relatively sparse. Considerations of medical but low-tech aspects of treatment and prevention, and of recalcitrant, difficult areas of HIV experience that have important but not necessarily dramatic effects on how people's three-letter lives are lived, also appear relatively meagre. For instance, in the prevention arena, microbicides, which have been shown to be reasonably acceptable and effective in preventing transmission (AbdoolKarim et al. 2010), are much researched and often discussed. However, there seems little policy will behind them, compared to that driving the more cutting-edge ARV innovations that define the contemporary HIV field. In the field of treatment, attention to chronic health conditions that are exacerbated by HIV and life-threatening even when ARVs are successful, such as high blood pressure and cholesterol levels, is becoming increasingly important for the health of people living long three-letter lives, and can be argued to have synergic or 'leveraging' effects on health care for these conditions generally (UNAIDS 2011b). These possibilities, too, currently attract less policy interest and press for development than possibilities of better ARV treatment.

To meet the HIV part of MDG 6 by the deadline of 2015 demands a raft of resource-intensive strategies: programmes for social prevention, economic development, and women's empowerment, as well as scaled-up and extended ARV treatment, better treatment for opportunistic infections, widened testing, and transmission reduction. Medical strategies are the most costly, requiring continuing, ever-increasing provision by governments, international NGOs and other donors of standard medications; cheaper generic versions; and second- and third-line treatments (Médecins Sans Frontières 2009). HIV treatment's expanding uses of ARVs will inflate those costs. At the same time, there are many difficulties and uncertainties around ARVs' long-term effects, their interactions with other medications, resistance, adherence, accessibility, and, given that many people requiring ARVs and with access to them do not take them, acceptability. These difficulties are the ones that tend to be bracketed off within a medicalised HIV field focused on treatment and incidence figures.

Extending ARVs to people at higher CD4+ T cell levels produces a new set of problems which HIV's medicalisation, again, tends to underplay. Expanding the number of people taking these costly drugs, perhaps by 30%, in, for instance, Ethiopia, has resource implications but also implications for medical practice and psychosocial understandings of HIV. Given shortages of CD4+ T cell testing equipment, decisions will often have to be made by doctors or nurses on the basis of observable symptoms. This is more difficult when people are at the 350 CD4+ T cell level rather than the 200 T cell level because they are likely to appear much healthier. The expansion thus also requires increasing infrastructure and trained staff for delivering it and dealing with the additional issues around ARV side effects, resistance, and long-term health conditions that prolonged use of ARVs generates. In delivering this expansion, people who are in urgent need may, in addition, be displaced as treatment priorities (Konings et al. 2012). For HIV's medicalisation involves not only its reduction to medical descriptions, explanations and practices, but also a focus on a particular set of these, prioritised in policy and as scientific and technical innovation.

Moreover, the medicalised mode of this ARV expansion may leave little room for the additional psychosocial issues generated. Uptake and adherence become more difficult for people who are less likely to be ill than at the 200 CD4+ T cell level. ARVs may make their health feel worse, may require food and transport resources they do not have, and will induct them into a life of illness for which they may be unprepared and stigmatised.

Treatment as prevention, formulated within a highly medicalised framework, also runs into a number of difficulties that tend to fall outside that framework. Beginning treatment at diagnosis is not necessarily medically optimal; is individual health being subordinated to population health in this framework? TasP also makes the large assumption that treatment will reduce infectiousness in real-world, non-trial situations, although viral load is not easily manageable or even predictable for everyone, long-term, when taking ARVs. In addition, many people become infected with HIV through people who do not know they are positive, and this is a very large group to bring into testing, let alone treatment. HIV positive people who do not know their status are around 50% of the total across the pandemic and much more in many other countries, for instance, 84% in Kenya, in one study (UNAIDS 2011a). But 'test-and-treat' strategies are thought to be effective for reducing HIV transmission in a population, only if at least 75% of people living with HIV can be reached. Even in those predominantly high-income countries which reached such a percentage many years ago, new HIV infections have remained stable throughout those years. TasP-related enthusiasm about an 'AIDS-free generation' (International Association of Providers of AIDS Care 2012), drawing often on studies of low infectivity among small groups of people with very well-controlled HIV disease, tends to background these medical and logistical complexities, as well as the psychosocial issues that often underlie them.

PrEP carries a similar load of psychosocial issues and has not always shown great medical effectiveness. Reaching people who are at risk of becoming HIV positive; providing new infrastructure for their prophylactic ARV treatment; maintaining effectiveness and, especially, adherence (which is suspected to have been poor in at least one study with women in South Africa showing no effects of the medication); and controlling the costs of the programme at a time when treatment for HIV positive people is under financial pressure (Morin et al. 2012; Van Damme et al. 2012): all these are going to be large challenges. In addition, PrEP raises medical problems about dealing with the uncertain long-term effects of ARVs, resistance, and side effects, in people who are HIV negative. There are also sociopolitical difficulties attendant on medicating away people's economic, social and psychological barriers to safer sex, and on medicating groups perceived as high in HIV risk implicitly in the service of protecting the low risk of the majority.

Nguyen and colleagues (2012), in describing the current moves as a re-medicalisation of the pandemic, look back to the 1980s, when medical approaches to HIV were distant from, and often opposed to, people living with HIV themselves. At that point, patients negotiated hard with doctors to bring about more equal settlements. As Oscar Moore described it in a 1995 magazine column, on the verge of the rollout in high-income countries of effective treatment, 'The great victory of the past few years has been the building of a sense of collaboration...patient-doctor partnerships...continue to play a key role in the development of treatments' (Moore 1996: 130). That collaboration may dissipate if medical discourse and practice pursue goals distinct from those of people living with HIV, and even those derived from evidence. Nguyen and colleagues suggest that the first danger in the new medicalisation is the inevitable incompleteness of biomedical strategies, which they associate particularly with early ARV treatment, though as we have seen this problem applies to all the extended uses of ARV. Second, Nguyen and colleagues point to the shutting down of debate about critical factors, like those considered earlier in this chapter, at conferences, and perhaps this point could also apply to policy reports like those I have been citing. Third, they point to how local and other contextual factors, which could include those I am calling psychosocial, are being ignored, 'surely only', they say acidly, 'to resurface as "culture" once much-heralded interventions fail to deliver' (Nguyen et al. 2011: 293).

Most international organisations, policymakers and activists emphasise multi-factorial approaches and caution against relying on medical technologies (Piot et al. 2009). Kippax (2012), for example, drawing on her knowledge of the Australian HIV pandemic in particular, repeatedly emphasises the need for social programmes to continue since trial efficacy often fails to translate to more general effectiveness. Even IAPAC's Consensus Statement, considered above (International Association for Providers of AIDS Care 2012: 4), places considerable emphasis on difficulties of implementing TasP and PrEP like those I have mentioned. UNAIDS (2011a) similarly takes care to enumerate the challenges attending early ARV use, treatment as prevention, and pre-exposure prophylaxis, and routinely mentions associated psychosocial issues.

However, the HIV pandemic is now definitively characterised not just by the possibility of effective medical treatment and expanded treatment access, but by growing and diversifying ARV uses and, in much medical and policy discourse, strong optimism about and commitment to them. These medical technologies promise (though as Nguyen and colleagues [2011] suggest, they may not deliver), clearly defined goals, implementation strategies, and evaluations. They provide quantitative models, albeit often overly simple, that predict the future, extrapolating epidemiological and cost trajectories from specific treatment scenarios. And they are supported by powerful commercial stakeholders, in the form of pharmaceutical companies especially, and professional and political stakeholders, searching for ways to demonstrate yearly targets met and progress towards MDG 6. Psychosocial HIV technologies are slower, as IAPAC points out; are harder to define and evaluate; are inevitably interwoven with other factors; and attract few powerful lobbyers. As a result, the contemporary medicalised field can work like an implicit override button on other fields, especially those of social HIV policy and practice (Kippax 2012). Consequently, institutional practices around HIV operate with medical treatment, prevention, education and care as their goals, but tend to roll the first two together and to neglect the last two (Van Damme et al. 2006). These latter, though featuring in policy discourse, are largely left to individual HIV citizens, NGOs and markets to sort out, a tendency likely to increase (Hecht et al. 2009).

As mentioned earlier, such medicalised skewing is not unique to HIV (Sanders et al. 2008). However, HIV's particularity, as an incurable and fatal condition only held in check by recently produced, powerful medications, which need to be taken daily, and as a condition whose transmissibility is reduced by treatment, means that the pandemic's medicalisation, and that medicalisation's problems, are especially intense.

Living with HIV's medicalisation

How does the medicalisation of the pandemic play out in people's lives, across HIV statuses? HIV positive people are educated at clinics primarily about medical treatment and safer sex, with occasional appended advice on lifestyle and nutrition. They receive psychosocial support predominantly around diagnosis, starting and adhering to ARVs, and having children. Unknown-status people are offered HIV testing antenatally; in sexually transmitted disease clinics; in public health clinics in high-prevalence epidemics; by targeted services, in low-prevalence epidemics, if they are perceived as at risk; and increasingly, via self-sampling and self-test kits. Despite the rollouts of testing mentioned earlier, it remains infrequent in general medical and in non-medical public contexts, especially in low-prevalence epidemics (UNAIDS 2009b). People of all statuses can access medicalised forms of prevention such as early treatment (if HIV positive), condoms, PEP, and in some countries and communities, male circumcision and PrEP. However, markedly fewer resources are devoted to the least medically complex of these, and still fewer to social technologies around sexualities, relationships and gender inequities. As the Health Protection Agency and UNAIDS remark, these 'psychosocial' aspects of provision are vital and take up relatively little of total HIV budgets, but they are underprovided and under contemporary threat from budget cuts (Health Protection Agency 2011a: 16; UNAIDS 2012a).

How does medicalisation operate for people around HIV treatment? At one end of the ARV access continuum, those who need ARVs but do not have access to them are aware of and campaigning for them. In these circumstances, psychosocial approaches to the pandemic take second place. However, such approaches are in any case less integral to contemporary ARV programmes than they were in earlier days of ARV scale-up, which emphasised treatment literacy and community decision-making (Abdullah and Squire 2010). Recent international treatment policies retain these elements (Health Protection Agency 2011a; UNAIDS 2010), but largely reframe them around getting and keeping people on ARVs, and ensuring proper adherence to all medications.

In the middle of the ARV access continuum are HIV positive people, in developing and developed worlds, who take ARVs and who are dealing with side effects and their treatment, resistance and the need for alternative medications, the implications of lifetime ARV use, and long-term HIV-related illnesses. Queenie, for instance, whose situation I described in the previous chapter, had good CD4+ T cell levels and low viral load thanks to ARVs, but also had many other health problems related to HIV, which she did not mention until very specifically asked about them. This was common among interviewees in both the United Kingdom and South Africa, who were happy to have ARVs and aware that they were in conventional medical terms doing well on them, and who seemed to some extent unable to talk about, or expressed guilt when talking about, other medical or non-medical problems they might have (see also Davis 2010; Fassin 2007).

HIV's medicalisation focuses on the clinically important aspects of HIV's manifestation and treatment, but not its other aspects, however annoying or troubling, either for medical professionals or for people living with HIV themselves. Interviews with John, a research participant in his 50s who has participated in my UK HIV study since the 1990s, provide useful perspective on the epidemic's ongoing medicalisation and its limitations. In 2009, John began not with HIV, but with the story of a common HIV-related pre-cancer condition, not susceptible to ARVs (Bower et al. 2004):

John: {The cancer specialist} looks, he says there hasn't been any change. It hasn't progressed to cancer/Right/ but it, but that will be the next stage if, if, that's the only way it will go if/Right/ if it gets worse, um, so that's quite worrying but I realise because I'm quite well read on HIV treatments and all the complications of it all, that the, um, you can have {precancerous signs} for many, many years and it never progresses/mhm/and you can end up dying of old age or of something completely unrelated but it is something that's got to be monitored fairly closely and, um, so I'm now going to go for six months without any treatment, because the treatment that they give you although it works at the time hopefully, if it hasn't worked it carries on working even when you stop which is quite interesting so hopefully over the next six months, there might be, you know maybe the {precancerous signs} will get smaller or go down a grade. So, um, I've just got to get on with my life really and try not to think about it too much/mhm/...so, um, so that's that, so in some ways that is a far bigger issue than the HIV which is, um, very well controlled/mhm/by the medications, I've been on my current regime now for certainly six years and I just had my CD4 results from three months ago, um, that was 1300 which is excellent, my doctor said 'could I have some please /(laughs)/ because you've probably got a higher CD4 count than I have'. A viral load undetectable again, apart from two viral blips over the last six years it's, um, it's been undetectable most of the time /mhm/so, and even when we had the blips it went back to being undetectable without having to change treatment which is handy because I'm very heavily pre-treated, so my options are somewhat limited/mhm/for future treatment so, um, that's, you know, going, quite, quite well.

John tells the story of his new HIV-related illness at length, saying that he has discovered the precancerous cells early, there is a likelihood they will not progress, he has gotten appropriate treatment, and his CD4+ T cell counts and viral load are good. This is a medicalised, naturalising narrative. John knows a lot about HIV-related illnesses, their risks, monitoring, and treatment. He says his successful ARV therapy means HIV itself is not a concern; he talks about himself and his doctor as 'we'. They are associates, even friends. John appropriates all this medical expertise for himself, often a positive move.

Yet John's story also denaturalises itself by putting HIV's medicalisation in question in some ways. Potentially fatal new medical problems arise around HIV, John suggests; sometimes they cannot be completely solved, and this is worrying. The only solution may be not to think about it. Even John's ARV therapy is potentially in jeopardy because of his pre-treatment earlier in the epidemic.

While the precise medical history that John delineates belongs to the UK epidemic, the narrated pattern of medicalised management increasing across the epidemic and over chronological time, yet continuously undercut by uncertainties, failures and new problems, appears in the South African interview data too. Interviewees such as Nicco, medically optimistic when they started their accounts, would often, like John, include their ongoing physical difficulties with ARVs, HIV itself, and other conditions, in the later portions of their narratives, after their pharmacological success stories. A few, tracing their lives with HIV chronologically, included such difficulty early in the story, from where, despite happier endings, it continued to resonate. Although recalcitrant physical problems take up less narrative, and perhaps also less personal, social and political space, in the South African interviews, their place within South African interviewees' accounts has grown as more interviewees spend more time living with HIV and ARVs.

It is often argued that the pandemic's medicalisation, particularly via ARV treatment, has depoliticised it, narrowing and marginalising the field of HIV citizenship, especially in high-income countries (Mykhalovskiy and Rosengarten 2009; Nguyen et al. 2011). More specifically, Davis (2009) has pointed out HIV positive people's contemporary difficulties in addressing their HIV-related problems in other than medical treatment terms, as with John, whose concerns are indeed framed almost entirely medically here. Davis discusses how difficult it can be to approach even clearly psychosocial issues, such as unprotected sex in relationships, outside of medicalised discussions of different HIV strains, viral load, and infectivity.

For people with concerns clearly outside of the medical field, there are now not just barriers to considering psychosocial issues, but practical problems in finding out about and getting access to psychosocial services, even in the United Kingdom, and sometimes in cases where they may still be in place. The epidemic's medicalisation exacerbates such problems. In a 2011 interview, Sean, a man in his 30s, doing relatively well, immunologically, on ARVs but with many accompanying physical and mental health problems, and his partner, Tyler, in his 20s, also with considerable health problems, described only hearing about non-medical HIV services incidentally. While this was not true for all UK participants, most noted that such services were reduced and much less easy to access than previously. Sean and Tyler explicitly co-narrated this decline as related to HIV's characterisation as disease, instanced through their clinic's focus on medically related services around trials and STIs (sexually transmitted infections). They made sense of this story of absence by co-evaluating what was available as 'nothing social':

> **Sean:** The services is out there but we, I don't think we've used as many as we could of, because we haven't had the information sent to us it's only what we've heard from other people...the hospital's brilliant, but I don't think for um, not for advertising stuff like that/I don't think they/It's like
>
> **Tyler:** They advertise like um when they're doing studies and stuff like that, nothing like social.

Sean: Nothing social, yes, and it's more like sexually transmitted diseases or stuff like that on the wall isn't it, stuff like that, or where you go to get seen about stuff like that.

It had also taken Sean, like a large number of other UK interviewees with marked mental health problems, an extremely long time to find psychological help for mental health conditions not related clearly to treatment adherence, or even perhaps to his HIV status:

Sean: I have counselling sessions weekly and find it helps me. It was very hard for me to get the support from a counsellor, the waiting list was about 18 months I had to wait. (E-mail follow-up to the interview)

It is obvious that the psychosocial issues affecting Sean, Tyler, and many others in this study, as well as in the epidemic more widely, are of major, ongoing significance in all epidemic contexts. Research on mental health issues among people living with HIV suggests levels of stress, anxiety, and/or depression are generally high, perhaps around 50%. This is true in low- as well as high-income settings. In Tanzania, for example, a study of patients taking ARVs long-term reported side effects, transport, food and wage costs, but also psychological difficulties with lifetime medication, as unaddressed issues that reduce treatment retention if non-medical, social support, both practical and emotional, is not available (Roura et al. 2009). In many sub-Saharan African countries where the gender balance of people living with HIV is roughly equal, twice as many women are accessing ARVs as men; it is unclear what psychosocial factors are keeping men away (Zungu 2012). Across Africa, Asia and South America, 'lost to follow-up' patients tend to be those who have to pay consultation fees, still standard in many countries; but such 'lost' patients are also impacted by psychosocial factors. For instance, they tend to be part of larger programmes, which are less able to follow up on their patients, and to be older and so concerned not to impose the burden on their families that ARVs might bring (Konings et al. 2012).

In high-income countries, such as the United Kingdom, 5% of people seeking medical care are lost to follow-up yearly, and one in ten at 350 CD4+ T cells or less are not taking ARVs (Health Protection Agency 2011a). The US situation is more dramatic: only 77% of people taking ARVs, and 28% of the total number of people living with HIV, show viral suppression. These figures indicate a high level of problems with encouraging people to test, to stay in regular contact with their doctors, and to take the medications, for what seem to be multiple reasons, including many of the same reasons that operate in low-income countries (MMWR 2011; Roura et al. 2009). The ambiguity of some people living in the United States with HIV about scientific accounts of HIV may, as we have seen, also play a part (Bogart et al. 2010). The unreliable access to good care and medication that characterises US health services could also be involved, for the medical resources supporting HIV's medicalisation differ markedly even within the same country.

What about medicalisation's impact on prevention? It has been suggested that the 'treatment optimism' of people living with HIV might disinhibit safer sex, particularly if expanded treatment steals prevention resources. There is, though, evidence from a number of epidemic contexts that knowledge of ARVs and openness about HIV promote condom use and HIV testing (Boulle et al. 2009) and that long-term ARV treatment affects sexual practices in complex ways not reducible to disinhibition (Davis 2009). Nevertheless, in situations where treatment has reduced viral load to undetectable levels, the low risk of transmission leads many HIV positive people in sero-concordant relationships, that is, relationships with other HIV positive people, to decide not to use condoms, and this can happen in sero-discordant relationships too (Mlambo and Peltzer 2011). Having unprotected sex while taking ARVs may not always be low-risk, and the guidelines require medical practitioners to spell out the uncertainties to their patients. However, efforts to negotiate condom use may be undercut by early treatment availability, treatment-as-prevention discourse, and, sometimes, by circumcision, if these practices medicalise away the salience of other forms of prevention. Discussions start to concentrate on risk levels in relation to specific viral loads and CD4 counts, or on the risk reductions achieved by circumcision, rather than on the complications of condom use. Even another medical area of prevention discourse, that around co- or super-infection by other HIV strains, becomes backgrounded by these medicalised, naturalised technologies of bio-prevention. Such shifts have implications for other STIs and for reproduction also. It is especially problematic for those for whom the negotiation of condom use is, for economic, social or psychological reasons, difficult, and for whom, therefore, TasP may reduce their access to this powerful prevention strategy.

There are other circumstances, too, where pharmacological medical HIV technologies may supplant, not complement, lower-tech medical or social technologies. Some HIV negative people who have access to ARVs through friends, family, health system leakage, or private commercial sources have been using them, unprescribed and before any official PrEP programme, as pre-exposure prophylaxis to reduce risk in situations of potential transmission, for instance, if they choose to have or cannot avoid having unprotected sex with people of HIV positive or unknown status (see for instance, Uganda Radio Network 2012; Zablotska et al. 2012). Here, questions about dosage, side effects and resistance may replace questions about the negotiation of condom use. In addition, such activities demonstrate how quickly and directly HIV's naturalising medicalisation passes into everyday practices.

Medicalisation and its undoing: doctors and policymakers, activists and citizens

Treatment possibility, expanded treatment access, earlier treatment and diversified ARV uses constitute a medical field which allows HIV to be lived with longer, with better health, and as a condition that is part of life. At the same time, accompanying naturalising, medicalised discourses and practices can over-determine HIV strategies. They can marginalise non-medical aspects of the pandemic, underplay the limits of medical knowledge, and constitute HIV as treatable disease rather than liveable illness. These moves can be read both within policy narratives, and within the stories told by people living with HIV themselves.

The medicalised HIV citizenship produced as a result is an emblematic example of the biological citizenship described by Foucault (1991), Rose (2007) and others. Citizens today are, Nikolas Rose suggests, defined and called into active existence by their biological as well as their conventionally political characteristics, and this 'politics of life itself' offers both possibilities and limitations. In the case of HIV, people are always citizens in relation to this viral condition, obliged to live within the pandemic but also enabled by this definition to take action as biological HIV citizens. Currently, it is becoming more difficult to negotiate ownership of this biological citizenship, and in the process translate it. Biological citizenship is also tending to crowd out other forms of HIV citizenship that constitute people's three-letter lives. Its contemporary determining character, and the history of its progression to this point, has a particularity which strongly inflects the lives of many people and affected by HIV, across the pandemic.

It is not clear how recent forms of HIV's re-medicalisation will develop. While HIV organisations and websites vigilantly report new treatment and prevention strategies, they are also careful to include qualifications and to note the experimental character of medicalised hope. Moreover, many HIV activists are still fully occupied in fighting for free, accessible, and good-quality treatment in both developed- and developing-world contexts. A recent report by NGO representatives to UNAIDS's programme board addresses not treatment or prevention advances but the straitened funding circumstances affecting existing medical services and the psychosocial resources provided by civil society (UNAIDS 2012b). Despite current mechanisms for and a considerable history of Greater Involvement of People Living with HIV and AIDS (GIPA) in the international governance of HIV programmes, a contested divide may be growing again between these demedicalising interests, and those of acronym optimists. As Chantal Mouffe (2006) describes it, even the most apparently univocal social or political movements, however uncontroversially progressive their aims, contain opposed, agonistic interests within them. The complexity of HIV's naturalisations, undoing themselves from the inside as in the case of medicalisation, will become clearer when we consider, in the next two chapters, the naturalising and denaturalising processes of normalisation and denormalisation, marketisation and demarketisation.

5
A Long-term Condition: HIV's Normalisation

Introduction: a citizen like any other

In early 2013, I visit a UK HIV organisation, some of whose service users have participated in my research, to give some feedback about what all 47 interviewees in my study of HIV support narratives have said. As is usually the case, the workers and volunteers, most of them living with HIV themselves, already know almost everything I tell them. Again as often happens, their apparently 'local' knowledge, accreted from numerous stories of practice in a specific city, turns out to have greater transferability than it is generally given credit for. At the end of the discussion, I mention how many interviewees positioned themselves ambiguously in relation to HIV. Interviewees narrated themselves both as citizens like all others, for whom HIV is just one aspect of their lives, and as people in whose lives certain three-letter acronyms are powerful, and must never be lost sight of. Once more, this ambiguity around HIV's normalisation is something that the group knows about very well. One member says that the organisation faces the issue all the time, especially with newly-diagnosed people. He wants to tell them the encouraging story of HIV's good medical management and the normal, happy lives that HIV positive people can live. At the same time, he knows that this is not how living with HIV always works out. So he must position his redemptive narratives (McAdams 2006) strategically, against all too common experiences of highly de-naturalising illness, as well stigma, discrimination, exclusion and isolation.

In the previous chapter's considerations of the epidemic's contemporary naturalisation through medicalisation, it became apparent that while people living with HIV and ARVs themselves negotiate medicalisation in complex, not always positive ways, medicalisation generates some over-simple positions within HIV policy. Such clear divisions between policy and personal narratives do not appear in the case of HIV's second major naturalisation process, which I shall call normalisation, and which also takes a very particular contemporary form, with commonalities across many national epidemics. Normalisation's complexities are built into people's everyday lives, as the volunteers and workers at the HIV organisation I have just described recognise very well. And so specific advocates of HIV's normalisation can rarely be posed 'against' other HIV advocates.

It might seem initially that HIV's normalisation is an entirely good thing, with no inbuilt disadvantages. However, this naturalisation process, like medicalisation, delivers both benefits and difficulties, and in this case they are very hard to disentangle. People's narratives of living with HIV enact the complexity of that doubled process especially clearly.

The treatment possibility era, and the growing emphasis on treatment-led prevention, has generated a tendency for the HIV pandemic to be, not just medicalised, but normalised (Green 2009), and medical normalisation is one powerful aspect of the process. The strong medicalising orientation just described is accompanied by a normalising integration and mainstreaming of HIV services within health and social services, for instance, within chronic illness services, or within advice on general healthy living. As shown at the beginning of Chapter 3, the United Kingdom's Health Protection Agency suggests that HIV is a 'long-term condition', rather than an illness, while the US Centres for Disease Control follow UNAIDS in treating it as a 'chronic' disease that can be addressed alongside others (Nigatu 2012; UNAIDS 2011b). Grassroots HIV organisations like the one I describe above have also taken on this medically normalised story of HIV, though they are aware of the difficulties it presents.

When HIV is normalised medically, it is seen as an ongoing, though reducing, and potentially defeatable, pandemic, to be considered in parallel with other important health challenges as part of the natural order of health and illness. The Global Fund, for example, makes this move, discursively and in practice, by addressing HIV in parallel with TB and malaria. UNAIDS's 'zero new infections' and 'zero deaths' aims suggest that the past decades of the pandemic can be brought to a halt, leaving us in a normalised, stable state within which the 'zero stigma and discrimination' goal moves people of all different HIV statuses into citizenly alignment. Living with HIV or taking care to avoid becoming HIV positive are, similarly, often presented as regular aspects of contemporary health, to be taken on by and assimilated to general chronic health and sexual and reproductive health services. The Terrence Higgins Trust, for instance, offers a 'LifeCheck' self-assessment very similar to the lifestyle self-evaluation provided by the generalist National Health Service, with the very broad aim of enabling online visitors to 'gauge where you are in your journey and find out what you need more information about' (see Terrence Higgins Trust 2011 http://www.tht.org.uk/myhiv/HIV-and-you/News/Positive-update/Issue-2-August-2011/Is-your-Lifecheck-completed_qm).

Normalisation operates not just medically but across all the fields of the HIV pandemic. As a general process, it has also been described, promoted and criticised in many other areas of diversity and difficulty, such as prison practices (for instance, Sloan 2005); discourses of social work, gender, class and 'race' (for example, Fahlgren and Sawyer 2011) and patterns of care for people living with mental health problems (Pinfold 2000). Stories of chronic illness, of which HIV is now an example, telling of 'life as normal', have been analysed to show greater complexity than at first appears, for these stories are always co-constructed and revised (Robinson 1993). The normalisation of disabilities, of which HIV is one, should, it is often said, involve not just mainstreaming or 'integration', which often gloss over the specificities of differences, but also changing the physical and social environment. Still, such normalisation's relation to emancipation and inclusivity is questioned (Perrin and Nirje 1985; Walmsley 2001).

The normalisation of HIV encourages some extremely important moves towards, for instance, de-stigmatisation, universal voluntary testing, universal and early treatment, the wide use of condoms, and rights and justice for citizens of all HIV statuses. The normalised HIV citizen is enabled to act socially and politically in association or alliance with other healthy citizens and other biological citizens, and to claim entitlements (Epstein 2006; Rose 2007; Robins 2009; Mbali 2005). S/he can test regularly with statutory health services, or as and when s/he wants by using self-test or self-sampling kits. If s/he is HIV positive, s/he is increasingly given HIV-related health and other services along with other services and other people, rather than separately. This should result in the holistic concern for the whole person which people living with HIV repeatedly say, as we saw in the previous chapter, that they want. They frequently say, for example, that they yearn to forget about their HIV status, to be treated as just another person with a chronic condition, an older person with some health problems, a person trying to get back into the labour market, a person struggling to establish her/himself in a new country after a difficult migration, or a parent striving to do the best for her/his children. However, such normalising integration is often undermined in practice by the simplifying medicalisation, intensified by the current reduction of non-medical services that Tyler and Sean narrated in the previous chapter. Moreover, like the mathematical process with which it shares a name, normalisation can work to 'fit' particularities into a pre-assumed shape. There is little room within normalising accounts and practices around HIV for the particularities, sometimes small-scale, sometimes very significant, associated with the epidemic. People living three-letter lives may at times find their HIV status irrelevant, best minimised. Yet at other times, it is vitally important for that status to be recognised in its physical, social, and psychological specificity.

One area where this contradiction comes into focus is that of primary health care for people living with HIV. Since the advent of effective ARV treatment in high-income countries in the 1990s, and the 2000s rollout of that treatment in low- and middle-income countries, care for people living with HIV has increasingly been normalised by its incorporation within primary care services. In low-prevalence countries like the United Kingdom, general practitioners are expected to be able to deal with non-HIV-related and even some HIV-related issues for their HIV positive patients. They are enjoined to offer HIV testing, particularly in high-prevalence communities and localities; to consider doing routine screenings, vaccinations and mental health and sexual/reproductive health care with their HIV positive patients; to be aware of diagnostic criteria for HIV and opportunistic infections; to be on the lookout for difficulties with ARVs; and to liaise with specialist HIV treatment centres where necessary. In all this, the United Kingdom's Medical Foundation for AIDS and Sexual Health declares that HIV care is much like primary care practice with other chronic diseases: 'In many ways, looking after someone with HIV is no different from looking after those with other chronic conditions' (Madge et al. 2011: 67).

In this account, HIV healthcare is indeed normal healthcare, part of the natural span of health and illness provision. However, in my work and that of many others, people living with HIV in the United Kingdom repeatedly talk about bypassing their GPs (general practitioners) and going straight to their specialist HIV clinics for even minor, apparently non-HIV-related conditions, despite being encouraged by their clinics to use their GPs. Sometimes, they do not tell a GP their status. They encounter large difficulties of inadequate or uncertain GP knowledge; discriminatory attitudes; failures of communication between GPs and their specialist clinics; and breaches of confidentiality and anonymity at their local surgeries, usually by receptionists. The situation has improved as GPs have become more experienced, and some GPs in areas of relatively high HIV prevalence are said to be knowledgeable and confident. However, the majority of my 2011 interviewees still used their GPs little, demonstrating the difficulties of normalising HIV primary care and people's resistance to that normalisation.

In other, high-prevalence and low-resourced circumstances, the normalisation of HIV services alongside other services has been driven much more strongly by resource requirements. The scale of such epidemics' demands means that all medical and social welfare professionals have to be involved in meeting them. Moreover, where HIV is a part of most people's normal lives, present in every family, its normalisation is inevitable and highly appropriate. At the same time, it has been important for what is often seen as the skewing bonanza of HIV funding, particularly from international sources, to have more generalised, cascading effects. Often, HIV is only one of the crowd of health, social, and economic needs with which people live. Thus, the normalising integration of HIV services is also a matter of avoiding what might otherwise be a divisive exceptionalism around those services, as discussed in Chapter 2. Such integration can still, though, allow space for the particularity of HIV to be addressed (UNAIDS 2011b).

For instance, the rollout of testing and treatment has of necessity involved the devolving of HIV services to primary health care and the integration and interaction of HIV services with other health services around conditions often found together with HIV, for example, with sexual and reproductive health clinics, and TB and drug treatment services. In such circumstances, normalisation can build wider skills and knowledge for professionals and for patients. South Africa's Western Cape ARV rollout, starting in 2003, was an early instance of such normalisation, since it involved task-shifting treatment services to settings and staff not previously associated with cutting-edge medical care, and work with community-based organisations which had many diverse focuses of their own. These aspects of HIV treatment's normalisation became integral parts of ARV and other HIV service expansions in South Africa and elsewhere (Abdullah and Squire 2010; UNAIDS 2009a: 119). At the same time, as with other policy and service mainstreaming, for example around gender, the integration of HIV can be too narrow, or it can homogenise or invisibilise the condition. Important specific issues may be lost sight of; the commitment to address HIV in every context may remain a mere declaration on paper, or something that is always said, rarely acted on (Elsey et al. 2005).

Within social care provision, many high-income countries used to have specific provision for people living with HIV, but now tend to mainstream such provision. In the United Kingdom, for example, publicly funded social care today requires all social workers to be able to deal with HIV issues. It is expected that those working with African-origin, migrant clients, intravenous-drug-using and gay male clients, and in high-prevalence HIV localities, will be particularly skilled and involved (National AIDS Trust 2011a). In South Africa, HIV care provision is also often associated with facilities for children, youth, and victims of sexual violence, providing a valuably holistic set of services (Killian et al. 2007). Once more, such mainstreaming can mean that the particular requirements of HIV positive service users get overridden, especially when resources are under pressure. Frequently, for instance, in the United Kingdom, but much more in South Africa and other middle- and low-income countries, social care services are expected to be provided by volunteers who cannot fully meet service users' requirements on a voluntary basis (Campbell et al. 2007; Naidu 2012).

Living like a normal person

What does HIV's normalisation mean for people themselves? If HIV positive people, HIV-affected people, and people at risk of becoming HIV positive can be treated and protected by Western medicine, served and given entitlements by social services and the law, they turn into regular, unremarkable citizens, just like anyone else. HIV itself becomes part of a broad group of medically treatable and preventable 'chronic' illnesses that allow regular participation within social life. It is thus doubly normalised, as itself a manageable, familiar health condition, and as a condition with features comparable to, for example, diabetes, heart disease, tuberculosis, and some cancers.

HIV's normalisation also operates through its constitution of people living with HIV as *self-regulating* citizens. More and more, these citizens are expected to manage their own condition. They see doctors much less than previously if their health is stable; they themselves evaluate, report and otherwise act on any potentially significant changes; they are enjoined to take care of their own health and pursue wellbeing; they should feel able to disclose their HIV status when they think it is necessary or useful; they find work and pursue relationships; they live like anyone else. As we have seen, taking and managing ARV therapy is becoming a normalised part of 'living with HIV' increasingly early after diagnosis, with those medications now much more likely than before to fit relatively seamlessly into HIV positive, healthy people's lives and to enable such lives.

As with other chronic but potentially fatal conditions, discourses and practices operating around HIV thus constitute its citizens as biomedicine's partners in a normalised enterprise of survival and, as far as possible, healthy, happy and productive living. These discourses and practices also give their citizens normalising self-care responsibilities in realms where medical and lay expertise overlap (Rose 1999). People living with HIV are induced, and induce themselves, to pursue good nutrition, exercise and stress management, and to deploy 'complementary' or 'traditional' treatments where these do not compromise Western medical approaches. They are expected, and expect themselves, to be citizens like any others, able and obligated to live healthily, and to work and love, Freud's requirements for a contented life.

At the start of Chapter 3, Nicco, interviewed in South Africa in 2012, described how she has come to terms with her HIV status. She also narrated how she has brought her family to accept her and now speaks out about her condition within her community, a citizen among other citizens, distinguished but not othered by her HIV status. She positioned herself as a normal person. Such accounts of being a person among others, just like anyone else, occurred throughout people's accounts in South Africa and the United Kingdom. Yoliswa and Queenie, for example, told similar stories. Among my South African 2001 interviews, Mhiki, a woman who at that point had ARV access through a hospital trial, began her interview with a tale of entwined medical and self-management, and healthy 'living with HIV' that already exemplified UK and South African interviewees' articulations of normalised HIV citizenship. Of course there were important specificities in Mhiki's account, related to the resources available to her, to gender, and to the epidemic's South African history. Nevertheless, many of the common requirements of self-regulating HIV citizens mentioned before make themselves heard here:

> **Mhiki:** With regard to things that are helpful to one living with HIV firstly, you must accept it. When you are told that you have HIV, accept that because that is what will make you live a long life. Secondly, it's good behaviour. If you were drinking and or smoking, you must stop all that. Thirdly, if you are taking medication, you must take your medication as prescribed. Finally, if you

have a boyfriend, you must condomise. ... Since I told my family, I'm feeling very well. ... If you've got a problem, you can share with the other people in the support group ... if I have a problem {with side effects} I can phone Sister {name} and go to {hospital}. If I don't have money I can borrow it from my neighbour and when I come back the sister give 20 rand to pay the neighbour back ... I try to eat good food and even exercise because, every Saturday I go to play a netball. We've got a netball club. So, I'm doing exercise.[1]

At the levels of personal, interpersonal and social relations, Mhiki's story articulated HIV positive, ARV-treated living as normalised. HIV positive citizens can, like anyone else, accept their health condition, behave healthily, take their medicines, and have responsible relationships. Later, expanding on her story, Mhiki provided snapshot examples of this life.

More recently, Yandiswa, a South African woman in her 40s whom I interviewed in 2012, described responses to her 2004 diagnosis. At that time, though ARVs were not universally available in her neighbourhood, treatment was a possibility: it was known about. Yandiswa's story of her family's response diverts to consider her own acceptance, and then returns to the family 'by my side'. She narrates both herself and them as strongly and deliberately positioned against historical and current stigmatisations of HIV, and tragic renderings of it as a literal or metaphorical death sentence. Instead, they normalise HIV into a condition that should not harm the people affected, and an illness like others:

Interviewer: So why do you think that your family did not have a problem, because other families do find a problem and make things difficult for a person, so since your family accepted you what do you think might be the reason for that?

Yandiswa: For them to accept I think it's because they know that, maybe since things have been spoken {in the media} about people living with HIV killing themselves because of HIV. So I think they saw me telling them that I am HIV positive, and I have accepted that I am HIV, so I don't want anyone crying to me because I am HIV positive, or someone avoiding me because I am HIV positive. Because HIV is something that we are used to now, it's like any other disease, it's like TB, all the diseases, when you take your medication you get well, so I never stressed about that, but my family was by my side.

People who view themselves as potentially HIV positive may also be naturalised as citizens by their normalised practices of self-governance.

For everyone sero-negative or of unknown HIV status is required to regulate their health and relationships, as are all contemporary subjects, via social and educational technologies around, for instance, abstinence and partner reduction, as well as health technologies such as self and partner testing, male and female condoms, male circumcision, PEP, and potentially, PrEP. More broadly, the HIV epidemic has become a normalised, manageable part of political, economic and social worlds, in both high- and low-prevalence epidemics, via health service testing and monitoring, education, popular culture, and international aid.

Perhaps, then, the normalised HIV citizen is just one specific form of the contemporary bio-political citizen (Rose 2007), with not much that is specific to HIV about it. Her/his citizenship is biological but concurrently and necessarily social and political. In being thus constituted, subjects are also, as Butler (2005) points out, ethical. To be called into being as a normalised HIV citizen is to take on certain responsibilities towards truth and life. Who we are in relation to HIV, like other socially contentious conditions, is also who, as normalised citizens, we ought to be. Social normalisation is also moral normalisation.

We can see this connection in the increasingly common framing of people living with HIV as legally responsible for transmission, in ways that differ from country to country but that always emphasise a responsibility towards the health of others. Parents who are HIV positive and who knowingly refuse or do not access treatment for their babies, for example, may be criminally culpable, as might be parents with religious beliefs steering them away from some forms of medical care for their children. However, this assignment of responsibility, or responsibilisation, of HIV positive citizens has some particular characteristics of its own. It is often said to position them discriminatorily in relation to sexual relationships, as morally pathological. They, but not people of unknown or HIV negative status, must take on the responsibility for safer sex. In the socio-moral world to which the normalised HIV citizen belongs, all are equally responsible in some areas, but in other areas, some are more responsible than others (see for instance, Cameron et al. 2008; Lazzarini et al. 2012; Monk 2009; Weait 2007). Some of our UK interviewees were very concerned about this disproportionate citizenly liability around disclosure. Like Quentin, who we heard from in Chapter 2, they cited legal difficulties as one of the reasons they avoided relationships with anyone who not declaredly HIV positive. Others faced the ambiguities of this kind of normalisation more directly, though they were still difficult. Robert, for instance, a man in his 40s who was very open about his HIV status, brought in the voice of an HIV negative friend working in the HIV sector to articulate his own frustration:

> **Robert:** I was treated really badly by someone, I hadn't disclosed my status, but didn't do anything risky, and he made me feel like shit, and what was really great was a friend of mine who works in {HIV organisation} I phoned him up because he's a wise old sage. 'I feel like crap' {I said}, he said like 'tell him to fuck off,' he said, 'if he's so concerned about staying negative he should have said "I'm negative", blah blah blah, from the outset'. He said 'I'm fed up with', he's negative himself, my friend, 'I'm fed up with these people expecting a positive person to disclose. If they're so desperate to stay negative then they should do it.'

Normalising may, then, conceal some very firm and discriminatory categorisations of the HIV positive citizen. It may also mean that you may in some ways not be an 'HIV' citizen at all. In South Africa in 2004, most of the female research participants from 2001 who had been diagnosed early, during pregnancy, were not easily contactable for a second interview. Still well, they no longer used the HIV NGOs through which they were recruited, though they attended clinic check-ups. They did not greet clinic workers if they met them outside, except by the subtlest of signs. Though most had disclosed their status to their families, they often lived, in their wider social networks, as if they were HIV negative. By 2012, a number of South African interviewees who had been heavily involved with treatment activism had moved on, or back, to other forms of work in which their HIV status was not remarked or necessarily even known. Similarly, in later rounds of the UK interviews, a couple of participants who had previously been engaged in providing voluntary or paid HIV services were no longer involved and declined further participation with the research, saying they did not want to focus on HIV in their lives. A number of new participants in the 2012 UK interviews noted that on diagnosis they had been surprised to find they had friends and acquaintances who were also positive but whose status had been normalised out of their social interactions. These people had never mentioned their status before, even when HIV was discussed. Now, to help their newly-diagnosed and disclosing friend, they were happy to talk about their status and experiences.

HIV's normalisation can challenge, or reinforce, the pandemic's medicalisation, for normalising educational and social HIV technologies may agree with or depart in important respects from medical technologies.

The South African edutainment charity *Soul City* (2008), for example, which has a widespread, normalised television and radio presence, ran an online 'OneLove' campaign, starting in 2009, foregrounding discussions about multiple versus single partners, sexuality and relationships, encouraging high levels of questioning and uncertainty that are unlikely to be part of mainstream health education campaigns. However, *Soul City*'s broadcast work tends, for good health-education reasons, to be more in tune with medical guidelines. Similarly, MTV's 'Staying Alive' television and radio campaigns, beginning in 2009, and in particular the extremely popular *Shuga* serial drama, shown and radio-broadcast in Kenya and later many other African countries, about young, sexually active urban youth, preoccupied with money, relationship and family worries, having fun and parties, operates to normalise HIV for youth in those countries. *Shuga* delivers relatively conventional medical messages about testing, antiretrovirals and the health difficulties associated with HIV. However, the community-based discussions around *Shuga*, which as with *Soul City* and other similar edutainment projects appear to constitute the most influential elements of the shows, tend to move outside of these conventional knowledge boundaries, exploring the more difficult intersections of love, sex, work and HIV (Borzekowski 2011). In both these cases, HIV's normalisation within psychosocial technologies of health, reproduction and relationships, as a difficult issue generating complex, dialogic narratives, can operate at a tangent to the simpler, medicalised form of its naturalisation.

The inscription of HIV within normalised biological citizenship also allows activist groups to work with or to challenge mainstream medical expertise, sometimes campaigning for accepted medical HIV technologies, sometimes demanding alternatives (Epstein 1996; Robins 2009; Rose 2007). For instance, in the South African context, treatment activists argue for third-line medications not currently available or second-line medications for which there is often a long wait, on the basis of the constitutional guarantee of 'health for all'. As mentioned in the previous chapter, NGO representatives have used their normalised, formally recognised position within UNAIDS to criticise medicalised treatment optimism's grip on policy (UNAIDS 2012b).

'Health' itself is framed more variably than in medicalised discourse in the popular discourses within which the normalised HIV citizen lives, which present it as a personally felt and judged entity. Nicco's own close association of herself with her successful medications, not through their medical properties, but through her ownership of health through them, is one example; John's arrogation of medical knowledge and authority to himself is another. The Terrence Higgins Trust's LifeCheck campaign aims at something similar, when it presents health for people with HIV as a self-assessed, self-directed, holistic matter: 'Taking a lifecheck empowers you to take control of your life with HIV, get a good understanding of the areas linked to it and get more in depth information and advice if you need it' (Terrence Higgins Trust 2011 http://www.tht.org.uk/myhiv/HIV-and-you/News/Positive-update/Issue-2-August-2011/Is-your-Lifecheck-completed_qm). If health is defined generally, as 'feeling well', HIV's normalisation may even act orthogonally to its medicalisation, an opposition of varying usefulness. Subjective convictions of good health can, for instance, work against the contemporary narrowing of lives lived with HIV and ARVs into disease stories, discussed in Chapter 4. However, they may also lead to health-threatening resistance to medical injunctions to start treatment.

Troubling normalisation

Despite its beneficial effects and its challenges to medicalisation, the normalisation of HIV citizens raises problems because of the many difficult aspects of HIV that cannot, in fact, be rendered wholly 'normal'. There are several reasons for this recalcitrance. First, HIV is not fully analogous to other chronic illnesses because of its associations with pathologised social states such as sex work; intravenous drug use; and gay, female and 'promiscuous' sexualities; and its potentially fatal, still difficult-to-treat nature. These characteristics, as well as the physical and social visibility of HIV illness, treatment side effects, and prophylactic actions like taking vitamins, eating healthily, having caesareans and formula feeding, generate continuing stigmatisation even in situations of accessible treatment and care (Flowers et al. 2006; Roura et al. 2009). The HIV organisation whose discussion of these issues I describe at the beginning of this chapter, found such insistent stigma, whether experienced or perceived, a sticking point in their attempts to draw people into a collective normalising narrative of three-letter lives. A number of our South African women interviewees in particular also suggested that, however treatable HIV becomes, however strongly discrimination is resisted, the condition's association with transgressive sexuality, particularly for women, will always render it socially stigmatised, unlike, for instance, TB.

Second, contemporary medical approaches to HIV do not always fit unproblematically with normalisation. In the previous chapter segment, we saw some examples of disjunctions as well as synergies between medicalisation and normalisation, in the fields of HIV education and action. More fundamentally, ARVs can be difficult medications to take, hard to incorporate into 'normal life'. Some have persistent side effects; they may not work consistently, or at all, for everyone, so ARV failures and changes may be involved. At the beginning of Chapter 3, an extract from the UK's HPA's latest report suggests a normal lifespan is available if living with HIV and that HIV is not even a chronic illness but a long-term condition. This does not jibe with the ways in which many people live with HIV. One participant in my UK study withdrew at the last interview round, despite clinically successful antiretroviral treatment, because of a disability related to long-term HIV infection. Many long-term participants, like John, have experienced new HIV-related illnesses as time progresses. Some recently and early-diagnosed participants have been very sick. They have not followed the currently dominant narrative path of prompt diagnosis, early treatment and living healthily with this 'long-term condition'. Medical uncertainties also trouble HIV negative people's 'treatment optimism' and any potential normalisation of treatment-led prevention, affecting people's understandings both of the health consequences of being positive, and of treated HIV positive people's infectivity (Davis 2009; Persson 2012). No participants in the United Kingdom or South Africa, for example, including the small number of HIV-affected partners interviewed, treated the transmission risks of unsafe sex as negligible in the absence of detectable viral load, despite their frequently expressed knowledge of the low transmission risks shown in these circumstances in some well-known trials.

Thirdly, HIV positive people are not always able to relate 'normally', that is, like non-HIV positive citizens, to work, parenting and relationships. Their health and experienced and perceived stigma set limits on such relations. They may not fully self-govern, as normalising discourses of HIV enjoin them to, towards healthy, risk-free actions. Nor do HIV negative or unknown-status people always conduct themselves in a normalised way in relation to HIV, treating it without stigmatisation and minimising their risk. For instance, they take – and, the law suggests, they are expected to take – much less care around safer sex than HIV positive people do, particularly in low-prevalence epidemics. In high-prevalence epidemics, the apparent contemporary 'normality' of three-letter lives may become embedded, for those who are HIV negative or of unknown status, in deeply pessimistic discourses of HIV as an inevitable concomitant of living a normal, pleasurable life; of HIV as a feasible route to practical resources and social fellowship; or of ARVs as a passport to an unwanted half-life within which people masquerade as healthy and happy (Lana 2010; Zungu 2012).

These limits of normalisation are of course true of other health conditions such as other STIs, TB, diabetes, cancer and obesity. But in the case of HIV, such problems are intensified by the virus's particularly stigmatised character and its relation to discourses of sexual transgression, irrationality and uncertainty. Nicco had to work hard to talk her family round, to talk herself back into normalcy with them, and to become a regular, unremarkable part of her family and community again. Mhiki describes a very deliberate process of struggling for a healthy lifestyle. Some UK interviewees, in particular those who had been living for more than ten years with ARVs, told stories of such fragile and critical health that 'normalisation' made no sense in relation to them. Often, too, HIV strongly disrupts dominant, 'normal' stories of sex, love and relationships. In both UK and South African studies, women interviewees told of times when 'love' or desire meant they decided not to use condoms, a normalised moment of abandonment for people unaffected by HIV that nevertheless violated the normalised self-management required at all times of HIV positive citizens. Such self-management technologies are themselves probabilistic and individualising, and on these accounts, they do not infallibly deliver normalcy. Several interviewees in the UK study told stories about becoming HIV positive that traced how their narrators, when HIV negative, had been very well educated about the virus, even in some cases working in the HIV field, and how they had either taken informed risks that did not work out, or had taken no risks at all, except in believing others whose trustworthiness seemed unquestionable, or who were themselves with good reason convinced that they were not HIV positive. Self-governance into normal life and health takes little account of such uncertainties of knowledge, emotion and viral transmission.

Mhiki's interview, which provided an emblematic story of normalised self-governance within this chapter, also indicated very clearly the limitations of HIV's normalisation because it went on to unpick this normalised life story. Later in the interview, Mhiki said, for example, that one of her sisters could not be told of Mhiki's status because she would gossip; her boyfriend did not know and could not consider his own status, and rejected her when she told him her diagnosis, causing her to leave him; her HIV positive child, who did not yet know about her own status, hated HIV positive people and was causing her serious problems on this account; and a friend had told her just to abandon this sick child in the hospital. Mhiki herself had been, she said, one of those who thought HIV only affected the promiscuous, the foreign, travellers like truck drivers, or those who had blood transfusions (see also Squire 2007). Mhiki's initial account sounds at first like the story of an unproblematically normalised, albeit perhaps extra-carefully detailed, life with HIV under treatment. Within this wider skein of difficult stories, it reads more as an effortful assertion of normalcy, against many stigmatising factors. Many of those factors are specific to Mhiki's context. The effort to oppose stigmatisation through normalisation, however, has more general significance.

Mhiki's narrative of her life with HIV exemplifies how HIV's normalisation can oppose stigmatisation. But the story is at the same time the tale of how 'non-normal' HIV citizens continue to be. HIV still produces very particular, often socially pathologised kinds of citizens. Its compromised normalisation in medicine and other fields points to the limits of seeing 'biological politics' as an undifferentiated field, and to the difficulties of configuring 'health citizenship' in generalised ways. This is not to endorse HIV or AIDS exceptionalism (De Waal 2006), a perspective that, as we saw earlier, can turn HIV into a uniquely tragic, and often implicitly low-income, African, 'othered' condition, that conveniently leaves little possibility of effective action because it would be difficult and expensive. Rather, HIV citizens' narratives counteracting normalisation, based in the ongoing pandemic's particularities, articulate the multipolarity and specificity of HIV citizenship, and can be a continuing resource for criticism and activism (Crimp 2002; Epstein 1996; Robins 2009; Watney 2000).

HIV's normalisation naturalises by undoing stigmatisation. It turns HIV into a regularised part of biological and social life. But naturalisation via normalisation tends to underestimate the power relations around the pandemic, and the uncertainties of HIV knowledge. A fully normalised HIV citizen would not, perhaps, be an 'HIV' citizen at all. Moreover, through normalisation, individuals become HIV citizens with human rights, but also individualised human responsibilities, including an unfulfillable responsibility to understand everything and act fully rationally about HIV. As Quentin's and Robert's stories and those of many other interviewees indicate, such responsibility is discriminatorily and heavily felt by people living with HIV. As others' stories of unsuccessful risk management or passionate risk disavowal show, this responsibility also continues to be hard to negotiate in sexual relationships.

6

Investing in the Pandemic: The Marketised HIV Citizen

Introduction: turning HIV programmes into investments

In 2012, I interview a woman of 40, Siyanda, at an HIV NGO near Cape Town, South Africa. She is HIV positive herself and has a child who is also positive. Because Siyanda is healthy, she does not receive a disability grant, and she has not been able to find employment. This means she lives off child support grants. Occasionally, she does not have enough money to give breakfast to her HIV positive child, and the ARVs are too strong to take without food, so she withholds them from the child, something that could negatively affect their health. She says she feels ashamed of this. At the end of the interview, I give her the standard fee and she is very pleased. She says she can use it to buy fruit for the children on the trip her church group is about to take, so that they will be like the other children, bringing healthy things along for themselves and to share.

If, as the previous two chapters suggest, HIV citizens cannot be completely medicalised into health or comprehensively normalised into sociality, perhaps they are more fully naturalised via marketisation, that is, by their incorporation into contemporary relations of consumption, as consumers of goods within markets. In the anecdote above, an HIV positive child's health is compromised by her family's exclusion from the waged economy, while that family's normalised social position within their faith community is enhanced by a financial payment. As Siyanda also repeatedly noted, paid work would naturalise her relations to HIV in a dramatic way.

By substituting economic technologies for medicalisation's knowledge-based and normalisation's ideologically based technologies, marketisation seems to operationalise HIV citizenship more thoroughly, turning citizens into manageable packages of buyable and sellable elements. The process applies to treatment and to prevention, for both of which cost-benefit analyses increasingly need to be made to justify funding, often now re-characterised as 'investment'. Within this framework, treatment has a double payoff, as prevention as well as health maintenance, while it is less easy to argue that psychosocial prevention strategies are effective and profitable. One consequence is that, in straitened economic times, psychosocial prevention budgets often suffer. The 2013 New York City mayoral campaign included a public narrative of this shift, told in the lesbian and gay mayoral forum, charting a three-year decrement in prevention funding and a shift in HIV funding towards treatment and to hospitals that do not do prevention work (ACT UP NY 2013).

At the international level, countries receiving aid for HIV services are increasingly being told to adopt more financial responsibility for their epidemics. Their own reports on their progress frequently emphasise the percentage gains they have made in internal budgeting for the epidemic (UNAIDS 2011a; Malawi Government 2012). Becoming a good citizen in the HIV context thus depends strongly, even at the national level, on attempting to pay one's way and being known to do so. That could mean, in the cases of individuals like Siyanda, trying hard to get paid employment, working on temporary projects for small amounts of money, and demonstrating these efforts publicly. Other framings of citizenship in terms of, for instance, social justice, care, rights, or collective political action, appear more and more difficult to make politically, in policy, and in the everyday contexts within which the pandemic is lived.

This marketised constitution of HIV citizenships, often called 'neo-liberal', seems to have strengthened, at all levels, since the global financial crisis. It inflects international NGOs and government policy, community-based organisations, and the discourse of people living with or affected by HIV and ARVs themselves. HIV funding is falling, for the first time, down by 10% in 2009–10, and budget contractions are having effects on all forms of services. There was a $4 billion Global Fund shortfall in 2010 because large funders reneged on their promised contributions, and US PEPFAR, (the US President's Emergency Plan For AIDS Relief) funding was not increased (Global Fund 2010; World Bank/UNAIDS 2009). Bilateral funding is also being heavily cut. The UK Department for International Development's funds will be cut, overall, by 32% by 2015. As UNAIDS said at the end of 2009, at the 25th Programme Coordinating Board Meeting, 'The global economic crisis is having a real and tangible negative effect on HIV programmes in nearly all low- and middle-income countries' (UNAIDS 2009c). Now, the impact is felt in high-income countries as well.

The financial-crisis rationale for cuts has been paralleled by some funders', policymakers' and doctors' concerns to divert funds from HIV in order to promote health generally, to act against HIV aid dependency in recipient states, and to avoid the HIV exceptionalism discussed earlier in this book (see Chapter 2; see also De Waal 2006; England 2012; UNAIDS 2012a: 4). HIV's normalisation and its marketisation thus work in synergy, inducing HIV services to compete for resources with, for instance, maternal and child health (to which some PEPFAR funds have been diverted), and requiring high-prevalence countries to prove they are good global citizens. Such long-standing policy tendencies seem to have drawn extra discursive strength from the need to justify the large extent of current economic cuts.

Claims of reneging on governance or accountability agreements may also lead donors to cut programmes, even for life-sustaining ARVs (Bernays et al. 2007), to guard against funding or drug misuse. And perceptions of resources needed and previously received may frame justificatory narratives of spending cuts. Funders told one Brazilian children's organisation, for example, that they were no longer interested in funding HIV projects, given the country's improved economic status (UNAIDS 2012b: 8). Again, these criticisms re-inscribe long-standing development discourses, this time around democratic and transparent structures, and sustainability. Sometimes, though, the cuts just happen without any other rationale than donors' financial difficulty.

It is clear that even with a condition as difficult to 'buy out' of as HIV, health markets exist at every level in the pandemic. Regions, nations and organisations purchase branded or generic drugs from national or international companies. They enter into contracts with international nongovernmental organisations and companies, and with developed-world governments if they are low- or middle-income nations. These contracts provide ARVs, other drugs, and other HIV services, on the basis of organisations', nations' or regions' agreement to make contributions themselves, to meet health and political governance standards, and sometimes to guarantee pharmaceutical markets to companies based in donor countries. Treatment and prevention initiatives are also researched, developed and implemented within a market frame. For example, US state departments of health now devolve some HIV testing to the Walgreens pharmacy chain, and Walgreens and CVS are among the stores offering HIV home sampling and self-test kits as for-profit products.

More generally, in deliberations over treatment and prevention, specific programmes are now also almost always judged against the putative costs of other actions, though often with little reliability (Granich et al. 2009; Nguyen et al. 2011). For instance, much debate over treatment as prevention is driven by financial models which operate alongside epidemiological projections, factoring in how cost-effective, as well as health-effective for individuals and populations, a particular treatment intervention or change would be. A similar narrative, albeit with different endings, appears in PrEP debates. Here, powerful financial arguments, derived from PrEP's projected logistical, behavioural and medical difficulties, often qualify clinical and policy enthusiasm (Morin et al. 2012).

These concatenations of market and epidemiological logics have become more common since the financial crisis. The marketisation of the HIV pandemic is now apparent, not just in policy negotiations about costs and value for money, but in policy discourse, when it turns market approaches into the hegemonic, 'natural' framework for addressing the pandemic. Such discourse converges with that of Hayek (2011 [1960]), a primary economic philosopher of what is often criticised as 'neo-liberalism', that is, the contemporary free-market-based approach to economies, societies, and even subjectivities. For Hayek, the 'natural order' of human living derives from the operations of the free market. As if applying such an ontology to three-letter lives, the UK Health Protection Agency's 2011 report included for the first time market-aware chapters on the cost-effectiveness of treatment and expanding testing, and a cost-benefit analysis of prevention activities (Health Protection Agency 2011). As the quote at the beginning of Chapter 3 on HIV services and 'value for money' indicates, UNAIDS has also moved towards such analysis. Its 2010 report included for the first time a chapter on 'HIV investments'. It now frames financial commitments to HIV care and prevention as payments now for payoff later. Such framings are paralleled by many NGOs reorienting HIV initiatives into market-friendly social enterprise or entrepreneurship. UNAIDS (2011a) itself notes that this approach has become more intense since the recession. Indeed, its own 'Strategic Investment Framework' was initiated as a better-management response to the HIV budget cuts of 2009–10, concentrating on targeting, local appropriateness and efficiencies. The framework factors in the 'efficiency gains' from getting more community contributions to HIV work, 'synergies' between programmes and the prevention budget gains of treatment, and it calls for at least 15% of countries' HIV budgets to be self-funded and therefore more sustainable (UNAIDS 2012a:

7ff). UNAIDS declares this a community-led and not a commodity-led strategy, but that still leaves it as a *market* strategy.

Marketised framings are always produced for particular audiences, they are not the only policy framings in existence, they are not necessarily what is happening in practice, and they are invariably contestable. The most recent Ugandan report on the country's HIV situation points out the impossibility of government funding making a significant impact now that ARVs must be extended to a whole new tranche of people living with the virus in order to meet WHO guidelines (Republic of Uganda 2012: 14). Even more pointedly, in 2012, the NGO delegation to UNAIDS's 30th programme meeting produced, as mentioned in previous chapters, a thoroughgoing critical account focused on funding cuts. The account, replete with case studies, enumerated the cuts' detrimental effects, particularly on civil society programmes, warned of dangerous consequences, and urged a more robust response to market-driven crisis and strong action from UNAIDS, in enhanced collaboration with NGOs, in order to 'get to zero':

> [T]he NGO Delegation expresses strong concern that – in this time of unprecedented crisis – the Programme Coordinating Board is failing to fulfil its leadership role, especially as it relates to leveraging UNAIDS' unique position as a convener capable of driving a more systematic and coordinated response, one that fully realizes the important role civil society can play. (UNAIDS 2012b: 9)

The report stays within the HIV sector's market logic in order to qualify it. It points out that 'the cost of doing nothing is far greater than the cost of doing something' (UNAIDS 2012b: 19) and that HIV programmes have many 'value added' aspects in their developments of civil society, an implicit counting-in of the local and security 'capitals' accruing from HIV programmes. That does not stop the report from having a considerable critical edge.

Similarly, in the United States, the resurgent ACT UP (AIDS Coalition to Unleash Power) movement, reinvigorated 25 years after it campaigned for destigmatisation and treatment, and now with several strong branches, has been campaigning since 2011, along with Occupy and a raft of other social justice campaigns (see http://robinhoodtax.org/whos-behind-it/endorsing-organizations), for a 0.5 cent tax on financial transactions, a 'Robin Hood tax' to fund people living with HIV in the United States and internationally. This move is closely aligned with the current investment-oriented nature of national and international organisations' thinking about HIV. However, it is also powerfully inter-national, particularly in its sense of the global economy and its appeal to transnational allies.

Living in the HIV marketplace

So far, I have described some notable and obvious aspects of HIV's marketisation. Often they are criticised, but they seem more widespread and accepted since the 2008 financial crisis than before.

Marketisation also operates in less explicit, 'undercover' ways. What looks like resilience and self-reliance is often, as with Queenie, whose situation was described at the beginning of Chapter 3, also a response to financial restrictions or cuts. The uncertainties of the global phar-macological market continue to impinge on the thoughts of many people living with HIV, even when ARVs are available and everything is going well. Yet they do not quickly or easily report their fragile posi-tion as drug consumers in a global ARV sellers' market as a concern. In Yoliswa's interview, her closing mention, almost an afterthought, of the global uncertainties overhanging her life with the virus exhibited both this concern and the importance of keeping it in liveable, minimised perspective, on the edges of life narratives (see Chapter 3).

The citizens of the HIV pandemic are committed to researching, culti-vating, finding, buying and using whatever will improve their own HIV-related health, whether or not they are positive or have access to ARVs. The very general finding that HIV positive people conduct their own self-care by buying traditional, alternative and complementary medical remedies, or the ingredients to make such remedies, alongside conventional Western treatment, indexes this commitment (Babb et al. 2007; Josephs et al. 2007; Langlois-Klassen et al. 2007; Milan et al. 2006). So does the consumption of prevention 'goods' such as condoms, male circumcision, HIV testing, PEP, and PrEP, which may all be bought from doctors, pharmacists or online, where not prescribed free (Uganda Radio Network 2012).

In my South African and UK research, many participants reported always being on the lookout for substances and products that they could use in health-promoting ways. This concern was at its strongest in the pre-ARV 1990s in the United Kingdom. For South African inter-viewees, it was most prominent in 2001, if they needed but did not yet have access to ARVs. For such participants, alternative products, which might help them maintain their health till effective treatment came along, were often prohibitively expensive. In the later UK and South African epidemic contexts of free ARVs, a concern with health promotion through parallel complementary product consumption remained common, though less pronounced, in both countries. Benjamin, for example, who was on a South African pilot ARV programme even in 2001, told a habitual narrative of continually seeking out and buying products said to enhance immune function:

> **Benjamin:** Like if, like I saw a catalogue of medicines and then I find that I do have money to buy that, {I do}, because I was told that my immune system is low.

Often such purchasing commitments were broader, tied to normalising discourses of nutrition and lifestyle, and also involving popular media consumption. Zukiswa's story of her successive attempts at healthy living, countering HIV-related weight loss, skin problems and thrush, demonstrates the imbrications of this progress with the purchase and consumption of goods and media:

> **Zukiswa:** When I (used to) buy veggies, carrots for instance I never cooked them, I don't like cooking them not unless I'm cooking for my baby. I usually clean them and eat them raw with er cayenne pepper I mix it with hot water. I heard that from the radio, but before I did that I was losing weight, it was going down, I even saw that my complexion was changing and then my tongue there was that white substance. That thing, like a baby who eats milk/Okay/I ate that, I used those carrots, I used cayenne pepper putting it in warm water. Alcohol, I used to drink alcohol and then I paused I was told that I must er, and then I realised that I am someone that has got the virus so I had to drop the pace. Even if I drink, I should drink less, but I gave up, I quit...I do my own investigations...I listen to the radio and take notes. If they say what helped someone, I write that down.[1]

Less discussed, because of their illegality, is people's purchase of 'recreational' drugs, usually cannabis, to deal with pain, stress, and appetite loss and sometimes for access to pleasures that provide a normalising continuity with pre-diagnostic lives. Several UK interviewees have described such purchases, across all the decades of the epidemic. For example, Sean, speaking of himself and his partner Tyler, both living with a difficult combination of ARV side effects and HIV-related illnesses, said in 2011:

> **Sean:** We both find it very hard to eat food. I feel sick and find it hard to put food {into my mouth...without smoking cannabis}. I feel {without it} we would not eat...Eating is one of the biggest struggles that we both find hard on a daily basis. (Email follow-up to interview)

Other examples of the ubiquity of HIV consumption economies are informal pharmacological markets. HIV positive people may divert or sell excess medications to others, for treatment or prevention (Zablotska et al. 2013). Many migrants in the developed and developing worlds send financial remittances home to relations living with HIV to ARV or other medication costs. Some with excess HIV medications or access to alleged HIV medications online send pharma-remittances. Though the expansion of ARV access worldwide has reduced these flows, medications that are branded rather than generic, or difficult to obtain in middle- and low-income contexts, may still be sent. Within southern Africa, Zimbabwe's political instability and economic problems led at one point to ARV supply problems with attendant profiteering, sales of fake ARVs, and cross-border importations from Mozambique and South Africa (Veenstra et al. 2010). Given the resource restrictions of sub-Saharan Africa in particular in relation to ARVs, such pharmacological economies are not surprising. Despite the dangers that attend unprescribed and unmonitored ARV use, some ARV access is always preferable to none.

HIV remittances have been, like the more general remittance economy, affected by the economic downturn and by concomitant reductions in migration (Sirkeci et al. 2012). In the longer term, HIV remittances are also strongly determined by histories of migration and HIV epidemics, as well as by economic gradients between host and source countries, and improvements in ARV access. In 2010, Nicholas, an African migrant living in the United Kingdom since the 1990s, related his shift from supporting family members back home living with HIV and other issues, to supporting his own family, partly to increasing ARV availability in his home country, partly to his family's increasing economic and social embeddedness in their new home country:

> **Nicholas:** What is happening, access to (ARVs) in Africa is becoming more and more available there is no doubt about that...you don't have to be in the big city...the country {of my birth} is saturated

with so many organisations ... And because of the cost of living you can't really afford to live your life here {UK} and then have so many {dependents}, it's not working anymore, yeah it's not working anymore ... personally when I came in the first two years I was able to live a basic life and able to support the people back at home but as time went on I have got my life here, my lifestyle here has established itself, I have responsibilities here by the time my (family), I don't have any money to spare to anybody, so for most people that comes have families here so you can't keep on looking after somebody who is not here when you have issues here, that won't be that way.

More broadly, we can see HIV citizens' self-governance through medicalised consumption as just part of a constellation of similar framings of health as consumption, particularly notable within health promotion in high-income countries, and within healthcare wherever free treatment is not available (Bunton et al. 1995; Noah 2012). In medium- and low-income countries, the first means tried to address ill health are usually traditional or non-prescription medicines, which may be more acceptable for some ailments, more effective, and cheaper, even where public health provision is free, if there are transport and clinic visit costs to meet. In developed and developing worlds, too, Western medications are frequently used in parallel with non-prescription, traditional, and, in the West, 'complementary' medicines for many health problems, not just HIV (World Health Organisation 2005: 17). People also address general failures of wellbeing in their lives, not just bodily illness, by buying traditional or complementary medical expertise and products.

Finally, three-letter lives are part of global consumption-led economies, perhaps most developed within high-income countries, though not exclusive to them. Within these economies, citizenship is constructed through sets of responsibilising discourses and practices, including particular forms of thinking and feeling as well as action, that can be bought, or bought into, through consumption (Rose 1999). These patterns may be acquired directly, through employing psychotherapists or traditional spiritual practitioners, for example; or indirectly, through, for instance, consuming psychosocial public services and media messages around HIV education, treatment and care, such as the *Soul City* (2008) 'OneLove' campaign, or MTV's *Shuga* edutainment series (Borzekowski 2011), both described in Chapter 5, or magazine advice on how to talk to children about sex and HIV (Wilbraham 2010).

HIV's marketisation is perhaps least obvious in high-resourced contexts, where the markets supporting medicalisation and normalisation are strongly developed but highly naturalised and little remarked-upon. However, budget cuts since the 1990s and the intensified austerity of the post-2008 period have sharpened awareness of this market structure, something strongly apparent in UK research participants' narratives in this period. Sean's story of the recent move within London ARV procurement to start new ARV users on cheaper drugs, and that move's effects on his own body, was typical of many participants' critical accounts of marketisation. After the cheapest drug combination caused an unresolvable rash, as it does in large numbers of people, Sean was given the second cheapest, jaundice-inducing combination:

> **Sean:** Everyone said 'oh you'll like it, you love a tan', they call it the tan drug and stuff, but the one that I really wanted was had no side effects at all, which is the next one down from if I had the reaction to this one I'd be on it, so yes, so I think they should give me the one that, okay, it's expensive, but you know, that's why they do all this research, to find out, take the better one, then a better one comes out, they say 'oh sorry, we're going to use this one because the better one is costing too much', what's the point of finding a better one if you're not going to use the better one, so we had no side effects at all, so that's, but yes, and that's what I learnt through, I didn't know how it worked, the drug choice, I thought they just put you on a better one. I didn't realise the doctor (said) 'I'll put you on this one, the cheaper one, and the Government says we have to start you on the cheaper one because we haven't got the money'.

At the same time, Sean and Tyler discuss not just the limitations of services and the limited amounts of psychosocial services, but also their concerns about using up or wasting these marketised resources. Given their histories of medical and other difficulties, including appetite problems, it was not surprising that both of them reported over-experiencing some acute-need medical and social services, and that nutritional resources did not work well for them. More notable was their concern that resources should be used well and fairly and not over-used. This highly responsibilised narrative of personal and fiscal restraint and equity, typical of many interviewees, also proceeded in this case from Tyler's and Sean's positioning as non-entitled, non-tax-contributing young people at diagnosis:

> **Tyler:** Sometimes you feel quite bad using them {services} as well/Yes/ Just because, I don't know, you always feel, I don't know, because I

was diagnosed quite young, I've always felt as if I'm not entitled to these services, because I've never really, I didn't have space where, I didn't have it, you know what I mean.

Sean: When Tyler come out of hospital two years ago, we was getting {HIV organisation's} meals, but the food was not to our taste, it was a waste so we cancelled, so someone else could get better use of the service. (Email follow-up to interview)

In low-resourced contexts where HIV treatment is possible but not always accessible, markets are more obvious and contentious. Obtaining and affording ARVs, prophylaxis and treatment for opportunistic infections, and food to enable the medicines to work are primary concerns, supplanting the broader, consumption-driven pursuit of healthy HIV life. People without ARVs may be consumed by the need to buy available medications and immune system enhancers, whatever their price and effectiveness. Nosizo, for instance, speaking in 2001, told of needing but not having access to ARV. She followed this with an account of the financial resources poured into her healthy food purchases, and a list of healthy foods that were at the same time items on the government's AIDS-denialist menu of nutritional 'treatment' at the time:

Nosizo: Yes, if you got that money you buy... {African potato} and garlic and is right for your food and then, the chillies is right when you are cold and fruits, drink with the water, and then the lemon and then if you eat the right food.

Even when ARVs are available, the marketisation of HIV remains in some cases in competition with HIV's medicalisation, when HIV citizens try to sell or buy alternatives to the difficulties of lifelong ARVs such as herbal medicines, curative diets, or religious or traditional spiritual remedies (McGregor 2007). Interviewees in both the United Kingdom and South Africa mentioned such oppositional consumption obliquely and critically, as a concern of others, not themselves. Prior to the 2011 UK deaths of several HIV positive people pursuing cure by prayer rather than ARVs (Dangerfield 2012), Nicholas, in 2010, told the stories of one friend who briefly forsook the clinic for a church that promised cure by fasting and of another who continually put his money into witchcraft antidotes:

Nicholas: I have a friend who has been using it {ARVs} for so many years, who still thinks that some of the things happening to them are based on witchcraft and it's sad though (inaudible). They spend their hard-earned cash and say they will go to Africa and have a witch-doctor remove it but it is something like an egg within the body, and they are getting too deep, start thinking that everything is done by witchcraft and all, and it is people's beliefs I guess, yeah.

In 2001, 2003 and 2004, South African interviewees, too, mentioned people on the radio, in the newspapers and in their neighbourhoods touting alternatives to ARV like herbal substances, vitamin regimens, faith cures and spiritual cleansing. Among these participants, living in a community with an active Médecins Sans Frontières clinic already running an ARV pilot, treatment literacy was relatively high. Non-medical products seemed to them to carry a price tag, but no signs that would contradict the growing evidence, before their own eyes, of very sick people's recovery through use of ARVs. Nevertheless, like Nosizo, they would, before ARVs arrived, try anything and spend everything while waiting for the drugs. In 2003–4 though, and again in 2012, the South African participants' market concerns focused on obtaining firstly enough food, and secondly, healthy food. ARVs might be physically difficult to deal with, but this and the stigmatisation bound up with them was no longer, as it was with Nicholas's friends, intense enough to drive them away from pharmacological and into herbal and spiritual cure economies. When alternative products compete with ARVs in the HIV marketplace, this competition has considerable personal, medical and policy significance. Such competition seemed relatively insignificant for the UK and South African interviewees when ARVs were accessible. However, as in Nicholas's case, several interviewees in both national contexts mentioned friends or family members who had opted to buy into other solutions because the financial or other, social costs of ARVs were too high.

It may be that within the naturalising era of HIV treatment possibility, the strongest market pattern is determined by the epidemic's medicalisation. Complementary products have a niche bounded by their pharmacological inactivity in relation to the virus, and reduced by ARV knowledge and access, and low HIV stigma. This account of the HIV market fits with the South African interviewees' shifting narratives between the first few years of the twenty-first century and 2012. It does not, though, have validity for people who are normalising their HIV citizenship in other, non-medicalised ways. Zungu's recent work (2012) suggests that a marketised HIV citizenship, oriented towards publicly funded Western treatment and activism to optimise it, can coexist in the same geographical area with a very different, attenuated citizenly relation to HIV, characterised by opting out of all HIV health economies, and into a cultural economy of moral blame, within which purchases can only go a small way towards spiritual salvation. Zungu has described such an economy in operation among older men of unknown or negative HIV status, in exactly the peri-urban South African area of intensive and long-term HIV service provision where I have conducted research. These men's characterisation of HIV as 'our disease' indicates acceptance, but also a fatalistic kind of normalisation, on which HIV's marketisation, still less its medicalisation, has little impact, even though they must all know people now successfully participating in the international economy of ARV-dependent health. In the face of these men's collectivised abdication into an, at best, ambiguous naturalisation of the pandemic, even the extensive power of global markets is limited.

Free and not-free markets

Marketisation means that HIV citizens are 'free' within markets. Their relation to the virus is simplified. This can be a liberating frame within which to understand HIV. The epidemic need not be thought of as a socio-political issue, an existential condition, a moral failing, or even an intractable health problem, if individuals and governments simply seek market solutions. However, markets are structured by power relations, and marketised HIV citizens are forced to pursue their own health and survival within markets they can never subjugate. This ambiguity undercuts discourses and practices of responsibilised, consuming HIV citizens from within. As has been recently highly apparent, markets also do not always work. Difficulties in funding ARVs and other programmes, as well as psychosocial provisions, have been acute since the 2008 financial crisis. Informal remittances and formal funding have fallen. As Queenie's extended social resource-sustaining responsibilities show us, and as Yoliswa's overshadowing concern indicates, the HIV citizen is operating within unpredictable markets that often fail. Nicholas's struggles with the transnational market across family diaspora, Tyler's feelings of disentitlement to 'too many' services, and Sean's accounts of the tussles between health and savings visited on his own body via his health authority emphasise the conflicts that are integral to markets. Siyanda's story, at the beginning of the chapter, demonstrates the potential large costs to children's health of small decrements in HIV support, and the social capital gains attendant on even a minor, one-off food supplement. Against such accreted qualitative data and much other evidence, problematising the 'three zeroes' aim of UNAIDS, a zero-sum game plays out within marketised health budget decision-making.

The marketised naturalisation of HIV simplifies the set of things that must be known and holds out the possibility of some resource-balancing via informal economies where the formal market economy fails. As we have seen, however, many limitations attend HIV's naturalisation by marketisation. The marketisation process overlooks the differential powers of market stakeholders, as well as markets' own shifting strengths, which render knowledge of them incomplete and non-predictive. HIV citizens themselves, defined economically rather than politically, also become only partly knowable. This makes marketisation a more obvious example than medicalisation or normalisation, of a naturalising process which denaturalises itself.

The failures of medicalisation, normalisation, and marketisation described in the preceding chapters are not unique to their operation around HIV; they appear much more widely within contemporary societies. In the next chapter, I examine in more detail the specific denaturalisations of these processes that happen within the HIV pandemic.

7
Being Left Behind

'Left Behind' was the middle movement of Hidden Legacies, a
seven movement set for four synthesizers, bass, drums, solo-
ists, and men's chorus ... a haunting lyric about the desolation
of loneliness – being left behind, and the guilt that that often
holds – [is juxtaposed] with the bouncy life-goes-on country
2-step in the music. During the first part of the song, couples
peel away from the chorus, two by two and begin 2-stepping
around the stage. By the time the instrumental arrives, all
collected dancers participate in a flashy line dance. When the
singers comes back in, one by one, the dance partners 'leave'
their partners, leaving them alone, dancing alone, until at the
very end, only one man is left dancing alone.

(Roger Bourland 2006)

Introduction: denaturalising three-letter lives

The problematic naturalisations and denaturalisations achieved by
medicalisation, normalisation and marketisation appear in acute
form around HIV, but they are not particular to it. This chapter argues
that the HIV citizen's formation by the naturalising processes of the
pandemic is also disrupted by factors highly specific to HIV, and that
these specificities are difficult but important to address. In my UK and
South African research, these factors created the strongest discontinuities in people's HIV narratives, positioning the narratives on the edge
of HIV citizenship, and the narrators as HIV citizens under erasure, on
the borders.

The naturalisation of HIV often involves medical, social, political,
even economic progress. The HIV-specific denaturalisations of this

progress script that I am going to consider, then register as being 'left behind', left out of the redemption script. I have transposed the 'left behind' expression from a title within Roger Bourland and John Hall's (1992) *Hidden legacies* song cycle, which refers to those in the United States, particularly gay men and their friends, who were living after the wave of deaths in the 1980s and early 1990s, and before the arrival of effective treatment (see also Odets 1995). However, the phrase has been used in many other contexts within the pandemic, also, to refer to breaks or discontinuities in people's experiences of living with HIV and ARVs. It can describe the gaps between the new realities of effective treatment and the problematic histories of ARVs with which people diagnosed earlier in the pandemic, like John, still live. It can apply to the fracture lines between the contemporary presentation of HIV as a 'long-term condition' and the much more fraught states of illness of even some younger people who became HIV positive relatively recently, like Sean and Tyler, as well as older research participants like Quentin, who have been HIV positive for a long time. It might refer to the distance separating persuasive prevention discourses and our more complex personal translations of them (Davis 2009). It could, too, describe the contradictions between living normalised HIV positive lives in some contexts such as the HIV clinic and support group and among like-minded friends, and lives characterised by stigmatisation, fear of stigmatisation, self-stigmatisation, silence, and isolation in families, at workplaces, and among acquaintances (Campbell et al. 2006; Flowers et al. 2006; Herek 2002). It can reference the social and health as well as economic marginalisation experienced by women such as Siyanda, described in the previous chapter, who live their three-letter lives in poverty, or the men in Zungu's (2012) research who at times actively abdicate all HIV's naturalisation processes, aside from their own, fatalistic version of normalisation. 'Being left behind' could also describe the disjunction within many of my research participants' interviews, for instance, as with Mhiki, between stories, often at the beginning of the interviews, of an accepting, proactive and 'living positively' approach to HIV, and more complex accounts, often later in the interviews, of persisting problems and uncertainties.

Such discontinuities put in question the completeness of the HIV knowledges that we most often encounter. The discontinuities also point to macrostructures of power and microstructures of emotion that can put brakes on improvements in HIV treatment, prevention and care to the levels that MDG 6 and UNAIDS's 'three zeroes' propose. These changes will not happen by ignoring the forces operating against them.

That is why this chapter focuses on these specific and persistent denaturalising issues within the pandemic.

The denaturalising issues I want to consider are first, HIV's biological mutability and the variety of its physical effects, which puts the medicalisation of the pandemic in question; second, HIV's place in low-resourced contexts where treatment access is not guaranteed and HIV itself is a significant resource, which renders the pandemic's marketisation particularly problematic; and third, difficult personal elements of living with HIV, which mean that there is often something idiosyncratic and important left out of normalised framings of the pandemic.

Not knowing about HIV

The naturalising possibility of 'knowing' about HIV is supported by powerful contemporary medical knowledge around it, and emblematised by the clusters of acronyms condensing that knowledge, most strongly by ARV or ART but also by TasP, PEP, PrEP, VTC, PMTCT, and all the abbreviations of drugs and organisations. But as we have seen, the medicalisation of the pandemic is often oversimplifying. Moreover, the nature of HIV itself makes knowledge about HIV unavoidably and continually uncertain. When you are HIV positive, the prognosis is not certain, the future effects and nature of treatments are unknown, and there is considerable unmapped individual variability in response, as well as differences between HIV strains. John's stories of his present problems with treatment and future uncertainties in his illness trajectory (Chapter 4) and Quentin's stories of his specific ARV difficulties demonstrated this provisionality in HIV knowledge for people who are living three-letter lives. Even when you receive testing, your HIV status may fall within a 'window period' that provides a false negative result; rapid testing produces false positives. If you are trying to avoid transmitting or contracting HIV, uncertainties also exist, not just at the level of social relations and emotions, but also around different physiological and genetic vulnerabilities, and the effectiveness of PEP, PrEP and TasP (see Davis 2009; Zungu 2012). The resultant states of not being sure about what will happen to you in relation to HIV denaturalise HIV knowledge.

Because HIV is unpredictable, it commits people who are infected or affected to ongoing vigilance about things they cannot fully know about, or alternatively, to a decision to abjure such vigilance and accept ignorance (Rabinow 2004). Both situations qualify the notion of a medicalised, normalised, self-monitoring and aware citizen. John, the UK interviewee quoted in Chapter 4, who was preoccupied with an HIV-related precancerous condition, was, as we saw, not just persistently vigilant but also consistently worried about this condition. He was in addition explicitly aware of medicine's prognostic limits: 'you can have {precancerous signs} for many, many years and it never progresses'. He also included the diagnostic limits for an asymptomatic condition in his story of his journey through the illness signs:

> John: [B]ut if I hadn't been on that screening programme, which I have been for the last 18 months now, they wouldn't have picked it up and I suspect probably the majority of gay men, long-term survivors, particularly with HIV, if you're not having any problems you wouldn't think there was anything wrong and there's no screening programme, I don't think.

In John's earlier interviews, similar concerns around ambiguous conditions appear, for example around lipodystrophy, in 2001. Many interviewees in both samples told stories about the difficulties of this side effect, from 1997 onward in the UK, and 2003 on in South Africa. While ARVs' side effects have lessened and lipodystrophy treatment has improved, these changes do not entirely remove the uncertainty. Long-term ARV treatment, usually at some point involving changing drug regimes, always has the potential to produce new uncertainties about side effects.

Related ambiguities arose around treatment interruption, which was a particularly intense concern for people taking ARVs in the late 1990s, when regimes were more difficult, side effects less manageable, and interruption effects little understood. Morag, for instance, a woman in the UK study who had lived with HIV for many years without severe illness, described in 2001 her early history of ARV or drug 'holidays':

> Morag: Well {in 1997} I had probably just tried one {ARV regime}, if I can remember... I think my T cells disappeared completely or went down to 40 um and I took three months off and nothing happened. It didn't make the slightest bit of difference... (my doctor) says they've actually done research in America and they've found that it's cheaper to send people on holiday for a week than it is to keep them on combination therapy {ARVs}, and the results are exactly the same... I've been taking drug holidays since I started, yeah. I mean it's not to be recommended, because I think the lower your T cells are the harder it is to come back. And maybe I should have

started this {ARVs} (earlier), but then I didn't have a choice, by the time I found out my T cells were under 200 there were 60, so I kind of missed out on that {effective and manageable ARVs, through not} taking them at 200 {T cells} which is maybe I think about the right time to take them.

Interviewer: So when you have taken {drug} holidays, has that been related to your T cells or was it just how you've felt?

Morag: No it's been related to the fact that I've felt um that the side effects didn't outweigh the advantages, I couldn't be in it any longer. Um, I don't know how you would cope with it, but diarrhoea is like, I mean I used to be in tears.

Morag's ARV story continues with a long account of the problems of diarrhoea.

This story does not entirely cut itself off from normalisation. It reaches out to the interviewer and to other potential listeners, those who are living with HIV and those who are not, by extending its pronoun address, '*your* T cells' (my emphasis), and by making a speculative parallel: 'I don't know how you would cope with it'. However, rather than resolving HIV's medical ambiguities, this inclusiveness draws those of us not living with HIV into its ambiguities, in this case, of ARVs that preserve your life while making daily life almost impossible; and perhaps, by extension, into the ambiguities around medical knowledge with which we all now live (Rabinow 2004).

The cost-benefit analyses of drug holidays Morag reported engaging in at different times in the late 1990s were multifactorial, their predicted outcomes imprecise for her and her doctors. ARVs' effects today are less debilitating, and there is more agreement on treatment interruption's disadvantages. However, people for whom ARVs are not working or are very difficult, a group that increases as ARV treatment scales up, remain involved in medically irresolvable dialogues on this issue. Moreover, as we saw in Chapter 4, the 'right' time to start ARVs remains a heavily researched and debated issue, even as it moves earlier and earlier from the 200 CD4+ T cell guideline with which Morag was operating.

The pattern of repeatedly facing new, possibly insurmountable medical conditions and treatment difficulties was, for research participants in both the United Kingdom and South Africa, a consistently denaturalising aspect of living with HIV, across historical and national differences in diagnosis and treatment, knowledge and resources. HIV is always leaving its citizens behind in this biological way, something that is less salient with less threatening and slower-moving health conditions. Perhaps, as Rabinow (2004) argues, we need to recognise these knowledge limitations as part of science, to accept the non-naturalisable aspects of the 'natural' world, in order to address them in life technologies like those around HIV citizenship and to understand such citizenships as predicated on ignorance as well as knowledge.

Knowledge about HIV is further denaturalised by the virus's positioning within broader discourses and practices of 'health'. 'Healthy living' has no agreed limits, and its content varies. The World Health Organisation's recent (2013, 2009b) guidelines for starting ARV therapy at 350 and now 500 CD4+ T cells per cubic millimetre (/mm^3) may avoid the fatalities associated with late treatment and reduce infectiveness among more people at risk of transmitting HIV. But the WHO recognises that in many countries, getting much less healthy people onto ARVs even at the 200 CD4+ T cells/mm^3 level remains problematic. Better-resourced settings, like, initially, the city of San Francisco and then, the whole of the United States, as we saw in Chapter 2, advise immediate treatment on diagnosis, regardless of CD4+ T cell levels, to maintain 'health', with transmission reduction a secondary, if welcome, possibility (Russell 2010). Work on the effects of early treatment, and on treatment as soon as possible after infection, suggests that such initiatives can preserve health and may even obviate the need for later treatment (Bacchus 2012; Kitahata et al. 2009).

'Well-being' is, like health, a slippery concept (Cameron et al. 2008; Conceicao and Bandura 2008). Encompassing definitions of wellbeing have been said to operate as divisive, consumption-driven, non-sustainable aspects of Western modernity (Carlisle and Hanlon 2008). However, it is also argued that holistic 'healthworlds' are well-established aspects of traditional health formations that need to be recognised by Western approaches to health, especially in the HIV case (Germond and Cochrane 2010). A notion of 'wellbeing' as involving, following Sen, opportunities or capabilities to pursue it, not just resources available or capacities achieved, may be useful for developing the multi-level approach the HIV pandemic requires (Barnett and Whiteside 2006; Seckinelgen 2012). At the same time, discourses of 'wellbeing' and 'healthy living' sometimes fail to address important specificities of HIV. For John, Nicco and Mhiki, and Sean and Tyler, for instance, 'health and well-being' are maintained by rigorous pharmacological and behavioural regimes whose strictures perpetually mark the possibility of their losing both. For many citizens not affected by HIV, and for some HIV positive people themselves, exemplified most dramatically by Nicholas's ARV-refusing friends, described in Chapter 6; by Quentin; and in this chapter, by

Morag, ARV regimes themselves significantly detract from health and well-being.

Being 'left behind' by the knowledges around HIV is, then, an inevitable if hard-to-tolerate feature of living with medicalisation. It is particularly likely to manifest itself in relatively new and mobile medical fields like those of HIV biotechnologies, which must, in addition, cope with the changes that HIV itself undergoes. Being left behind by 'health and well-being' happens across social as well as historical differences in the pandemic, as Yoliswa's and Nicholas's transnational concerns make explicit. However, it is important to remember that being left behind also characterises discourses and practices of 'health and well-being' generally. These categories are more fluid, over time, than their contemporary definitions might suggest; but they are also more normative than their apparently unproblematic extension to 'long-term conditions' such as HIV might indicate. This means that the difficult features of would-be healthy, happy and open lives lived with HIV and ARVs, which appeared in interviewees' discussions of unrecoverable physical health, mental health issues, criminalisation, disclosure and safe sex in relationships, remain partly but recalcitrantly outside dominant individualised technologies of health choice and responsibility.

I want to consider now another denaturalising unevenness within the pandemic which underpins many of the limitations of naturalisation already mentioned, and which might seem the clearest and the simplest to address: that of resources.

Not having resources

Where the multiple and extensive resources required for HIV's naturalisation are not available, many people, currently around 6.8 million (UNAIDS 2012a), live in the treatment possibility era, but without appropriate treatment access. Many of those living with HIV and ARVs lack cash, nutrition, transport, social support, and other resources which affect treatment viability. Such constraints also limit HIV testing. Resource shortages thus undermine naturalisation very directly by constraining HIV's medicalisation. In addition, they limit HIV's normalisation, when people living with HIV must fight for resources, often from positions of disempowerment; and HIV's marketisation, since the people, communities, and countries most affected by HIV often have few resources to participate in, let alone govern, markets.

Within the HIV pandemic, naturalisation, as social theory understands it, is a process that erases the significance of power relations.

Yet HIV's naturalisation is continually undone by material evidence of power imbalances and their deleterious effects. The most broad-based and successful HIV activism over the last decade has operated around treatment, where resource disparities are glaring. It has taken on existing power relations by campaigning for cutting-edge, 'first world' treatment for a pandemic concentrated in the developing world. In these campaigns, 'treatment' is often formulated in a way that takes account of broader power relations. Not just the medical resource gradient between countries of the north and south, explicitly used by Yoliswa to end her story of contemporary three-letter lives, but also intersectional, gendered, classed and racialised power relations within countries, and global inequities outside the health field, are part of the campaigns' analysis, as the new actions of ACT UP (described in the previous chapter) demonstrate. Treatment is framed democratically, as community-owned and organised. It is integrated with HIV education and prevention. It is allied with other campaigns around, for instance, 'human rights', poverty, xenophobia and gender-based violence (Farmer 2001; Mbali 2005; Robins 2009). However, access to ARVs is still a major demand. And as Althusser (1998) might say, the economic – in this case, the economic constraints of low- and middle-income countries – determines the determining, resource-intensive, medico-pharmacological field.

The fight for treatment is never a one-off campaign. Once ARVs are obtained, it is still necessary to campaign for frontline drugs, second- and third-line treatments, and the next generation of drugs (Médecins Sans Frontières 2009) to be made available to resource-constrained communities. UNAIDS's (2012a: 23) current 'strategic investment framework' budget demand is for an increase from $15 billion to $22.4 billion by 2015. Treatment, alongside prevention, social care for people with HIV and others affected such as HIV-affected children and other pandemic-related expenditures, if met fully, will, estimates suggest, cost up to $35 billion yearly by 2031, even assuming 50% fewer new infections (Hecht et al. 2009). Difficulties in modelling 'human capital' losses (Lamontagne et al. 2010) mean this too may be an underestimate. Recent recession-driven difficulties in maintaining treatment exemplify resource precariousness. Even in developed countries with full ARV provision, there is unevenness, particularly around less-common illnesses and new modes of diagnosis and treatment. John's evaluation of medical provision for HIV-related conditions in the small city to which he moved from London came at the end of his story of his ambiguous illness indicators which we saw in Chapter 4, and provides an example:

John: I mean it just makes me think, 'God help anybody who's being treated in the provinces' because if I had been going to {hometown hospital} for my HIV treatments, well you know they are very good at doing the bloods and giving you the medications and all that sort of thing, anything like Kaposi's Sarcoma or, um, anal neoplasia, they are not very knowledgeable, shall we say…I am sure that a lot of the people that are treated there are in the same position that I am but they don't know because there is no way they are ever going to find out until it's too late.

In the area of psychosocial services, the effects of HIV's increasing medicalisation and the financial crisis were viewed by UK participants in recent interviews as exacerbating a longer-term reduction. Nicholas, for example, whose negotiations of transnational HIV markets we heard about in the last chapter, has run a small HIV support organisation since the 1990s. He began his interview with the tale of its decline, tracing the mainstreaming of HIV within social services and the dispersal of its advocates:

Nicholas: What I feel is that HIV has gone off the agenda and not deliberate, it wasn't a deliberate {thing}, it's just that people have grown now and moved on. People who are so keen and fighting the HIV battle have gone and moved into different areas, they…are at different roles within different organisations, not that they don't have the HIV agenda in their heart but because of their roles they kind of moved on and some unfortunately stop to think about it today.…And because of the funding, the last couple of (years)…it has become much harder yeah for example {for} this organisation.

Even in some high-income countries, resource constraints are so powerful that they seem to drive epidemics. In the United States, for example, HIV among heterosexuals in poor urban areas is more than double the 1% level in pregnant women which the WHO characterises as a generalised epidemic (Denning and DiNenno 2010). However, in the global south, resource shortages are much more comprehensive and intense. In South Africa in 2012, for instance, many interviewees like Zukiswa, Benjamin and Nosizo, describing their efforts to eat well and bolster their immune systems, accompanied these stories with qualifications of their financial ability to maintain such efforts. And Mhiki's narrative of obtaining ARVs in the early 2000s needs to be situated within the longer story of the hard and contingent struggle for treatment which appears elsewhere in her interview. At this time, ARVs were not freely or widely available. Mhiki was on a hospital trial only because of an insistent clinic nurse and family members who could lend her money to get minibus taxis to the hospital. Her treatment was compromised because she was too healthy to have a disability grant but unable to get a job in a local 50%-unemployment economy. Mhiki herself summarised the positioning of HIV within scarcity economies, and the ways in which HIV organisations must fight social injustice as well as HIV and poverty:

> **Mhiki:** So, I've seen that the most pressing thing is poverty. When there is nothing for consumption in the house, no paraffin and the like, that is affecting {us}, particularly since I'm the only one who looks after children. ... I also came across the movement called {Organisation 1}. This movement helped clear my mind because, if you go there you see and hear everything. Yet at first the movement called {Organisation 2} also found me. It took me under its banner and showed me that I was not gonna die of the disease that I had. I had to make things with my own hands. {Organisation 2} showed me that this was not the end of life. It taught me how to do bangles and ribbons. The problem however is that the stuff was never bought. The government also withdrew its grant from me. {Organisation 1} also showed me that I was not gonna die soon. I had to rise, go make up my mind {to live} and then I would be fine.[1]

HIV citizenship often involves making strong connections with broader forms of health citizenship to advocate for resources. HIV's biological citizenship can thus be not just collectivised and effective in the HIV field, but integrated with politics at varying levels. For Mhiki, the analysis she presented led her to work with the activist Treatment Action Campaign (TAC), which centres on HIV but also relates to broader concerns around health, poverty, gender-based violence and xenophobia. Many of the South African interviewees involved with activism, such as Yoliswa and Mhiki, had transnational connections through the NGOs and CBOs (community-based organisations) with which they worked. HIV organisations have also increasingly made broader thematic connections that have expanded their concerns. In South Africa, the AIDS Law Project's wider reframing as Section 27, aiming to pursue the 'health for all' guarantee of this section of the South African constitution, and the development by members of TAC and other civil society organisations of the Social Justice Coalition, are clear examples. In the United Kingdom, Nicholas's organisation had responded to HIV's naturalisation in the developed world by establishing projects in his country of origin at a time of severe HIV resource constraints there, and a number of other African-origin migrant participants within the UK study were similarly transnationally involved. John's concerns about unevenness in UK HIV medical services had led to his involvement in educating doctors about the realities of illness experiences. Both the 'theoretical' and lived, 'experiential' analyses that interviewees narrated (Scott 1991) thus performed complex positionings of HIV citizens in relation to resources and power over them that went considerably beyond the resource gradients associated with HIV and ARVs. As interviewees' narratives developed through the course of the interviews, such complexities deepened.

HIV has some particular resource requirements that make its naturalisation within general community activism or mainstream politics difficult. First, the scale of resources demanded by the pandemic is enormous (Hecht et al. 2009). Second, in low-resourced contexts, HIV itself brings resources. HIV organisations and HIV positive people receive goods that other organisations and individuals do not. For instance, as Mhiki mentioned, they may gain craft skills from income generation projects. In South Africa, if their CD4+ T cell count falls below 200 cells/mm^3, or they are otherwise severely ill, they can apply for a disability grant, a grant-in-aid for home care, and housing benefit if necessary (Western Cape Government 2012). As we saw in the previous chapter, large external and, increasingly, internal resources are devoted to HIV epidemics, especially, in the contemporary context, in view of MDG 6 progress assessments. Third, even with the promise that the epidemic is reversing, these resources come more and more into question, particularly in times of fiscal crisis.

To mitigate the skewing which such resource provisions generate, policymakers often now 'mainstream' HIV within their action plans. HIV programmes in low-resourced, high-prevalence contexts may try to address the situation by focusing on health and social needs generally, as well as on people's HIV-specific requirements. Nevertheless, HIV programmes' drugs, food supplements, donated clothes and toiletries, information workshops, employability skills trainings, childcare and education are specific goods. They are commodities that the non-HIV-affected as well as the HIV-affected want, and sometimes take, use or sell. Even the social and cultural capital created by HIV services for their clients can be an object of envy for people with little family or social support. Lana (2006), for example, reported resource-constrained young South Africans saying they wanted to be like the HIV positive people they knew who helped each other in support groups and developed direction in their lives, to the extent of wanting to become HIV positive themselves. Similar HIV resource envy has been reported in other circumstances, from Cambodian people living with diabetes, for instance (Men et al. 2012).

HIV's resource skewing does not just happen in low- and middle-income countries. HIV services create resource gradients in high-income countries, too. In some of my 1990s UK interviews, for instance, HIV positive ex-drug users reported their non-HIV positive friends envying their HIV status for goods such as free meals at HIV services organisations that accompanied it. By the 2012 interviews, the social requirement to provide evidence for HIV resource claims was strong. For the first time, several new participants spontaneously offered to show me letters from their clinics to confirm their HIV status and legitimate the interview fee.

As policy imperatives within the pandemic succeed each other, they generate resource conflicts between themselves. The medicalised approaches to prevention now said to be taking financial resources from socially oriented prevention initiatives, for instance, may also be undermining the capacity building and skills transfers that such initiatives have promoted. Women's moves towards determining their sexualities and negotiating condom use, documented in popular media like *Soul City* and *Shuga,* and men's moves towards a sexual decision-making less constrained by hegemonic masculinities (Higgins et al. 2010; Robins 2009), are resources that may seem of less value in the contemporary 'HIV economy'. Contemporary moves in HIV services run the risk of 'leaving behind' people and programmes doing this kind of work.

Paying attention, not just to markets' internal failures, but to wider formations of power, shows up resource lacks and lags across the HIV pandemic. These denaturalising discontinuities cause many citizens 'living with' HIV, particularly HIV positive people, to be structurally 'left behind'. It is important to recognise these multiple, often disempowering dimensions of HIV citizenship. It is possible to address if not entirely remedy such structural disjunctures, as many HIV treatment, prevention and education and care campaigns have done and continue to do, despite economic limitations and political constraints (Campbell et al. 2009; Epstein 2006; Farmer 2001; Rachlis et al. 2012). However, some subjective denaturalising elements within the HIV pandemic are less susceptible to change. The next segment of this chapter turns to these denaturalisations of personal understanding.

Not understanding HIV

This segment considers HIV as not just biologically and economically, but also psychosocially non-naturalisable in its particularities. This non-recuperability was, again, something that emerged in John's account of his 'cancer scare'. John's story contained, interspersed with its qualified account of medicalised HIV citizenship, a description of more personal ambiguities: his long period of living healthily with HIV after diagnosis, amid the deaths of friends; and his getting screening and treatment for his precancerous condition, amid continuing fears about that condition:

> **John:** Because I'm a long-term survivor and I've outlived so many of my friends who died in the 80s and early 90s I think well I've done extremely well to get this far, so if anything happens now, you know, I've had an awful lot of borrowed time compared to a lot of people and so, um, what will be will be... I'm fortunate that it {precancerous condition}was spotted fairly early on... but if I hadn't been on that {screening programme}... {HIV treatment is going well} so really this is why this cancer scare, I suppose I call it, is, is far more frightening now than the HIV itself.

Not being able to know exactly what HIV means for you, personally, continually undermines HIV's normalisation. Such inevitable denaturalisations appeared elsewhere in John's interview too: for example in his grief when a longstanding HIV positive acquaintance died, for the loss of the history this person carried as well as the person him/herself; in the ARV side effects that he no longer minds but that he thinks mark him out, at least to many gay men, as an HIV positive person of a certain treatment generation; and in his lack of understanding of some recently diagnosed people who in the treatment possibility era feel none of the fear that he remembers at diagnosis. In these and many other ways, John describes being historically and socially marked and marked out as an HIV citizen, shadowed by the epidemic's particularity. Although he is HIV positive, unlike those 'left behind' in the Bourland song described at the beginning of the chapter, he is, like them, often alone, intimately connected to death as well as to life, called on by 'shadows of former selves' (Bourland 2006). Quentin's narrative of his difficult social experiences, at the beginning of Chapter 2, and those of other UK interviewees for whom disclosure was difficult or impossible, mark in addition how HIV citizens are left behind or cast aside by HIV's continuing, isolating stigmatisation. Siyanda's sadness in the face of her triple jeopardy, as someone HIV positive, poor, and a mother who cannot care properly for her sick child, registers the psychic, 'left-behind' effects of resource shortages within the pandemic.

Such marks of personal, historical and social particularity qualify broader notions of health and biological citizenship, as well as more specific framings of HIV citizenship. First, they register the expressible limits of citizenly understandings, a qualification that also characterises Mouffe's (2006) understanding of citizens' identities. John's, Quentin's and Siyanda's stories of HIV citizenship are all necessarily and importantly incomplete, in ways that constantly induce us, as well as them, to question and try to extend our understandings of the pandemic.

Second, and more specifically, such stories fold an inescapable past into the present, as the song 'Left Behind' indicates: the former selves with whom the protagonist lives continually 'beckon and call' to him. For Morag, for example, who in 2001 had recently lost several people close to her for whom ARVs did not work, her own longevity and relatively successful ARV treatment naturalised her as a healthy, productive citizen, who could often forget about HIV. However, it also isolated her in a position which only she could, albeit imperfectly, grasp:

> **Morag:** It doesn't get any easier. In fact it gets a lot more difficult in a lot of ways. Um it was easy earlier on, because the support was there. But the longer I've been around it's um. You know who's going to support me? There is no one who's been diagnosed longer than me really.

Third, and relatedly, grief and loss are powerful elements in many HIV narratives, undoing normalisation (Long 2009). In the 2001 South African interviews, people talked repeatedly, with difficulty, about their dead partners, siblings and children. These are losses that few HIV programmes and indeed few people living in the middle of a generalised epidemic are able to address comprehensively. Busisiwe, for example, a young, recently diagnosed South African woman, told of her discovery of her HIV status just before the death of her child, in a story exemplifying the disjunctions produced by loss:

> **Busisiwe:** I was pregnant. I went to {hospital} and the baby came out when the child was four months old and s/he was as small as this radio {voice recorder}. I discovered that I was HIV positive.

I accepted it in that way. I realised that I had to accept it since I had seen both the tummy and the baby and there is nothing I can dispute.

Interviewer: Was the child alive?

Busisiwe: Yes, I was also having dreams at night and when I was dreaming, I saw people showing me (lifts her beads, those of a trainee sangoma, a traditional healer, into the shape of an AIDS ribbon) 'it's okay'.[2]

Here, Busisiwe linked her own enlightenment about HIV, which happened when she was tested during pregnancy and then had a still-born child, to her ancestors, the 'people' who reassured her about the condition in a dream. Dreams are a common way to communicate with ancestors for some South Africans, particularly for those who, like Busisiwe, are training or being 'treated' in order to be traditional healers, or sangomas. This is, therefore, a story about both personal grief and religious faith. In this story and thereafter, Busisiwe presented herself, not just as a moral HIV citizen, but also as someone called on, by her ancestors, and also by Christianity, to testify about, educate, and even to try to cure the condition, on behalf of herself and others.

It was more difficult, however, to understand Busisiwe's ambiguous talk about the child who died. Her comparison of the baby to the mechanical object on the table, the voice recorder, was distinct from the interactive pattern of the rest of the interview (see also Squire 2007). It took the baby out of a story of the past and brought her into the present. At one moment, as the interviewer's intervention suggests, Busisiwe even seemed to be saying that the child was born alive. The narrative kept the child in the world, as did Busisiwe's subsequent invocation of her ancestors, with whom the child was trans-historically linked, in the story, so that they could care for her.[3] A kind of benign haunting thus took over Busisiwe's HIV story, reconnecting her with the child her story brought into the room. The comparative connection Busisiwe made between the baby that died and the new technological object, the 'radio', also moved the story and Busisiwe herself, who was keen to talk about HIV, even to talk to the media, towards the future. However, her melancholy connectedness was not to be undone by such moves or by improvements in health or passing time.

The haunting element of living within HIV epidemics is perhaps an inevitable disruptive subtext of any apparently normalised HIV state. For many naturalised HIV citizens, who understand and manage the condition medically and socially, and consume appropriate products, information, attitudes and feelings, are themselves consumed, by an illness with strong resonances with an earlier tubercular meaning of 'consumption' (Sontag 1988) and linguistically marked, pre-ARVs, by names such as 'slim' that described its wasting effects. Many are also to some extent consumed by 'unproductive', unending grief. Stuart Marshall (in Bad Object Choices 1991) noted in the late 1980s, when qualifying ACT UP's appropriation of the phrase 'don't mourn, organise', that in the context of the deaths of many people to whom you are close, mourning is inevitable and ignoring it can generate paralysis. People who live with HIV, particularly in high-prevalence circumstances and over a long time, are living, in Odets's (1995) resonant phrase describing HIV survivors, 'in the shadow of the epidemic'. They cannot avoid it, and they find many different ways to address it, sometimes, like Busisiwe, indirectly. The treatment possibility era cannot naturalise the disjunctions of grief that it leaves behind.

The anchoring object in Busisiwe's story also broke up the story in an unresolvable way. We all looked at the 'radio' when Busisiwe named it. As a clearly new object from the developed world, it was unique in the room. It seemed nothing like a baby; but perhaps an HIV positive baby like Busisiwe's is also something that arrives from outside or the future, something new, strange and unfamiliar, even un-familial. At this moment, the story seemed to be generating the 'autoimmune' undecidabilities about selfhood and relations that Derrida (2002) has described as a psychosocial correlate of biological autoimmunity. In both cases, he points out that autoimmunity is a liminal condition. It is not just self-destruction, but life lived on the borders of survival (Bhabha 2011), moving forward and back. The mournful lyrics of 'Left Behind' were performed to the back-and-forth music and dance of a country two-step, relational and jaunty, that did not just make mourning bearable but that insisted on the possibility of pleasure alongside it. Bourland (2006) wrote of it, 'There is a "you-had-to-be-there" factor in this movement. The greatest impact this song had was in context of the rest of the 7-movement work. Excerpting it...diminishes that effect greatly'. Within the 'Hidden Legacies' cycle, it lies in the midst of angrier, more desperate, and also more hopeful songs.

This psychic experiencing of HIV citizenship as 'left behind', traversed by 'autoimmune' undecidabilities, appears across UK and South African research participants' interviews, at all dates. Busisiwe's narrated imagining of her baby, still with her, moving her towards the future yet still-born and strange, emblematises such experience. So do the successive narratives of HIV told by Michael, another South African interviewee. In

2001, Michael qualified the attack from within of his internal, unbidden guest by welcoming the virus as something to be lived with: 'I talk to it, psychological'. By 2004, this ambiguity had shifted. With a long and more or less stable cohabitation with HIV guaranteed by ARVs, Michael narrated the virus as a guest of whose habits he was literally, weary. His health was good, but he was always tired, a common aspect of the health of people living with HIV and ARVs. In the United Kingdom, a number of the research participants described present or past ambivalence about safer sex in the context of partners and friends already living with HIV. As one woman, Carol, said in 2001, for example, of her relationship with a very ill HIV positive man who had recently died, 'sometimes you just want it'. Carol's HIV positive status also kept her lover close to her; she narrated the parallels between his and her own illness progression, for instance. Christian, speaking of his relationship with his HIV positive wife in 2012, described himself with deliberate doubt as HIV negative last time he tested, within a story of his wife's well-treated low levels of HIV, their intermittent use of condoms, and consistent references by both of them to 'our condition'. Such stories, in which safer sex may deny people desire and through it life, or in which safer sex, and even sero-negativity, may distance you from people you love, also perform an 'autoimmune' psychic precarity.

Of course, such ambivalences must also always be read within a context of ambiguous or inadequate knowledge, perceived or experienced stigma, and unavailable or uncertain resources. Certainly, all these factors may have impinged on Carol's, Christian's, Michael's and Busisiwe's precarious positioning. However, it remains important to address these ambivalences as they affect the subjectivities. Such doubled readings will appear throughout the next chapter, in which I examine the particular characteristics of naturalisation and its undoing within the contemporary UK epidemic, drawing more extensively on the latest UK interviews in my HIV support study.

Conclusion

Being left behind is an inescapable aspect of the HIV pandemic, and perhaps of any health condition that distances the subject from much of the social world, especially if the condition is highly stigmatised. Considerable, important work is devoted to remediating the state of HIV citizens by medical treatment, by social inclusion programmes, and by campaigns negotiating associations between HIV positive people, and across people of different HIV statuses. But it is valuable at the same time to bear in mind the particularities that resist such improvements, inclusions and associations.

Throughout Section 2, I have argued that the ambiguities of a 'naturalised' HIV pandemic need to be acknowledged if the difficulties of that pandemic are to be addressed effectively. Such acknowledgement involves attending to the contradictions within naturalising processes such as medicalisation, normalisation and marketisation, and to the persistent denaturalisations generated by HIV itself in relation to its uncertain biological characteristics, its demanding resource implications, and its psychosocial difficulties, all of which can 'leave behind' HIV citizens.

Naturalisation is, I think, a useful concept for analysing the complexities of HIV citizenship and perhaps of other health citizenships, partly because of its progressive aspects, partly because of the denaturalising ambivalences it carries within its own meanings. In everyday speech, 'naturalised' citizens are not just unmarked citizens; they still bear the traces of the naturalising process, as do HIV citizens. In social theory, 'naturalisation' references ignored power relations, but also the possibility of understanding those relations. Such understanding is crucial for addressing the HIV pandemic. Again, in epistemological accounts, 'naturalised' routes to knowledge are messy and multiple, and such accounts of incomplete, revisable knowledges are important for addressing HIV.

The naturalising process of medicalisation appears, within the studies considered here, to allow HIV citizens to live and to be part of a wider biological citizenship. However, it also constrains them within often imperfect, sometimes coercive medical technologies. Normalisation makes HIV into just one aspect of citizenly existence; but the pandemic's complexities cannot all be normalised. Marketisation integrates HIV citizens into transnational consumption economies, with some gains in citizenly power; but this integration is unstable, and reduces citizenship to the economic.

HIV citizenship operates in a very particular context, characterised by the virus's fatality, medical intractability, social stigmatisation and emotional embeddedness. Nevertheless, the ambiguous processes of naturalised citizenship described here may apply to some extent to other less-stigmatised, less dangerous, but still health-threatening and high-prevalence conditions – for instance, in high- and medium-income countries, cancer, diabetes, heart disease, hypertension and obesity; in medium- and low-income countries, also, malaria and TB.

This section has also argued that denaturalisations of HIV citizenship arise, not just from the instabilities of medicalisation, normalisation and marketisation, but in addition, and to some degree independently, from the epistemological intractability of HIV as a biological condition, the enormous resource demands of the HIV pandemic, and the failures of understanding attached to HIV's troubling histories and emotions. Again, these processes depend partly on the specificities of the pandemic, that is, HIV's biological characteristics, its immense social, political and economic as well as medical impact in high-prevalence situations, and the psychic effects of its fatality, unpredictability and abjectification. However, these denaturalising discontinuities may still exhibit some parallels with processes operating around other medical conditions, such as those mentioned earlier.

Section 2 has suggested that naturalisations and denaturalisations appear often, and with useful complexity and depth, in people's HIV stories. The narrative data reported here are limited in extent, and in the epidemics from which they are drawn. HIV narratives gathered at other times and places in those epidemics, or within other epidemics in the global south or north, might diverge from the ones analysed in this chapter. Nevertheless, the patterns of naturalisation and denaturalisation in these data are often strongly evident, and are multiply interlinked, to an extent that may be less true in other forms of HIV representation. Indeed, naturalisation and its ambiguities, and the denaturalising processes of 'being left behind', are elements of HIV lives that policy and political formulations of HIV citizenship may gloss over, in order to generate useful collectivities and coalitions, to operate in the present and future rather than the past, and to act unambiguously. It is, though, important to recognise and work with the difficulties of naturalisation and denaturalisation processes, perhaps more than the onrush of contemporary priorities generally allows. They act as forms of knowledge about what is left out of HIV discourses and practices. And they mark the multiplicity and complexity of HIV experiences (Scott 1991), especially those elements that have not been acknowledged or that are just coming into existence.

Section 3

Living on and Living with HIV and ARVs: The Particularities of Epidemics

8
Living on: Three-letter Lives in the United Kingdom

The Government should recognise the scale of the HIV and AIDS challenge in the United Kingdom. Not enough is being done to respond to a steadily growing risk to public health. There are potentially huge cost implications in both the short- and long-term in failing to deal effectively with the epidemic. At a time when public health in the United Kingdom is subject to major reform, the Government should ensure that HIV and AIDS is a key public health priority.

(House of Lords 2011)

This year we're asking you join us in Standing Up and Standing Out for the 100,000 people living with HIV in this country right now and telling the world that people with HIV need support, not judgement. Thirty years ago Terry Higgins lost his life to HIV. Since then Terrence Higgins Trust has helped thousands of people living with HIV and hundreds of thousands at risk of sexual ill health. A lot has changed in 30 years, but the fight against stigma has never been tougher. Our centres all over the country still routinely come into contact with discrimination, disownment and prejudice. This isn't acceptable, and that's why this 1 December we're asking you to do whatever it takes to raise vital funds and awareness. Together let's send HIV stigma back to the '80s.

(Terrence Higgins Trust World AIDS Day page 2012)

Olive: But with me now, I feel like I'm empowered now. I always do counselling on my own yes, especially with other newly diagnosed, yeah, helping them.

Interviewer: Oh really, so how do you do that, with a group or –

Olive: No, it's individually yeah, because sometimes we have got a lot of friends, so sometimes you hear so and so is really down, she can't cope, she's got problems, yeah. So, we try to contact her, if she wants to come in and talk to us, then we will go and have a friendly talk with her, then he or she can ask questions, so. 'Are you really', because some of them they ask 'are you really positive?' I tell them 'yeah, we've been there before', and we tell, we share our own experiences, yeah. That is how it helps, it helps because it's a long journey from that moment when you used to cry, and now accepted it as normal life, yeah... some have got relatives who are dying, children who are dying, they can't go home, they are still grieving here. They are dealing with people's issues, it is difficult, it is difficult. I can put myself in that position. I've got a friend who is dealing with that same issue. She went through, she is going through a lot, she is now depressed, yeah. Sometimes I will go their house, sleep over, two days or three days, yeah. I will sleep over then I will invite her, I have told her 'you are welcome to my house, come anytime, if I am not there then my children are there.' Because, sometimes I got my grandchildren, 'feel free, don't be on your own' yeah 'come I will cook for you – if you want to cook anything, sleep on my bed' (laughs) yeah, because I know what she is going through, unfortunately, it's difficult.

(UK interview 2011)

Introduction

In 2011 I re-interviewed Daniel, a white British man in his 50s who in 2001 had just been coming to terms with his new HIV diagnosis. Ten years on, Daniel was doing well medically. His viral load was low and his CD4+ T cells were looking good. He had supportive family members and friends, though many friends from his youth had died. However, he did not feel well, and he had ongoing health problems related to his long-term HIV illness and ARV use. His family was far away; his remaining friends were working and many were too young to understand the life he had lived. He had retired early, when his health was poor, from a job he found tedious. Now, every day, he had to work out what to do with his life, on a small income. He had found new things that absorbed him, but he described often feeling very alone. Several of the HIV-related drop-ins he used to attend had closed. He decided to come to my university for the interview, largely because this was a different experience for him, and it would occupy his day; not much else was going on that week, for him.

Round about the same time I went, with students taking my 'HIV in the world' module, to an event for World AIDS Day at a sixth-form college where students come largely from South Asian backgrounds. We put up a display about HIV in South Africa and some postcards the students had made, which we were going to sell to raise some money for a South African women's HIV group. We were in a hall ringed with stalls dealing with sexual health issues, crammed with students taking time off from lessons. Terrence Higgins Trust, the oldest HIV organisation in the United Kingdom, was running the neighbouring stall. We were surprised by the students' engagement. Some were just hanging out with their friends; many others, especially young women, were making a serious tour of the stalls. They were picking up all the leaflets and generous supplies of condoms. A group of young Muslim women, wearing hijabs, spent a lot of time at the stalls. One of them told us, laughing, that none of them would have sex before marriage. Nevertheless, they took samples of everything.

This chapter explores contemporary lives lived with HIV and ARVs in a high-income, well-resourced country, the United Kingdom, which has low HIV prevalence and universal ARV treatment access. It examines the conjunction of the United Kingdom's relatively successful medical and policy addresses to HIV, and its continuing difficulties with the condition, as they are intricately expressed in research participants' stories, told during interviews in 2010 and 2011. It develops the analysis presented in the previous book section, of HIV's medicalisation, normalisation and naturalisation, and of the condition of being 'left behind', to pay attention to the particularities of these processes in the contemporary UK epidemic.

Both this chapter and the succeeding chapter in Section 3, which addresses the South African epidemic, draw, more heavily than previous chapters, on personal narratives from my interviews with people living with HIV, about the kinds of support that they use and want. These extended and fine-grained narrative accounts work well for exploring the commonalities and particularities of HIV's naturalisation in and across national contexts. They, more than the generalised and smoothed-out narratives that appear within media texts and policy documents, progress through complexities, contradictions, and new, exceptional aspects of HIV experience.

The current HIV situation in the United Kingdom[1] is complicated. It is characterised by low prevalence but stable levels of new cases; high levels of cases among men who have sex with men (MSM) and people of African origin; and high levels of late diagnoses, which have less good prognoses. The epidemic is generally not as visible as in higher-prevalence countries, despite some recent governmental and local policy initiatives aimed at renewing prevention efforts. Knowledge of HIV transmission prevention is relatively good, condom use relatively low, including in population groups where prevalence is higher. Medical and social services are in the midst of fiscal crisis and its political and policy fallout (House of Lords 2011).

As the quote from the House of Lords report that opens this chapter suggests, the rising number of people thought to be living with HIV, especially those untested, untreated and most likely to be transmitting HIV themselves, are, in the TasP (treatment- as-prevention) era, a particular focus of policy and popular concern. The report also suggests that HIV prevention education needs further campaigns, something that so far seems to have been subordinate to the push simply to increase testing. Perhaps, as suggested by our experiences with sixth formers who say HIV is nothing to do with them but who are nevertheless prepared to engage with it, there is more openness to such initiatives than is often assumed.

The House of Lords report says relatively little about people living with HIV themselves except as infection vectors, particularly if they do not know their status; as stigmatised and discriminated against; and, in an important but short section, as needing and themselves providing peer support. Although the report acknowledges considerable input from organisations of and for HIV positive people, its imagined audience seems mostly to be an undifferentiated HIV negative public, the at-risk public of 'public health'. On the other hand, the THT's (Terrence Higgins Trust's) emphasis for World AIDS Day 2012 on the third of UNAIDS' 'zeroes', that is, less stigma and discrimination and more openness, tries to build commonality between people of different statuses. By implication, stigma reduction among non-HIV positive people will also have good effects on the testing and treatment agenda for people who are HIV positive. Nevertheless, THT is still asking its readers to stand up for 'people living with HIV', a request that makes it sound as if all those readers are negative. Such orientations towards an assumed HIV negative public who must be kept that way ignore the fact that HIV positive people are already the most involved and effective preventers of HIV transmission themselves and treat HIV as something that, despite all the talk about its liveability, cannot be included within everyday citizenship. Assumptions like these were something that interviewees in my study, like many others, often remarked on in HIV education materials. Neither of these public accounts is able fully to address some of the important, continuing and specific difficulties of living with HIV and ARVs in the United Kingdom that Olive's and Daniel's stories exemplify. HIV positive asylum seekers must frequently, as in Olive's account, live on the borders between their own health and illness, and those of others close to them, as well as between citizenship and illegality, social inclusion and exclusion, optimism, guilt and loss. Many times, as in Olive's case, they have come from high-prevalence situations with little treatment access where HIV remained a death sentence well into the first decade of the twenty-first century. People who have lived three-letter lives for a long time often describe feeling pushed 'to the side of their own lives' (Larkin 1964), like Daniel in his long story of a life lived alongside or, as discussed in the last chapter, 'left behind' the life he expected to have.

When I was interviewing the research participants for this round of my UK research, they talked often and extensively about the recession and social welfare cuts. Indeed, I sometimes got the impression that I was researching people's responses to the global economic crisis, as much as their strategies for living with HIV and ARVs. The chapter delineates research participants' frequently resistant and in some cases explicitly oppositional positioning as HIV citizens, within a situation which is often described as one of intensifying 'neo-liberalism', that is, of growing economic, political and policy orientations towards free market solutions. However, to describe participants' accounts only as responses to neo-liberalism would be an over simple, reductive interpretation. I try here to give a more specific analysis of people's accounts of how living with HIV and ARVs intersects with austerity living or 'living with the cuts', and living within 'neo-liberal' economies more generally.

The previous chapter explored being 'left behind' as an integral aspect of living with HIV and ARVs, experienced alongside HIV's naturalisation, constituting three-letter lives as perpetual efforts at survival. This chapter examines more specifically how people now living with HIV in the UK narrate 'living on', the literal meaning, in French, of surviving or '*survivre*' (Derrida 1979), which in French also has the sense of living precariously on something, rather than just living on through time. How do people living with HIV and ARVs in the UK survive liminally, on borderlines, as we saw them doing in the previous chapter, especially on the borderline of health and illness? How do they do this in a situation where such survival is often medically, socially, economically and emotionally fraught?

To explore these narrative positionings, the chapter explores how the stories in the UK study engaged in specific ways with medicalisation, normalisation and marketisation and their contradictions, as well as with the difficulties of knowledge, resources and understanding that also characterise HIV epidemics. First, however, the chapter provides a brief outline of aspects of the UK epidemic relevant to the research and of the research process itself.

HIV in the United Kingdom

The HIV situation in the UK is, as mentioned, not simple. Around 96,000 people were thought to be living with HIV in the UK at the end of 2011 (UNAIDS 2012a). The year 2011 saw 6,280 new diagnoses, a number that is close to incidence over the past decade, despite targeted prevention initiatives aimed at people seen as at highest risk. A declining but still-high number of diagnoses, 47% in 2011, were made late, when people were already ill and likely to do less well with ARVs. Deaths among people who are HIV positive remain around 500 a year, with increasing numbers (now 46%) among those over 50. Most HIV tests are in antenatal and STI settings. Coverage in those locations is 97% and 70% respectively. Policymakers are urging improvement, 'so that no-one leaves the (STI) clinic without knowing their HIV status' (Health Protection Agency 2011a: 5; see also 2011b). Since about 24% of people living with HIV do not know their status, testing is clearly needed in new situations. Testing initiatives have been widened to cover GP surgeries and general hospital admissions in high-prevalence areas, as well as to provide increased emphasis on African communities and MSM. These initiatives aim to bring people who are positive but who do not know their status into contact with HIV services quickly. At the same time, HIV organisations have combined to issue positive though still cautious advice on TasP (British HIV Association and Expert Advisory Group on AIDS 2013; see also Lancet 2011).

As mentioned in previous chapters, treatment in the United Kingdom is said to have 'transformed HIV infection from a fatal illness to a chronic manageable condition'. The HPA says that 'people diagnosed with HIV can expect a near-normal life expectancy, particularly if diagnosed promptly' (Health Protection Agency 2011a: 6, 4). ARVs are universally accessible. In 2011, 84% of people receiving care were on ARVs and 87% of people receiving care were virally suppressed. These figures are relatively good among high-income countries, much better, for instance, than those in the United States. The numbers will rise as people continue to survive and as a result of people moving onto treatment earlier, as World Health Organisation (2013) guidelines advise. However, some patients are not as stable on medication as might be predicted (Thomson et al. 2013). HIV clinicians are also being enjoined to work with those whose low CD4+ T cell counts are below 350, with those not receiving ARVs, and with patients 'lost to care', who tend to have higher viral load and infection potential (Krentz and Gill 2013).

Internationally, only 57% of pregnant women who are HIV positive receive treatment (World Health Organisation 2012). In the UK epidemic, as in most other high-income countries, the situation is much better. A full 99% of diagnosed women's babies are negative. This represents a very good level of treatment to prevent 'vertical' transmission, though many children who became HIV positive perinatally before such treatment was available are now living with the condition as young adults.

In a number of places in the world, particularly in Eastern Europe, the Russian Federation, and Asia, still-increasing incidences of HIV are being driven by intravenous drug use. The United Kingdom's prevalence is 1.5 per thousand, that is, 0.15%, similar to the rest of Western and Northern Europe, less than Eastern and Southern Europe where HIV epidemics are bigger, mainly because of larger numbers of non-safely injecting drug users. Only 2,300 people are thought to have become HIV positive through intravenous drug use in the United Kingdom; for drug users, harm reduction programmes have been generally effective though transmission continues, at a low level.

Despite repeated attempts to address gay men's high incidence of HIV, gay men remain a group who are disproportionately affected in many HIV epidemics. Within the UK epidemic, around 40,100 of the people living with HIV in the UK are thought to be men who have sex with men (MSM). Among gay men in the United Kingdom, HIV prevalence is around 1 in 20, and 1 in 12 in London. There is high and increasing incidence among 15–44 year old MSM. 3010 new cases were reported in 2011, the highest number ever. Gay men are less likely than other groups to be late-diagnosed. However, their drug resistance is higher, overall. This may partly be because many gay men diagnosed in earlier years – men like John, whose story we read in Chapter 4, or Daniel, whose current situation I described at the beginning of this chapter – were pre-treated with drugs that did not work but that conferred resistance on these or related substances now used in combination therapy.

In the 1990s and the following decade, increasing migration of people from high-HIV-prevalence sub-Saharan African countries to Europe, often to countries that had previously colonised them, radically changed the epidemic in those countries. However, among the 2990 women and men whose HIV infection, diagnosed in 2011, was probably acquired heterosexually, though, over half became HIV positive in the United Kingdom. This number is going up, while diagnoses of people who became HIV positive outside the United Kingdom are going down. Nevertheless, of the 51,500 heterosexuals living with HIV in the United Kingdom, 30,600 were born in African countries. Of that number, two-thirds are women. Thus the epidemic among women of African origin in the United Kingdom is highly feminised. Black African men are particularly likely to be in the late-diagnosed group, and patients lost to follow-up are especially likely to be female, young, black African, not on ARVs, recently diagnosed and infected outside UK. There have been small increases in prevalence among UK-born women.

As people living with HIV survive longer, the percentage of people over 50 living with HIV has risen. This 'greying' of the epidemic is seen in other high-income countries that rolled out treatment in the late 1990s, and it is something that is starting to affect countries with later ARV rollout such as South Africa, too. People over 50 are also particularly likely to be late-diagnosed, and 46% of deaths now occur within that age group. HIV is also sometimes said to be associated with faster ageing. Living long-term with the virus, its associated illnesses, the treatments and their side effects, all have negative effects on age-related conditions such as hypertension and cholesterol, stroke, cognitive impairment, kidney disease, bone disease, and diabetes (Health Protection Agency 2012; Madge et al. 2011; UNAIDS 2011b).

Many people living long-term with HIV and ARVs are also living with what the United Kingdom's National AIDS Trust (2011b) has called 'fluctuating symptoms'. People with good levels of CD4+ T cells and undetectable viral load may still be dealing with ongoing symptoms and side effects, such as fatigue, headaches, nausea, skin conditions and neuropathy, or with the legacy of earlier illnesses and side effects, as well as with continuing mental health issues. This description applied to some people in the study who were doing well on their medications and to some who were relatively recently diagnosed, such as Sean and Tyler, as well as to those from earlier 'treatment generations' like John and Daniel, or to those who, like Olive, had gone through serious illness before getting treatment. A frequent interviewee story was of the unpredictability of physical and mental health associated with living with HIV and ARVs.

The UK HIV support study

In order to explore these patterns of difficulty within the UK epidemic, I wanted both to re-interview people who were part of previous study rounds and to bring more participants into the study. I had a number of interests in doing this. First, increasing numbers of people in the United Kingdom, as in other national contexts, are living long-term with HIV and are contemplating such long-term survival at diagnosis. In the United Kingdom, the number of people for whom this happens is rising. The amount of people diagnosed yearly is now around double that in the previous peak years, the 1990s. Large numbers of people who are HIV positive are still not diagnosed, despite extensive testing initiatives. I wanted to explore the complexities of this experience with the increasing numbers of people who will be living for a long time with HIV in the UK.

Second, long-running attempts to mainstream and at the same time reduce psychosocial and, to a lesser extent, medical HIV services have intensified since the 2008 financial crisis. These attempts are likely to have greater impact as social welfare restructuring and cuts bite deeper. Major reorganisation of health care started in the first decade of the twenty-first century. As in many other high- and middle-income countries with public health systems, the United Kingdom's National Health Service (NHS) is being reoriented, even more than in its 1980s and 1990s reorganisations, towards external as well as internal markets (Lister 2013). The 'neo-liberal' restructuring of the welfare state towards the voluntarism of Prime Minister David Cameron's 'Big Society' means that people living with HIV, who have been able to claim Disability Living Allowance if appropriate, are all now having their disability status reassessed for a new allowance, the Personal Independence Payment. If they are thought able to work, they will be asked to search for full-time employment in a now relatively high-unemployment economy. These moves have caused widespread protest and concern within health and social services, in NGOs, and among patients and claimants, including people living with HIV. Without focusing explicitly on this issue, the study registered its current salience.

Third, pilot work for this fifth round of interviews suggested moves away from the narratives of entitlement that appeared frequently in my UK research participants' accounts of living with HIV and ARVs (Squire 2006), towards a much more economistic emphasis on what can be afforded nationally and internationally, and towards personal rather than collective responsibility for HIV citizenships. These moves suggested that citizens living with HIV were adopting some very particular narrative strategies in the current UK context, which merited investigation.

Fourth, in this pilot work, as well as in the field of cultural representations, the epidemic appeared to have little current visibility within the United Kingdom. This low visibility seemed to underline HIV's contemporary double presence in the country, either as a high-profile condition afflicting faraway poor countries and migrant communities secreted within rich countries such as the United Kingdom itself, or as a treated, liveable, unmarked condition among high-income countries' own citizens (Patton 1991; Squire 2007).

Lastly, when addressing the most recent interview materials, I wanted to determine how and to what extent the current narrative patterns of naturalisation and denaturalisation (Squire 2010) that I traced in both UK and South African data in Section 2, could be given a more specific and contextually embedded articulation in the UK context, given my contemporary concern with the particularities rather than the exceptionalities of HIV epidemics.

The study was the most recent of five interview rounds in my research on HIV support in the United Kingdom. It involved 47 semi-structured interviews with people living with HIV, covering topics of medical, social, family, friendship, work, online and other media, and faith support, as well as self-support, each lasting generally between one and two hours. None of these categories were asked about specifically, unless they had not been covered by the end of the interview. Even then, they were not all always asked about, since I stopped interviews after around two hours. This was so that some interviews did not become life story interviews, for which consent had not been obtained, and also because, however enthusiastic, participants often got tired. Indeed, some interviewees had considerably shorter interviews for this reason.

Fifteen interviewees had taken part in earlier interviews, some starting in 1993.[2] Other interviewees from these rounds have in some cases died, many are untraceable, and a couple do not want to continue participating in HIV-related research. New participants were recruited through HIV-related community organisations in and outside London, announcements in a national HIV-related online publication and chain referral.

The interviews did not ask participants to tell stories. They were designed not to entrain people into personal specificity of any kind. Rather, they elicited participants' own accounts of support, as the interview announcement said. However, it was expected from previous interview rounds, as indeed transpired here, that many of those accounts would have a narrative form (Squire 2013).

About a quarter of the interviewees were from outside London. Participants included 14 women, one of whom was bisexual, one lesbian and 11 heterosexual. Four women interviewees were white European, and 10 were black African/Caribbean. Of the 33 male participants, there were eight men of African or African Caribbean origin. Three white British heterosexual men were in the group. The 26 gay and bisexual men in the group were of varying ethnicities and nationalities including Asian, African, African Caribbean, South American and other European.

Re-interviewing 15 people after ten years meant that the study was skewed towards older people living with HIV. Indeed, over 50s comprised about a third of participants; more were in their late 40s and a group of others were in their early 30s. The youngest interviewee, 22, became HIV positive at 16. Other research participants had also been diagnosed or become positive in their teens or earlier. Years of diagnosis ranged from 1986 to 2011; no participants were diagnosed more recently than six months.

Almost all participants (except for three) were taking ARVs. Those not doing so saw ARVs as a definite part of their future; in this sense, they were already living three-letter lives. This was a new characteristic compared to 2001 when guidelines for taking treatment were set at a lower level, treatment was more difficult, and people were less likely to be encouraged to take it, or to report, as they now do, the benefits of starting early. In addition, many new participants had been diagnosed when ill and had had to start ARVs immediately.

A large number of new participants who were on ARVs were doing well and said they had little contact with HIV services. In some cases they were told about the research by friends, but more often they were fairly regularly looking at HIV websites and magazines and saw announcements about the research there, indicating a quite high and continuing level of engagement with HIV information. All interviewees were paid a fee equivalent to an hour's research assistant wage at the University of East London, a sum that in a highly polarised economy has multiple meanings. For participants on benefits, and those who were asylum seekers, receiving vouchers, the cash payment was far more significant than for participants in paid work of any kind, a number of whom donated their payments to HIV organisations with whom they worked or which had helped them.

The interviews focused on how people living with HIV in the United Kingdom perceive the support they get for living with the virus, what works for them, what does not, and what forms of support they might like that they do not get. These results were fed back to HIV service organisations. Because the interviews were semi-structured, people talked openly and largely on self-determined topics, and so the material also provides a broader picture of how the epidemic is lived within the United Kingdom.

As the interviews are open enough for people to talk at length, continuously, about themselves, they include many narratives, which are the focus of this chapter's analyses. For attending to narratives' extended and mobile representations allows for some understanding of how people articulate complex technologies of medicalisation, normalisation and marketisation in the specific UK context.

HIV and living with the cuts

The interview material from this study provided many instances from almost every participant of the processes described in the previous book section: of narratives of naturalisation via medicalisation, normalisation, and marketisation, and of denaturalising narratives that countered or were 'left behind' by these forms. At the same time, the material displayed a number of specificities tied to the current UK epidemic. There were highly technical medicalisation narratives that were at the same time counteracted by participants' 'holistic' narratives of themselves as people, not patients, however 'expert'. There were narratives of normalisation alongside a 'responsibilisation' that could be constraining but also enabling. And there were narratives about the powers of markets within three-letter lives that were powerfully tied to medicalisation, creating an excluded class of the ill and poor, but that were also counteracted by participants' own subversions or reinventions of markets.

There were, then, considerable subtle and explicit counteracting narratives to what seemed to be the dominant narratives of HIV in the United Kingdom. However, many stories in the interviews qualified or ruled out action or activism, through their extensive accounts of what is often called the neo-liberal restructuring of health and welfare services, of recession and cuts, and of the reframing of the Disability Living Allowance. The uncertainties of HIV knowledge, resources for living and understanding, which I described in Chapter 7, also operated in people's stories to foreground the ongoing difficulties of stories about 'living on' with HIV.

These uncertainties and qualifications indicated a move away from the numerous narratives of entitlement that appeared in earlier rounds of this study (Squire 2006). In addressing interviews done in 2001, I analysed ways in which research participants articulated a shifting set of entitlements to services, knowledge, and care, in the quite difficult situation of treatment drugs that worked much less well than those now used. However, to focus on entitlement stories in these recent interviews, though they do appear occasionally in the material, would be to ignore the large majority of the interview material. This material can be read as counteracting dominant narratives in various ways, but it says little about entitlement.

Ten years thus seem to have changed the cultural narrative currency for participants. Narratives have moved, in the current political and policy climate, towards preoccupations with rationing and responsibility. Counteracting narratives focus on particularity and personhood, small-scale collectivities, and sometimes, a strategic social, rather than political, articulation of voices of people living with HIV. The story with which this chapter starts, from Olive, is atypical of the interviews in its explicit talk of empowerment and its account of how Olive enacts it. That story does, however, exemplify the narratives of local, socially embedded actions and activism within the current restricting contexts of the UK epidemic which appear frequently in the interview material and which are not simply either an enactment of market thinking, or a rejection of it.

The neo-liberal, exceptionality and borderlines

Contemporary health and social policy in the UK, as well as the interviews' extensive material on the cuts, might suggest that experiences of the UK HIV epidemic are today largely determined by contemporary neo-liberal discourses and practices. However, as the above description of the 2011 interview narratives and discussions in previous chapters may suggest, explanations framed around neo-liberalism cannot give full accounts of the study material. Participants' fine-grained stories of everyday HIV living contained a lot of material that neo-liberalism could not adequately explain. The concept of neo-liberalism had both general and specific limitations in relation to this material.

'Neo-liberalism' is a term used to describe free-market-dominated, deregulation-oriented approaches to economy and society. Such approaches have a powerful recent history in the US, Europe and Australia, where they have come into prominence after the 1970s dominance of Keynesian economic policy (Harvey 2005) and tend to be associated with moves from national to global free markets. 'Often, "globalization" functions as a master narrative of crisis, and neo-liberalism provides the

discursive solution to this crisis' (Barnett et al. 2008: 6). Neo-liberal policies may be seen either as promoting prosperity for all and, as we saw in
Chapter 7, a Hayekian natural human order, or as increasing economic
inequities within countries, concentrating wealth (Bourdieu 1998) and
reducing public welfare provision.

More broadly, neo-liberalism is often viewed as a form of governmentality, both ideologically and in practice (Bourdieu 1998; Wallerstein
1995). Such neo-liberal governmentality does not need to be driven by
the nation state. It is often implemented by larger international organisations, as when it was promulgated by the World Bank and International
Monetary Fund in the 1980s and 1990s to low- and middle-income
countries from its US and to some extent UK homelands, via 'structural adjustment' restrictions on government public spending and free
trade rules. Neo-liberalism is also performed locally within states (Jessop
2002), by individuals, perhaps even by narratives.

Neo-liberalism is said to extend into our social lives (Foucault
2000) and to turn moral individualism (MacIntyre 1984) into the basis
for all judgements and policies. At the most intimate level, subjectivities become neo-liberal (Elliott 2013; Gill and Scharff 2011). Individual
subjects are responsible for their own well-being and for evaluating and
maximising their position within markets. Aspects of lives previously
deemed personal (such as family and romantic relationships) or social
(for instance, social welfare and voluntary sector provision, health and
education), as well as work, become increasingly framed by marketised
frameworks. At the extreme, we could argue that neo-liberal 'subjects'
do not exist, since they are simply constellations of rational cost-benefit
analyses and decisions.

There are a number of problems with this mode of understanding.
Within it, the forms of neo-liberalism are homogenised. It takes little
account of regional or national histories (Jessop 2002). Neo-liberalism's
characteristics in middle- and low-income countries, many of which do
not have long histories of large-scale industrialisation and later social
welfare, are more complex. There, neo-liberalism may, for instance, act
progressively, against long-established patterns of resource ownership
or control, inequity and patronage (Ong 2006). Neo-liberalism is also
complicated by its interrelations with international companies and
organisations such as the World Bank and the International Monetary
Fund, and with varying economic and political situations. For nation
states still play a role somewhat independent of marketised governance.
Histories of democracy, other arrangements within countries such as
welfare states, and smaller histories of, for instance, social movements,

do not just disappear but are in dialogue with neo-liberal forces. Moreover, neo-liberalism is not as dominant or uncontested as it often sounds. The history of welfare provision in the UK (Barnett et al. 2008), for example, generates a particular and powerful resistance to current attempts to voluntarise social care.

Concepts of neo-liberalism also do not separate local initiatives from the overarching structure they propose. As a result, small-scale initiatives such as those narrated by Olive at the beginning of this chapter, or Queenie's stories of informal support networks described in Chapter 3, could seem individualised and palliative at best, collusive at worst, and pointless within the overall sociopolitical framework. Understanding contemporary HIV narratives as 'neo-liberal' thus means that the potential for effective action appears much restricted.

In addition, accounts centred on neo-liberalism do not acknowledge that the features they describe as neo-liberal always also exist alongside features that ameliorate the effects of neo-liberalism, addressing those who fall outside it (Ong 2006). Some such moderation is always necessary (Barnett et al. 2008). The United Kingdom, South Africa, as discussed in the next chapter, and many other countries, regulate citizens according to markets, but they also disburse benefits to enable people to live in varying balances of social inclusion and exclusion, to some degree independently of their market role. This dualism involves a changing constellation of policies, such as, in the HIV case, criminalisation, migration legislation and welfare reductions, on one side; but also welfare provision, aid and remittances. These latter ameliorative features frequently draw on discourses and practices of rights and responsibilities that do not align with markets. Their unmarked undoing of the 'neo-liberal', from within as well as outside its borders by its exceptions (Ong 2006), parallels the undoing of HIV's naturalisation which we explored in Section 2. It is not, therefore, surprising that stories of living with HIV and ARVs in the UK today perform a similar troubling of the neo-liberal as well as the naturalised contexts within which they are told.

Since 2008, the United Kingdom has been in a recession whose end is not clearly in sight, and cuts whose social effects will intensify over the next few years. This situation has intensified economic and social features associated with neo-liberalism. In what follows, I pay continued attention to how people articulate living with HIV and ARVs in relation to 'living with the cuts'. However, rather than talking about three-letter lives' alignment with or opposition to neo-liberalism, I want to convey this quality of 'living with' as well as 'against' the contemporary situation in interviewees' stories. These are stories of something more like para-liberalism, perhaps, operating tangentially rather than in opposition to neo-liberalism.

Explanations of interviewee narratives in terms of neo-liberalism would also tend to flatten the differences between and particularities of the stories. All difficult aspects of experiences would become side effects of neo-liberalisation. The notion of the 'para-liberal' works against such erasures of subjectivity, as does the idea of 'borderline' explored in the previous chapter and shaping this one. The title for the chapter refers to Derrida's (1979) essay, 'Living on: Borderlines', which turns on the double meaning of '*survivre*': both 'survival', and 'living on'. All stories about 'living on' with HIV, and living on, '*survivre*', on borderlines, are stories about the precariousness and persistence of surviving, 'survivre'. Despite the contemporary treatability of HIV, and its liveability, many of the stories in this research material are in very obvious ways, survival stories. They are told about a potentially fatal condition, still often late-diagnosed and difficult to manage even in the United Kingdom, and with a recent history, still well-remembered, of being a 'death sentence'. Derrida points out that narratives are not told or lived in the same places and times where a particular story is articulated, and also that a survival narrative is a kind of overseeing or over-living, *survivre* in yet another sense, melancholic and triumphant at the same time. If a story of 'living on' with HIV is about survival, it is also implicitly about the 'what-if' story (Sools 2012) of not surviving. One is never only on one safe side of the border, and this involves social and fiscal as much as medical navigations. The interviews are full of stories of the difficult contemporary UK context of surviving, 'living on,' and para-liberal negotiations of the borders of medical, social and economic citizenship. The stories cross and recross these boundaries, a process that itself can operate as part of a strategy for living with HIV and ARVs.

Medicalisation and HIV in the United Kingdom: fluctuating three-letter lives

The quote from the House of Lords report which begins this chapter characterises HIV as a public health risk, ignoring the public health of people living with HIV themselves. At the same time, the young people with whom I and my students talked at the 2011 World AIDS Day sixth-form event treated HIV as an important health consideration, though many were not in recognised risk groups. Most of these young people engaged with HIV, blurring what could seem relatively firm boundaries of risk and concern, showing no signs of 'othering' the condition. So how do people living with HIV themselves experience UK health citizenship, in a policy environment vacillating between service improvement, patient regulation and austerity, and popular narratives ranging from pathologisation and neglect to HIV's mainstreaming as a health issue? This segment of the chapter examines what the interview narratives in my UK study say about HIV positive people's own health: their relation, with considerable initial positivity, to the medicalised 'HIV as a chronic illness' storyline; their moves towards strategically critical, particular narratives, the distinct but overlapping stories of two treatment generations; 'health narrative' fluctuations within interviews and their complex management of uncertainty; and the shift away from expert and activist patient stories towards stories of holistic medicine.

Medical success stories, and what they leave out

As we saw in Chapter 4, the medicalisation of HIV destigmatises it, recognises it as an illness rather than a moral condition, and promotes treatment provision and effective education and prevention. It also frames HIV as almost entirely a bio-scientific issue, shifts responsibility onto 'expert patients', makes it very difficult to talk about non-medical HIV issues (Davis 2009), and can become problematic when medical services are cut. These ambiguities were a constant feature of interviewees' stories.

In these interviews, much more than in earlier interview rounds, almost all research participants talked first or early on about how well things were going medically and were, overall, very positive about the medical services they received. Olive, for example, started off describing her medical support by saying, 'Yeah, it has been very good, um, I can't complain. It has been very good, yeah, from my consultant to the GPs, yeah.' However, given time to continue, Olive also told a story of how difficult it used to be with her GPs, before she found an informed one, to be able to protect confidentiality; of her ongoing headaches which were taking her back to her consultant the next week; and of continuing diarrhoea, as with Morag in Chapter 7, and disabling neuropathy:

> Olive: It's only before, erm, years back, it was very difficult with the GPs/Oh, OK/I think I changed about three GPs/Mhm, because?/ You can tell that they don't want to, because of, yeah, once they know you are HIV positive, you have to disclose, every time you go they say 'what is it this time Olive'. Then I go back to my consultant, 'what can I do, this is what is happening.' Sometimes

you can see your (self) with a red mark/Mhm, in the GPs?/Yeah, he used to do that yeah...Yeah, the {ARV} side effects are diarrhoea, neuropathy. One day, sometimes I am OK. Sometimes, oh, I can't even walk/Is that neuropathy?/Neuropathy, yeah neuropathy, yeah. Diarrhoea is, yeah, the side effects are, yeah. I'm always dealing with side effects every day (laughs). Every day is like, you say 'I'm OK, I'm fine', if anyone asks, 'I'm fine'. Every day there is something (which is inside), but you have to deal with it/inaudible/ yeah, living with it.

Participant narratives, as they developed over the interviews, tended to progress towards problems with medications, side effects, or incompletely treated HIV-related conditions such as neuropathy, lipodystrophy, fatigue, poor sleeping, depression, anxiety and stress. Some had digestive problems, like Sean's and Tyler's, or HIV-related cancers, like John's, as described in Chapters 4 and 7. Many others had known or suspected cognitive deficits, cardiovascular and diabetic issues, and kidney problems like Quentin's in Chapter 2. Interviewees also often mentioned that treatment does not always work, and that people taking treatment do not always have 'a near-normal lifespan'.

Although these enumerations were less common with more recently-diagnosed and treated participants, they still occurred. Many recently-diagnosed participants reported, for example, ongoing psychological difficulties which had not always started in a medically expected way. Several told stories in which they became depressed around a year after diagnosis.

A number of interviewees told long stories of the difficulties of getting help for mental health issues which were said to be under-addressed unless they were affecting ARV adherence or causing suicidal ideation. Jana, for instance, a non-UK European woman in her mid-40s, taking ARVs since the early 2000s, with serious ongoing mental health problems only partly addressed, started with a very positive evaluation of medical services. She progressed to her difficulties accessing help for mental health only towards the end of the interview, when asked what other kinds of support she might want, again, only after first praising existing services:

Jana: I don't know because what I want now I kind of have it {everything I need} really. I mean the only thing I would say you know maybe that I can complain about my situation is the waiting list of things like having to wait a year to start the {psycho}therapy, you know, it was a bit long, yeah.

It is probable that this research underestimated the severity of mental health issues because it relied on participants who were able to volunteer. At least one of the two previous participants who did not want to participate again may have been depressed, and that could have had some impact on their decision.

In some ways but not others, HIV's medicalisation did indeed seem to rule out other kinds of talk about HIV (Davis 2009) for these participants. On one side, HIV's medicalisation did not seem to have strong effects on interviewees' stories of relationships and condom use. Many interviewees were aware of TasP; some debated how it might be affected by instabilities in viral load. But in stories about condoms, this issue remained secondary to interpersonal factors like the value of specific relationships and sexual practices. Psychosocial issues around living with HIV and ARVs did, nevertheless, seem difficult to talk about, particularly when they did not need clinical attention. Jana's mental health issues were being appropriately medically treated, and her consultant was perhaps more likely in this case than in others to be attentive to her psychological state because of her history. However, she, like many other interviewees, wanted to discuss aspects of her life with her consultant beyond her CD4+ T cell count and viral load but said she did not and could not because the appointments seemed time-geared to deal only with medical issues. Late in the interview, she told the story of her typical appointment a number of times, as here:

> **Jana:** I don't tell {my consultant about my life} because I just feel like, I don't have much time {in the appointment}. I'm not going to start 'oh by the way do you know I'm doing', you know, I feel 'let's get to the point' you know and I leave quickly/ Yeah/It's taken a lot of time realising that how I feel about it I because I'm used to it, I know it, where in the past I have but now I'm thinking, as I'm listening to myself, I'm thinking 'this is not right', you know.

The strongest limits on medicalisation's success appeared for interviewees who were very sick or in constant pain. For example, Penelope was a 55-year-old black African woman diagnosed in 2002 shortly after being made redundant and coming to the United Kingdom as a visitor. She had taken ARVs since then. Like Olive and several other interviewees, her interview contained a number of habitual narratives about symptoms that could not be treated adequately, especially neuropathy, for which she was using morphine patches. This was a situation of being 'left behind' with the pain, yet still living on with and speaking out about it in a determined, everyday way. It was not helped by three-letter lives of this kind being neglected in the dominant medical picture of chronic, manageable HIV illness:

> **Penelope:** Yeah, living with this condition I've seen people writing {about living a normal life with HIV} and it's not a, ok you can live a normal life, but you often get sick, everybody's different, I don't know, maybe people speak for themselves but they shouldn't speak for everybody yeah because it's different yeah, you know it is different, like at times I get a sharp sharp pain, it can be anywhere it can be here it can be on my toe, very sharp pain and I feel it and once it starts that day I won't sleep, the whole night will just go, like a needle, then it stops, then again, I don't sleep you know and I don't know what it is…it's very painful sharp sharp pain, it starts around five, I'm not sleeping that day it will go on the whole night like that and there's, I haven't found a solution for it yet.

The stories in the research are not, therefore, of unalloyed medical progress; they are highly qualified. They move between the successes of medicalised three-letter lives, and their constraints, particularly the constraints of living with the cuts. However, they are to some extent stories of more long-lasting 'difference', as Penelope put it, that is, stories that separate out *different* kinds of three-letter lives. It is to these medically based differences that I now turn.

Illness groups

A medicalised division seemed to operate in some interviews, as it does indeed in some policy discourse, between treatment generations. If living with HIV is a different kind of three-letter life medically than it used to be, with HIV and ARVs intimately associated, it is not surprising that more recently diagnosed and treated people register that difference, while people diagnosed and treated in earlier years tell stories about a history that current treatment optimism can seem to exclude or leave behind. Some interviewees in the first group distinguished their experiences strongly from those in the second group, particularly in relation to early-generation ARV and side effect difficulties and to long-term health problems which they thought they might not experience. Participants like Zack, the most recently diagnosed interviewee, in his early 30s, emphasised the contemporary good health of HIV positive people and the ease of medication, posing these factors against older accounts of HIV, and storying HIV today as something of ever-diminishing medical significance:

Zack: OK, I made the test, I know, and a week later I started taking medicines./right/ But, I mean, people think that when they see you 'yes, you should start treatment', and people think that you are ill or. I mean, people call it, like, a chronic disease but for me a disease is when you have symptoms, when you are, I mean, impeded, I don't know. My aunt has lupus. That is a chronic disease... she needs a lot of support, medicinal support. So, I only needed tablets, I still do everything, so I think they should change it from chronic disease to, I don't know, another name/ Some people say a long-term condition/A long-term condition. Yeah, but it is a 'condition' again, it's only something which is in my blood and it's contained and it's monitored, well monitored. And, they don't need to make me feel sick when I am not sick, I'm not ill. Some things need to change, as with the perception of HIV positive needs to change. And, I said before, um, before we recorded (laughs) that scientifically, we are miles ahead of the people's perceptions of HIV, I think there must be a lot of work to be done there.

By contrast, John, positioning himself within the earlier treatment generation, contextualised the illness uncertainties he lived with as happening within 'borrowed time', decades after his projected death. He referred repeatedly to his extensively 'pre-treated' health status, resistant to many ARVs, which derived from his use of the drugs singly and at doses not now used, and which limited his current treatment options.

Such categorisations of illness did not just apply to treatment generations. Many interviewees described contemporary living with HIV and ARVs as simply one of many 'chronic illness' experiences. They also often categorised themselves alongside others who grow more ill with age, pointing sometimes to 'accelerated ageing', as does some contemporary medical discourse around HIV and cardiovascular illness (Power et al. 2010). Zack, for instance, interspersed his narrative of how he managed his own drug regime with a brief description of his mother's age-related but early-onset illness, minimising his own condition by this comparison:

Zack: I'm really fine with taking my four tablets a day and once in the evenings /yeah/. It's not, it doesn't really bother me at all. My mother started taking treatment; she suffers from high blood pressure so she since the age of 36, she's been taking one tablet a day, now she is 60. Now she is taking more tablets, more than that, obviously, because there is other conditions when you get older, you know. And, that's the good thing about new treatment; there is less and less interaction with other drugs, and that is really good.

Though modified by the contemporary HIV treatment situation, these are not new ways of storying HIV lives. Oscar Moore (1996) described the commonalities between his and other chronic illness experience in the mid-1990s. Adam Mars-Jones's (1992) early story 'Slim' noted sarcastically how shortened lifespans were being presented as 'normal-in-the-third-world' by HIV organisations trying to turn drastically shortened lives into something bearable. Living with HIV has therefore involved for a long time these mobile identifications with health as much as illness, general illness as much as a particular condition.

It is realistic to take into account different treatment histories in analysing narratives of three-letter lives, in addition to the relations between HIV, chronic illnesses, and age-related illnesses. At the same time, these medicalised subdivisions and expansions, fuelled by the contemporary optimism that attends living with HIV and ARVs, can leave out some narratives of HIV. Optimism about the current 'treatment generation', however warranted, can, when over-generalised, position people recently diagnosed and ill as if they are doing something wrong and leave longer-diagnosed people outside of the medical present, artefactually excluded by progress-oriented medical and policy discourses. Unhelpful and sometimes discriminating divisions may start to appear between different kinds of narratives of living on or surviving with HIV and ARVs. Older-generation interviewees in this study who were living with considerable health problems did indeed say that they felt left out of HIV organisations' discourse of HIV as a 'long-term condition'. Younger-generation participants often mentioned that they had previously associated HIV with older people, and with a certain illness or treatment 'look'.

Over the course of the interviews in this study, however, research participants of both 'generations' produced highly nuanced stories, recognising individual differences in HIV illness progression and the uncertainties of ARV treatment and making no absolute distinctions between treatment generations. We have already seen Penelope note the variations from normal health involved with living with HIV and ARVs: 'ok you can live a normal life, but you often get sick, everybody's different, I don't know, maybe people speak for themselves but they shouldn't speak for everybody yeah because it's different yeah'. John's account of 'borrowed time' and his 'pre-treated' status was accompanied by stories of extreme attentiveness to new treatment opportunities.

Zack, before his narrative of good health, told a qualifying story of his prior poor CD4 + T cell count, high viral load, and early onset of symptoms and treatment.

It is possible for the naturalising inclusion of HIV-related conditions within 'chronic illness' or 'faster ageing' to make such conditions sound like regular, expected fluctuations in health status. Many interviewees, even those that made such comparisons, also qualified HIV's commonalities with 'chronic illness' or 'ageing'. Some participants explicitly rejected medical comparisons of HIV with, especially, diabetes, claiming that either HIV's medical control or its social normalisation, or both, had not progressed far enough to make such comparisons workable. Sometimes, interviewees posited futures in which better drugs or a cure would render even these relatively optimistic comparisons obsolete. Medicine might completely erase HIV as illness, as in Zack's story of where improvements in HIV positive people's health are going:

> **Zack:** I think because we are living longer and longer someone will say that we will die of old age, so it's getting better … I hope that finally there will be a cure and then, you know, I always imagine, like, in ten years or twenty years there will be a cure, and then, OK, and then I'm rid of the HIV virus.

These were narrative moves that are not often found in standard medical or NGO accounts of HIV, whose storied optimism depends on existing medical solutions rather than cure in an uncertain future. And such stories seemed to derive from HIV treatment activism rather than from medical knowledge itself, a tendency this chapter will explore more later.

Research participants' stories thus worked against homogenising and often minimising comparisons of HIV with other conditions, and against dilutions of it into a 'chronic illness' or 'long-term condition', as well as sometimes endorsing these moves. Such differences in medicalised positioning operated strategically to allow people to narrate different aspects of three-letter lives, by turns establishing and erasing differences across HIV illness, and across HIV and other conditions. The usefulness of such variability becomes more obvious when one considers the fluctuating nature of HIV as illness.

Fluctuating lives

In 2011 the National AIDS Trust published a report, 'Fluctuating symptoms of HIV' (2011b), pointing out the extreme difficulty with a chronic condition such as HIV of making definitive judgements about health statuses, like those needed to assess rights to disability benefits. Naturalising medicalisation processes operate to define HIV positive people at any particular moment as healthy or sick and as success-fully or unsuccessfully treated. These categorisations do not work well. Both for HIV positive people who experienced illness before treatment and for the increasing numbers of HIV positive people always in good health but living long-term with ARVs the physiological effects of the virus and the medications can be hard to predict. Commonly, inter-viewees explicitly described their health as 'up and down', or qualified their stories of healthy everyday lives with an underlying subtext of fatigue. Olive, as we heard earlier, narrated dramatic but not unusual health variations: 'One day, sometimes I am OK. Sometimes, oh, I can't even walk.'

At the same time, research participants' framings of their identities also fluctuated, including many aspects that were not related to HIV. Sometimes, participants rejected HIV-related illness as an aspect of their lives, regardless of symptoms. A number defined themselves as symp-tom-free when I asked them about health at the end of the interview, while in the interview itself they narrated high levels of symptoms such as depression and neuropathy, which would register on any medical assessment, as well as aspects of ill health such as fatigue and stress, to which HIV medicine might pay less attention.

It is unsurprising that following their 'fluctuating symptoms', partici-pants' stories moved in and out of HIV citizenship within the same inter-view. Zack, for example, though refusing all three-letter definitions, also told stories of his earlier health problems and his insistence on getting good treatment, the best doctors and ARVs, and HIV-specific services whenever he needed them. Medicalisation itself thus operated as a stra-tegic element in participants' stories, which alternately backgrounded and foregrounded HIV status, health generally, HIV as a chronic condi-tion, and HIV as a specific condition. These stories addressed, without being overwhelmed by, the fluctuating letters defining HIV lives, and the changes and uncertainties swirling around the condition.

Undeniably, 'living with the cuts' was one pressing determinant of these narrative strategies. Participants might at different times position themselves as 'healthy' in relation to the current economic climate, in which others perceived as much worse off were suffering, or as 'sick' in ways that demanded HIV-specific medical services, regardless of cost. Below, I examine participants' shifting 'para-liberal' positionings in rela-tion to HIV's medicalisation within a recession.

The limits of the expert patient, medical activism, and health as care

Participants in this study expressed high levels of knowledge about HIV and good treatment literacy. They told extensive stories of being 'proactive', as several called it. Like Olive, Zack and John, they researched and sought out the best clinics, doctors and medication. They challenged inadequate medical provision and demanded HIV-specific provision where appropriate. Some participants told stories of being more expert than the experts. At times they were the first to present drug interaction data to their GPs or trial data to their consultants. Their expertise included, as we have already seen in relation to 'treatment groups' and 'fluctuating symptoms', high levels of uncertainty about particular features of HIV such as strains and viral load, and about ARVs around resistance, that fit with the ongoing uncertainties of HIV medical science and practice and of medical discourses more generally (Rabinow 2004). Zack, for example, said he had medical discussions with his HIV positive friends in which they weighed up conflicting evidence, without expecting to reach firm conclusions.

While these continuing ambiguities are essential aspects of contemporary professional HIV knowledges, their place within HIV positive lives was narrated as difficult. Even the less contentious elements of HIV medical knowledges could be problematic for 'expert patients' by virtue of their amount and their highly technical nature. The policy demand that people living with HIV and ARVs engage continuously with such knowledges is also troublesome. It does not take account of the considerable resources of time, energy, emotion, knowledge, and other technologies, especially internet access, required.

In this interview round, such issues were much more prominent than a decade earlier. There were fewer 'expert patient' stories than before, not because participants lacked knowledge, but because they said they did not always want to be in a responsible, 'proactive' position in relation to medicine. Many interviewees said that they were tired of devoting themselves to topics for which their doctors should have responsibility, in which they were not professionally trained, and that emphasised an HIV identity to whose existing effects on their lives they did not want to add. Some very HIV-knowledgeable people were happy to forget their CD4+ T cell counts from appointment to appointment. Other participants had little internet access or found the medical and technical aspects of HIV knowledges difficult.

In this and previous chapters, people living with HIV and ARVs, like Nicco and Yoliswa in South Africa, and John, Zack, and Jana in the

United Kingdom, position themselves as HIV citizens within the broader context of health or biological citizenship in order to reiterate or remake claims on national and international medical service providers (Robins 2009; Rose 2007). But this variety of citizenship is not contested on level ground. Clinicians, particularly perhaps HIV clinicians, are often highly dedicated to patient involvement and decision-making. However, the structure of current medical technologies means that 'expert patients' validate, without really having the power to challenge, medical expertise. Sometimes their involvement in negotiations which they are bound to lose merely obviates any requirement for medical discourse to engage further with its non-professional constituents. In this study, narratives of patient-consultant discussions about treatment sometimes ended with the participant describing ceding the decision because they were simply exhausted by the unequal contest between professional and patient expertise.

It is important to recognise that participants' involvement with medical discourse as HIV and biological citizens was as much activist, as 'expert patient', in character. This activist engagement provided them with counteracting narratives that articulated criticism and alternatives. For instance, their medical knowledge often filtered through the interpretive lenses of HIV organisations such as THT, the National AIDS Trust, i-Base, The Body and Aidsmap. Many interviewee stories of 'proactive' engagements driven by such knowledge put them in direct conflict with medical practitioners, rather than in the conversational but implicitly subordinate place of the expert patient. Such stories might involve, for example, participants persisting in using specialist HIV clinics rather than GP practices, delaying or accelerating starting treatment, or demanding more expensive medications before cheaper ones.

Participants' medical and activist knowledges intertwined especially clearly when they were asylum seekers. Penelope, for example, told a story of not being prescribed ARVs that worked well with her other health conditions because they were not available in her country of origin and her consultant thought she might be deported. When given the first-line treatment of her country of origin, she had to change consultants to get better treatment.

Participants often strongly asserted activist over medical knowledges within their stories of mental health issues, thought to affect over 50% of people living with HIV in the United Kingdom (National AIDS Trust 2011b). While some participants separated off mental health as a concern outside of HIV medicine, many more questioned or asserted its relation to the lack of medically linked psychosocial HIV services, to

ARVs or to HIV itself. Jana, for example, referred to her current mental health problems as rooted in her own personal psychopathology, but her stories about it repeatedly and critically also related it to her experiences with ARVs. However, this account did not work with her consultant. As with other participants, her story of difficulties in getting psychological help suggested that mental health issues had to be presented to consultants in a very particular, medicalised way, as related to suicidal ideation or non-compliance with treatment, to get some consultants' attention. Jana did not do this. She related telling her doctor she was not feeling good; he told her that everyone gets depressed. She had, she reported, looked up her medication's association with mental health problems. She tried to deploy that knowledge by talking to her doctor about the 'research' around the medication, but to no effect.

More directly, Gerry, an interviewee of North American origin, in his 40s, again drew on HIV community knowledge about the effects of ARVs when he criticised the hiving off of his anxiety symptoms into non-medical care by his doctor, telling the story of his response: 'Why have I got to see the psychologist? Isn't it a side effect?' Finally and perhaps most importantly, participants' counteracting narratives of health care had strong links, not so much with larger HIV organisations' contemporary policies, as with their own face-to-face and online discussions with friends, and with community-level organisations and practices.

Participants also drew on narrated experiences of 'alternative' or 'complementary' health care for this counteracting narrative of medical care as human care, holistic and centred on interpersonal contact. Their criticisms focused on medical professionals who treat you as a set of viral load or CD4+ T cell numbers or just as a research subject; who look at the computer screen, not at you; who make you feel like they do not know you or that they are too busy; who insist that you go to your GP all the time, even though the GP always says they do not know what to do; who give you the sense that they are responding to the cuts in time or medications when they meet and treat you; who only care about your mental health if it might make you suicidal or an ARV treatment failure. In response, participants' counteracting narratives of a de-medicalised, 'holistic' HIV medicine focused on clinicians listening and spending time, integrated medical and social care, awareness of and provision for psychosocial issues at HIV clinics, direct people-to-people referrals rather than just leaflets, and more attention to the voices of people living with HIV. Participants gave examples within these counteracting narratives of consultants who sent monthly emails, nurses who gave out their mobile numbers, clinics where 'even the cleaners', as one woman said, seemed to be part of the HIV treatment endeavour. Interviewees were determined to name good consultants, clinics, and hospitals, even though they knew the names would be taken out of the transcripts. They also articulated doctors', nurses' and their own parallel HIV life trajectories, going beyond professional and patient stories, part of a shared effort to manage HIV.

These counteracting narratives could be qualified, subtle, and slowly developed, appearing in long and often fragmented storylines. Jana, for example, started out talking very positively about services available to her and then addressed cuts in services generally, rather than the medical services themselves:

> **Jana:** Obviously I think the main thing which you've probably heard it hundreds of times it's about the financial situation, so because of their money cut, other services are providing you know fewer things, less things in general, even things like in hospital, you know, in the clinic before um the doctor could give you things that you needed, now it's pure medications, nothing else, you know, where before, if you had a skin rash, they would give you special soap or you know things like that, now suddenly the medicine they will provide us and nothing else.

It was only when I asked if there was anything else to say about medical services that – hedged with non-entitled, gratitude-filled caveats about free treatment and having everything she needed – Jana described her long wait for psychotherapy and the consultation time limitations resulting from current service pressures. These expressed limits to medical treatment led to a critical narrative, including her own irritated, almost parodic approach to consultations, which often focused on physiological markers and involved skipping appointments if they were good:

> **Jana:** But you know, at the end of the day I think well I'm getting it for free so it {time} cannot be there and then so I kind of, and maybe {I would like} the doctors to have a bit more time because that I do nothing you know and I did feel at some point, I think I even missed one appointment because I could not be bothered. I wait three or four months to come and see my doctor and he say the results, I know them already, because I ring them. The results is okay, the prescription, 'okay, take this to reception for the next

appointment', I thought, I cannot be bothered to do that, you know.

Jana is reporting changes in a medical system that, when interviewed nine years earlier, she did not report as showing such signs of strain. She has in some ways a good relation with her doctor, whom she chose. He is the doctor of choice for many people, including a large group of patients of African origin. He gave her his telephone number, though she says she would never use it. Nevertheless, she skips appointments because she 'cannot be bothered' and reports feeling that she has no right to ask questions or have problems if all her physiological indicators are good.

Later, when Jana talked about the alternative therapies she used, she continued this counteracting narrative. She drew on her experience of alternative therapies as a model and took off from her earlier, what-if, hypothetical story ending, 'it would be nice not to feel like that {intimidated about using up time}', to produce a more emphatically critical story of what was wrong in her meetings with her doctor. It is notable how much she had to say during this third, most particular and most critical narrative of her hospital appointments within the interview, compared to the generality, brevity, and studied neutrality of her first:

Jana: And sometimes it's a stress like you leave the doctor like tense, I'm thinking, 'my God, he made me so tense', because, if he's like he cannot find this, his desk a mess, with his things, sometimes I'm (rushing) out, 'okay, sorry I'll go now!' And then you leave thinking that was a bit of tension there./Yes/It's only now thinking about it...And you know sometimes I have a good relationship with him, but you know, I try, I try to take as little time as possible you know, anything that I don't think is very important, I am, you know, I don't want to waste his time, that's how I feel. I know that it's a big queue, I know everybody's running late, everybody's stressed, my doctor is stressed, let's not make things any worse you know. I shouldn't be feeling like that obviously.

Participants with greater HIV-related illness experience often produced more direct counteracting narratives of the problems of HIV medicine. Gerry, for instance, HIV positive since the mid-1990s and recovering from a serious illness at the time of the interview, started off, like Jana, emphasising he did not want to complain about medical services.

He returned to that point many times. Nevertheless, he articulated a strongly critical story that moved towards possible integrated care, an ideal that appears frequently in HIV community discussions, though it is less foregrounded in larger HIV organisations' policy thinking:

> **Gerry:** One of the concerns I have without, the treatment or the approach to treatment is just that, there seems to be situation things, there appear to be a bit disjointed um. For example, I have a separate HIV doctor. I have a liver doctor. I have a separate haemo doctor and I have a separate GP doctor. So I have about five or six doctors, and it has actually occurred that all five of them have requested, for example, a liver ultrasound so I have five appointments within a week, for a liver ultrasound, so there seems to be, I find it frustrating that it's not a single authority to, point of contact, that I can go and feel comfortable there getting answers about and that person is the point person for all the other doctors. That probably adds a little bit to the general stress um, but apart from that it has to be said I appreciate the expertise of each individual doctor. Um and I feel somehow confident by that perhaps it upsets even more than the fact that I have to put up with this merry-go-round of doctors, that kind of thing. But it is sort of the one area that frustrates and causes a bit of tension, which is the one thing I often, try to avoid stress and tension (laughs) um, so I, I, so I think if I was designing an HIV support system or whatever, I would design it so that the patient has a point of contact, er, a super-doctor, someone not necessarily, someone who specialises themselves in every area. But that was almost more of a manager to look at that kind of thing.

Gerry's criticisms here, albeit qualified by his 'appreciation' of medical expertise, lead directly to what he wants: specialist but also joined-up care. He later adds to this counteracting narrative the requirement for more emotional care. He comes to the conclusion that cutting-edge care, even in the case of serious illness, might not always be the priority:

> **Gerry:** I don't want to appear to be complaining...but I would maybe actually trade the medical side for a little bit more support.

Many participants did indeed tell stories of medical practitioners already practising a counteracting narrative of HIV health care as care, despite intensifying constraints. Interviewees often said they had close relationships with their doctors emerging from their long professional-patient intertwined histories: shared histories of obstacles, possibilities, disappointments, renewed hopes, reversals, and ongoing struggles. Here, doctors, analogously to patients, had progressed from working with HIV to working with HIV and ARVs. Interviewees told stories of these doctors' strong opposition to a medical practice recuperated by 'numbers': CD4+ T cell counts, shortened consultations, cost-benefit analyses. They told these stories within their construction of a medical practice of health care, not health counting.

Such engagement was also narrated as part of a professional history. Good new doctors learned from older ones how to give the best care. They explained this process to their patients, so that patients would not feel they were losing out with younger staff. For such HIV medical practice in the UK is itself strongly imbricated with HIV activism and a commitment to the GIPA (Greater Involvement of People living with HIV/AIDS) principle. While the medicalisation of the pandemic may indeed be increasing (Nguyen 2011), this local history connecting medicine, care, and community remained strong in many interviews.

The 'health as care' counteracting narrative articulated by research participants did not clearly align with features of medical marketisation such as cuts, cost-benefit analyses and individualisation, often described as 'neo-liberal'. Despite such features' strength, they did not fully determine how interviewees told about or went about their medicalised lives. At the same time, people living three-letter lives still have to engage with contemporary cost-benefit structured medicine in a 'para-liberal' way in order to insist, like Gerry, that psychological services could be bartered for less physical medicine; or to know, like Penelope, that a particular ARV has dangerous and potentially costly interactions with another health condition; or to argue, as many participants did, that cheap, inappropriate treatments will end up more expensive in the long run. A 'neo-liberal' health economy must itself be responsive to resistant exceptions that define its boundaries: the treatments that do not work, the need for non-medical 'psychosocial' services. At these boundaries, para-liberal narratives like interviewees' stories of 'health as care' can indeed have counteracting effects.

The ways in which interviewees framed their counteracting 'health as care' narratives is also interesting related to the 'neo-liberal'. This narrative might itself seem like a technology of heavily marketised societies. We could view it negatively, as involving a personalised responsibilisation of medical services, and a form of 'patient involvement' that requires people living with HIV and ARVs to contribute large amounts of unpaid practical and emotional work to monitoring and pursuing their own care. However, in this UK study, the stories of interpersonal relationships that expressed this responsibilisation were often framed as larger, politically inflected narratives of how things should be. This happened when Jana said, 'I shouldn't be feeling like that obviously', or when Gerry started off the story of his fragmented care experiences by saying that 'things... appear to be a bit disjointed'. HIV activism in the United Kingdom may have more personalised voices than previously. The successes of treatment, and concerns about migration, criminalisation, and current market models of health, hedge the claims made by those voices. HIV organisations, particularly larger organisations, position themselves less as campaigning organisations and work more closely with government and policymakers than before. In this study, participants rarely seemed to be supported directly by such organisations in their often difficult and exhausting negotiations with medical authority. However, they drew extensively on the medical knowledges, often filtered through an activist lens, that such organisations provide. Moreover, for many interviewees, the histories of HIV activism that had formed them, and the present-day, smaller-scale community activism with which they were involved, helped them tell their counteracting, denaturalising, 'para-liberal' medical stories. Penelope's story of refusing medications prescribed on the basis of suppositions about her upcoming deportation, and Olive's account of her rights-supported practice of changing GPs, drew on the knowledges exchanged within informal support networks of the kind Olive herself described at the beginning of this chapter and Queenie described in Chapter 3. Gerry's narrative move from service fragmentation to a care-oriented holistic practice harked back to his experience of prior practice of this kind, itself produced by intense early HIV/AIDS activism.

In this segment of the chapter, I have described stories of medical failures and uncertainties around new long-term HIV issues, the limitations of medical solutions to symptoms and side effects, and service cuts, in the most recent interviews with UK study participants living with HIV and ARVs. Living medicalised three-letter lives means, it seems, constantly living with the cuts. But while participant narratives trace how health markets cannot now be relied on, they do not shift all solutions to the individual. 'Personal issues' are not siloed. 'Responsibility' shifts from the individual to the social in these interviewees' narratives. The stories move from a collective HIV history to the present-day narrator and then they shift back, via the larger claims made, to a shared political articulation. These oblique counteracting narratives could indeed be called 'para-liberal' strategies for 'living on' as medicalised HIV citizens. They appear in participants' negotiations with and opposition to marketised health, which is itself necessarily heterogeneous and responsive to claims from outside its borders; and in participants' assertions of 'health as care'. They also appear, as we will see, in participants' negotiations of HIV's normalisation.

Normalisation: HIV as the new normal

Self-management? UK HIV policy and normalisation

Contemporary UK HIV policy is directed at normalising HIV in several ways. Despite treatment successes, high hopes of TasP, and stories told by HIV organisations and many people living with HIV themselves about HIV's individual manageability, policymakers face widespread concerns about increasing HIV incidence, the 24% of people living with the virus who do not know their status, and low levels of testing overall. Health, social and voluntary sector policy try to normalise testing and present HIV as a treatable, normal condition in order to address these concerns and to undo fear-provoking 'death sentence' or minimising, 'nothing to do with me' significations of HIV. Such normalisation can work against stigma by positioning HIV as an illness or as a 'condition' that, like many others, is just a part of people's lives.

As Chapter 5 argued, however, normalisation may also gloss over the differences between different HIV statuses, and between HIV and other health conditions, making these differences, and HIV's own particularities, difficult to address. It may also turn HIV – not getting it, treating it, living with it – into a condition of pure personal responsibility. The United Kingdom's contemporary normalising HIV campaigns navigate the borders between normalising and destigmatising, and minimalising, invisibilising and responsibilising HIV. The Terrence Higgins Trust's LifeCheck project, for example, offers how-to narratives of self-sufficiency and anti-dependency that fit with contemporary neo-liberalism, but that also hold out the possibility of health and life. The African Health Policy Network (AHPN) has a name which hides its HIV remit, but which by foregrounding broad health concerns, allows AHPN to address African-origin people's concerns holistically, normalising HIV as part of health. AHPN's Do It Right campaign, encouraging condom use, and seen all over the London underground in 2011, presented HIV as a quiet, small-letter message within the posters, associated with 'sexual health' generally. This was such an effective normalisation of HIV within 'health' that, in a context of general silence about the epidemic, 'HIV' might not be noticed at all. My informal poll in that year's 'HIV in the world' module suggested many students had seen the posters' 'condoms' message but few had associated it with HIV. That might not matter too much, since the strong message from all the posters is about confident people of African origin, talking and acting positively, in ways that promote sexual health. The ambiguous character of such normalisations is, though, important to keep in view.

HIV normalisation as a way of living

Interviewees' own stories provide a fuller articulation than policy or media discourse of the complexities around HIV's UK normalisation. Most of my UK research participants, however positively they evaluated their own health, and whatever useful comparisons they could find between HIV and other age-associated or chronic illnesses, strongly resisted any extreme-case normalisation of HIV as always 'just like' other chronic or age-related conditions. Like Penelope, they refused to let this equation stand for everyone. At the same time, normalisation could operate, as we saw in Chapter 5, against medicalisation, and as a support for stories of 'normal life' outside of illness. Moreover, as in policy, and as with the medicalisation processes in the UK epidemic examined in the previous section, interviewees' stories of and against normalisation often operated via a responsibilisation of the narrator, this time, in both normalising and counteracting, denormalising stories. This move is not surprising, given that normalisation operates on HIV citizenship at the level of subjectivity, the 'personal'. Such responsibilisation could be read as a constraining co-option of narrators' subjectivities by 'neo-liberal' market concepts of subjectivity. However, it could also be understood, as in the prior chapter segment, as a kind of borderline, 'para-liberal' attempt to 'live on', on the edge between normalisation and de-normalisation: a para-normalisation, perhaps, that offers some possibilities for action and activism.

Throughout the study, interviewees' narratives articulated both HIV's normalcy and its particularity. This doubled approach displayed normalisation within the current UK epidemic as a strategy, always in question, rather than a fixed reality. Stories of the 'new normal' in the interviews charted it via commonalities with chronic illness generally, and also through 'normal' life alongside HIV, in relationships, families, friends and meaningful work. These were thus narratives of normalised three-letter lives lived paradoxically apart from HIV, except in relation to HIV's medicalisation. They articulated HIV's general sociality. In addition, though, the interviews narrated particularity through stigma in everyday living, isolation, uncertainty and the importance of HIV-specific psychosocial services. They valued HIV positive socialities specifically, against the constraints of cuts. HIV citizens thus narrated a socially rather than just individually responsibilised citizenship on both sides of the normalisation border.

Zack's shifts in narrative positioning are a good example. Zack returned often to the importance of treating HIV like other conditions. He even, as we saw in the previous chapter segment, normalised it medically to the point of removing it from the category of 'condition' or 'illness'. At this point, his normalising story of living with HIV and ARVs pursued medicalisation's success to the point of erasing the three letters from his life. This created an extreme case version of normalisation contradicting medicalisation, or perhaps of medicalisation falling into contradiction with itself.

Zack wanted everyone to be able to talk about HIV and HIV testing to be 'routine'. However, he also wanted disclosure to be entirely a matter for HIV positive people themselves. He assessed HIV positive people as the most understanding, 'been-there' service providers. He repeatedly noted the current pathologisation and silencing of HIV. Indeed, he said the interview was his first long conversation about his status. He had disclosed to and been rejected by potential partners, although sometimes disclosure had worked well. He wanted an HIV positive partner; sero-sorting, that is, choosing partners with the same HIV status would make things 'easier'. He had been depressed at times. He had been ill; his early dramatic recasting of HIV positivity as healthy has to be read retrospectively in the light of this later element of his story. He acknowledged another, non-normalisable HIV illness group, the earlier 'treatment generation' described in the previous chapter segment, experiencing severe and long-term HIV-related illness and ARV side effects. Yet his account of his earlier illness history challenged the boundary between himself and that group. Moreover, being asked to test all the time when you go to STI, antenatal and many London clinics, as now happens to the undifferentiated 'public', is not, Zack said, 'normalisation' for HIV positive people. It ignores them and forces them to explain themselves every time.

Zack's is a complex story of a newly conditional, socially situated HIV 'normal', in which people of all statuses can and should know and talk about HIV. Positive people, though, should not *have* to talk about their own HIV status, should have access to particular services and should be explicitly recognised as members of the health citizenry, as well as living normalised, unmarked, healthy lives.

Participants also provided many narratives of non-normalisable aspects of three-letter lives, such as mourning and depression, uncertainty and anxiety, that seemed, especially in the contemporary context of cuts to psychosocial services, to leave them behind emotionally, as the previous chapter described. There is a great deal of unexpectedness and loss to deal with around HIV, for instance in relationships and through deaths, separation from children, unemployment, and physical limitations. All these things tended to strike people unawares and to leave a legacy of what Gerry called emotional 'disconnection':

> **Gerry:** There is just a disconnection between um, where medically I supposedly I am and emotionally where I feel down, there needs to be some kind of support...I mean I can remember from ten years ago, living in {London borough} there used to be all these, 'come sit down, have a cup of tea'. I think that the people that get left behind are really the people who are medically well enough to not really need that much support but emotionally may be not quite so secure, um and again it comes down to the fact that they have to design our programmes around this target, um, you know fair enough reason to limit the supply of money and you I mean, you can maybe have a drop-in centre, I don't think that there are drop-in centres any more (laughs), years ago kind of thing that's kind of, I know if I would if I got a leaflet in the post tomorrow I would see that a new drop-in centre, I would be there on day one, I would be there making cupcakes (laugh)/(laugh)/ a day centre kind of thing. That was the beauty of the {local organisation 1} I can walk there and do some exercise, I would go there and come back home, I would talk to my new friends, just feel good about myself for the day...when you're home you feel very tired. Because it was a drop-in centre, it attends to without forgetting about HIV positive, kind of put it in perspective and not dominate kind of thing.

Gerry ended his stories of past HIV-oriented support by suggesting he could personally start a drop-in for socially disenfranchised HIV positive people. The strength of this suggestion, given his very demanding health situation at the time, testifies to his felt need for specific provision.

However, normalising again, Gerry's narrative went on to articulate the stresses around benefits for HIV positive people as similar to those that people with, for example, mental health and other long-term health conditions, have to deal with, and as themselves exacerbated by HIV's 'singling-out':

> **Gerry:** So I think there's a bit of a problem with this whole singled-out HIV being a specific kind of illness, this is, I think

maybe it happened before identifying, in people being identified, I don't want to be identified as being HIV, I want to be identified as having a chronic illness, because there is always going, every generation there's going to be a source like stigma attached to HIV and responsible for contracting HIV, this and that blah blah blah, there was going to be a source of stigma, whereas if I just be referred to having chronic illness, to stress, these problems, that I can be like anybody else, I feel guilty, and I don't have to worry about them spending tens of millions of pounds because, and I think that would be a good starting point, um, you know, why does it have to be a separate HIV illness? Why can't (there) be chronic illness clinics?...So there has always been that slight separation, that slight distinction, it has always been very distinct that you're always HIV, um (stammer), this and that illness in itself having prolonged and pronounced stigma, this identifies a place somewhere different on the map but it does have the effect of facing it. And that is what stigma is, that sort of you where there, um, so that's got to be something too late but that's historically.

Seeing the moves within this story enables us to read the strategic shifts between particularity and normalisation involved in Gerry's 'living on' the borderline of HIV normalisation. Normalisation as chronic illness is related as working against stigma. It is also in dialogue with a responsibilised guilt now intensified by HIV's cost within cash-strapped markets. Framings of luck and privilege, here and in the majority of interviewees' stories, constrain particularistic claims. Lastly, normalisation's stigma reduction also has a 'what-if?' storyline here, since HIV's history shows that normalisation did not happen

Later again, Gerry developed this dialectic between the particularities of living with HIV and ARVs, with anecdotes of important medication discussions specific to his HIV positive friends, and his normalised, non-HIV-specific good times with his non-HIV-involved friends.

Interviews thus generated long narratives of relationship to HIV that fluctuated strategically between declaring commonality with others living with and without HIV, particularly those with other long-term health conditions, and a strong sense that HIV is not just any other condition, because of its links with sexuality, the particular history of the pandemic, and the continuing stigmatisation and self-stigmatisation that many interviewees reported.

It is worth emphasising that around half the interviewees told stories of significant recent experiences of stigma and discrimination. Penelope

reported having two very scared sisters who made her feel unwel-
come, no longer borrowed her clothes, bleached the bath, and kept the
windows open when she stayed, as well a potential partner who 'ran
away', all working against what she called 'normal life'. She too said that
other HIV positive people were special to her, particularly in the absence
of the generalised friendship and family support woven through Gerry's
stories. Penelope also went to church with her HIV support group friends
and visited them during the week. Again, her story valued the specific
services that enabled this HIV sociality, her alternative HIV 'family', and
lamented cuts in them:

> **Penelope:** Yeah (inaudible) because I dunno if it will, I dunno what
> word to use, because you try and tell people they don't want to
> know, they don't want to know and if you fall out with somebody,
> they think that they know you but they don't you know you want
> to be open they don't want that, so you find yourself, like isolated
> /sure/so it's not easy mhm I try by all means but at times it does
> get to me, you know it will just live like a normal life but it does
> get to me mm yeah ... but I'm afraid most of them, support groups
> have closed down because of funding so there's not really, much
> to do you know and it's very difficult to to, like I've got my sisters
> and brothers they don't understand like when I'm feeling sick
> most of the times I'm feeling not well, if you tell them they don't
> understand but if you talk to somebody in the same situation they
> would understand you know so I am more closer to people, who
> are in the same situation, as I am, yeah.

Apart from stigma, illness and emotional pain, interviewees narrated
a range of other non-normal aspects of three-letter lives. Sometimes,
requirements to eat well, exercise regularly and be very sexually careful
were pointed out as not normal, an imposition of hyper-responsibility. A
number of interviewees were upset that HIV negative people, particularly
heterosexuals, were less often described as 'barebacking'. The one area
where HIV is clearly not socially normalised but criminalised is indeed
around sexuality. People living with HIV and ARVs are 'normal' in popular
discourse except that they are required to disclose their HIV status in
sexual relationships, whatever the activity, as we heard in Robert's story in
Chapter 5. The move from responsibilising to criminalising HIV positive
citizens was a particular concern for the heterosexual people in the study,
especially for people dealing with citizenship issues, for whom criminal
charges might mean deportation. Moreover, the multiple meanings of

silence around HIV status, what it means about HIV status in relation-ships, and whether to use or not use a condom, appeared in stories told by gay and heterosexual interviewees. It even showed up in some inter-viewees' own silences about not using condoms until quite late in their narratives. HIV citizenship is heavily socially as well as legally policed when it involves sexuality. Perhaps for that reason, interviewees 'living on' the borders of normalised relationships made many attempts to define those borders. For instance, they tried to specify the appropriate range of HIV citizenly responsibilisation in terms of when and how HIV status should be disclosed to actual or potential sexual partners.

Other 'normals'

'Normal life' involves many factors other than HIV, and so did the interviews. Participants very often marked the larger significance of, for instance, work issues, relationship issues or, for migrants, citizen-ship status and loss of contact with their children in countries of origin. Penelope had been in detention, treated 'like a convict'. She did not have citizenship status. She had left her children in her country of origin and, she said, in the process had betrayed them. One had died there, one had been abused by a carer. Her grief about this was paralysing. Her own survival, and her ability to send money to her children, which other women in similar situations cited positively, appeared across her narra-tives as relatively unimportant. By contrast, women migrants who had gained citizenship and brought their children to the United Kingdom through 'family reunion' programmes, like Olive, often directed their narratives towards this salvational conclusion rather than towards any other aspect of their HIV experiences. Good relationships (sero-concordant or sero-discordant), satisfying work and economic stability similarly shaped many narratives of redemption, relatively independent of how 'living on' with HIV was going. Moreover, as Olive said, when you are doing well on the medication, you sometimes wonder if indeed you have HIV. This indicates the degree to which HIV can move to the side of UK three-letter lives. You can 'live on', at times, as if viral status borderlines have been erased. You are normalised into a non-HIV-defined citizen, with normal responsibilities. However, you must still engage with the possible self-care responsibilities of HIV's particular illnesses and side effects (severe in Olive's case) and with the exceptional other-care responsibilities that attend sexual relationships involving HIV (though Olive was not looking for a relationship).

The 'normal' is also social. Across people's intersectional lives, some categories are more normal than others. Unmarked social normality involves middle-classness, maleness, heterosexuality, middle adult-hood, able-bodiedness, health and mental health, citizenship, educa-tion-generated cultural capital, family and friendship social capital, and resources of time and possessions. HIV stigma relates to these social differences too (Parker and Aggleton 2003). Many interviewees indi-cated how relationships, friendships, children, work or other activities you love, and access to psychosocial service support protected normalcy. One emphasised that living long-term and in a relatively manageable way with HIV depended on his having his own house and some savings. Another participant, Peter, a man in his 50s, narrated his life difficulties in relation to career disappointments rather than HIV status. Several more described their relationships as central to 'living on' happily. For one female interviewee who refused to re-interview, not HIV but another illness now defined her relationship to the world. 'Normal' is not homo-geneous, and its coordinates shift. Several young gay male participants normalised their own relations to HIV by contrasting themselves to an older generation of under- and poorly-treated gay men. At the same time, they told stories of cross-age friendships with older gay men that erased these normalising boundaries too.

Strategising the para-normal

How do these responsibilising stories, both normalising and denormal-ising, move away from an individualised focus on what each narrator, separately, 'ought' to do? As with research participants' redefinition of 'health as care' in the previous chapter segment, many interviewees' stories broadened their orientation during the course of their telling, moving from being stories of 'me' to stories of 'us', groups or collec-tives defined by historical or social coordinates. Such moves enabled the stories to trouble the boundaries of normalisation, turning HIV's 'new normal' into a para-normalisation. Gerry, for instance, remembering his own and others' experiences of earlier local psychosocial HIV care, suggested, as we have seen, micro-social support solutions of similar kinds: drop-ins with cupcakes. Later, after narrating the ambiguous value of separating off HIV from other health and social conditions, he formu-lated a kind of 'para-normal' role for employment services for HIV posi-tive people whose health is managed by ARVs. These services would be sensitive to positive people's particular requirements, here specified as them saying 'it's ok to go do this', but they would not be HIV specific:

> **Gerry:** There was a problem with people feeling th, that their lives were being defined by HIV with a wrong approach, but it {HIV} does

exist, but let's find the way to deal with it, but you don't want to be defined by HIV, so! So it still exists. It does exist, I am living with it. I have it so, I would like to find a way of, dealing with that, but making a parallel of, something else, I had to go on the internet on a web design course. I found that very useful and that was something I could do and there have to be this kind of things. I would like to be a cook for example, if there is any other place I can go. It does not have to be on HIV or positive people, it doesn't have to be like that. I need to, someone to tell me, it is okay to go do this, you know!

Within contemporary 'neo-liberal' market economies, Gerry's suggestions constitute allowable exceptions. Psychosocial as well as health services like drop-ins may indeed be required to keep the unemployed mentally as well as physically alive. Some workers need investment in their skills, knowledge and self-belief if they are to be employable. However, the neo-liberal subject is fundamentally market-determined: Potentially, all subjects are effective, productive parts of the whole. This means that the neo-liberal subject is a kind of sophistic construct. As a subject, riven with conflicts and uncertainties, it does not really exist at all. But Gerry's and many other interviewees' normalisation stories of 'living on' created very different kinds of HIV citizens. The stories operated in at most para-liberal ways, accountable to and taking account of markets, but not fully determined by them. Gerry's memory of the early days of HIV social support begins one story: 'I can remember from ten years ago, living in {London borough} there used to be all these, come sit down, have a cup of tea'. The story immediately above ends with a call for social recognition as an HIV citizen: 'I need to, someone to tell me, it is okay to go do this, you know!' These are strong counteracting narrative elements; marketised HIV discourse has no necessary relation to them.

Such para-normalising narrations of HIV and ARVs are not easy to produce. In the interviews, they often took place over long passages of talk that moved back and forth across borderlines. They did not emerge straightforwardly as rational arguments or persuasive conversational turns. Similarly, some interviewees who told stories about their own normalising practices, such as Olive, Gerry and Zack, who spoke about being open about their status, recounted not so much normalisation, as efforts at normalisation. They described doing hard work towards normalisation, and against a secrecy that both results from and generates stigma, and that they thought would, like HIV, destroy you from inside (Squire 2007).

Such para-normalising efforts also worked both with and against marketisation. Olive, for example, was keen to take her informal support services into the welfare market as some male interviewees from migrant backgrounds had done. Perhaps her gender inhibited such a move, for markets are not gender-neutral in practice as they are in discourse. More importantly, however, the marketplace does not operate with the kinds of subjectivity that Olive's negotiations of HIV's para-normality repeatedly insisted on. In the account quoted at the beginning of the chapter, her commitment to emotional empathy for people who are not just HIV positive but also migrants, parents missing their children, and grieving family members, and her taking social care into her own hands and home for people who were depressed, anxious and isolated, acted independently of any market rationale.

The next segment of this chapter examines perhaps less subtle strategic narratives of 'living on' HIV borderlines, in this case, on the borders of marketisation processes as they currently play out within UK three-letter lives.

Marketisation: does the HIV citizen exist?

The narrative of HIV and ARVs' cost-effectiveness

As we have seen in previous segments of this chapter and in Chapter 6, health and social welfare provision around HIV are increasingly formulated according to marketised logics. This last segment of Chapter 8 describes some more specific aspects of 'living on' in the United Kingdom's current marketised epidemic, and what this means for HIV citizens like those involved in my HIV support study. It starts, however, with some attention to marketised policy around HIV.

The 2011 edition of the United Kingdom's 'HIV in Primary Care' document (Madge et al. 2011) is a good example. In the United Kingdom, the rationale for shifting more HIV care to the primary health sector is partly about access, especially to testing, partly about increasing staff resources, and very largely now about cost-effectiveness. In its foreword, this document states, 'evidence is clear that early diagnosis has long-term health benefits and allows for cost-effective management of HIV as a long-term condition, preventing expensive and distressing major medical interventions further down the line'. Such prioritisations of cost were much less common prior to the global financial crisis. Later, 'timely' ARV treatment is foregrounded as 'cost-effective' ARV choice is likely, the document says, to be determined 'increasingly' by cost, and GP-based universal testing for new registrants in particular high-prevalence areas is advanced on the basis of US cost-effectiveness studies (Madge et al. 2011: 5, 13, 46).

Marketisation can seem to naturalise HIV into a problem whose solutions are openly accessible if paid for. In the current UK context, this narrative of how to deal with HIV is also now concerned with following a plotline of cost-benefit analyses to a budget-consistent conclusion. Again, though, this narrative frame has perpetually to deal with exceptions: aspects of personal and social lives that are not profitable and often, not even susceptible to a marketised framing. Certainly, cost-benefit analyses are only part of the narrative on GP HIV care presented in the document on primary care quoted earlier, and they are often at odds with other accounts, focused in this case on, for instance, social welfare or professional standards. This document and other, similar ones move across the borders of incommensurable explanatory frameworks all the time.

Marketisation narratives of HIV have other policy implications. Open markets give PWLAs rights as consumers. The 42% of people receiving HIV care who are in London have resources to choose from. Many London-based interviewees reported shopping around for consultants or, like Olive, GPs. Some interviewees also presented a cost-benefit analysis of the relative advantages of London-based resources, cutting-edge but often under pressure, versus the resources available in other cities, perceived as less expert by, for instance, John, but for others, as more available. A 2008 study suggests 25% of people travel for their HIV care, choosing the professionals that suit them best (Huntingdon et al. 2008). The UK epidemic thus provides many examples of patients operating as consumers within health markets. These marketised aspects of policy, as lived by patients, interact with other, incommensurable frameworks for storying care. They may be based, for instance, in the case of travelling for services, on habit, stigma avoidance and the desire for anonymity, as much as quantifiable expertise.

The 2011 interviews from the UK HIV support study provide, as has already become clear in this chapter, many instances of the marketisation of three-letter lives in the particular UK context of fiscal crisis and health and social welfare cuts, as well as examples of people's counteracting stories. In previous rounds of this research, participants told complex stories of biomedical understandings and interventions, social and cultural formations and subjective positionings in relation to the epidemic, and their changes. However, the latest interviews were the first to be structured so strongly into market-framed narratives. In these narratives, some of the constraints operating on market frameworks because of HIV citizens' limited resources, and the counteracting narratives operating against marketisation, became clearer than in policy materials.

The interviews contained some very thoroughgoing marketisation stories. These stories, like those of Jana, Penelope and Gerry, shown earlier in the chapter, traced drug restrictions and cuts, and reductions in time, goods and services in medical and psychosocial care. Several interviewees described being notified of drug prices by doctors or pharmacists, strong instances of contemporary cost-based framings of treatment which they suggested would not happen in the case of other illnesses. Many participants told of purchasing self-care through alternative or complementary therapies. Such stories often explicitly criticised market approaches to services. Zack presented himself as forced to pay for psychotherapy to avoid the long NHS waiting times. As we have seen, Jana's criticisms built up across the interview to refute 'time is money' pressures on consultant appointments.

The availability of general resources also constrains participation in health markets. Interviewees closely linked their narratives of HIV's medicalisation and normalisation to socioeconomic factors such as employment, pensions, property ownership, citizenship, and other social, cultural, and educational resources. In these stories, marketisation shut off non-wage-earning people living with HIV in the United Kingdom, especially migrants with only voucher income, from a variety of goods: psychosocial services that were in short supply within the NHS; benefits that required initial 'iinvestments' of travel, visits and phone calls; social networks that required similar 'investments' to stay active; support and leisure activities that necessitated travel; and good food, for food insecurity affects HIV's prognosis in developed as well as developing countries (Weiser et al. 2009). Sometimes, the economic situation of one's country of origin can continue to affect ways of living with HIV and ARVs within the UK, as with Penelope's initial prescription of cheaper, less-suitable ARVs on offer in her home country.

It was in relation to such resource-driven exclusions that interviewees' stories were most critical. Sometimes, the stories simply opposed their narrators' marginalisation. More often, told from the sharply analytic standpoint of those excluded, they brought structures of inclusion and exclusion, and the borders between them, into question. Living as an HIV citizen outside of marketised participation in socioeconomic life was often recounted as a highly determining and difficult aspect of 'living on'.

In addition, many interviewees' counteracting narratives operated, as in the cases of medicalisation and normalisation, around the edges of neo-liberalism, rather than in any direct opposition to it. As we have seen, Gerry and Olive formulated 'para-normal' strategies for people living with HIV and ARVs' support and integration into training and work that were intimately connected to people living with HIV's ability to make economic contributions. But sometimes, merely articulating the problematic marketisation of health and social life, as Penelope did when she laid out the economic restrictions with which she lived, as an asylum-seeker subsisting on vouchers, could be a counteracting narrative. At a time when explicitly activist and politicised forms of counteracting stories of HIV were less common, resistances got expressed, as we have seen around medicalisation and normalisation, in more personalised but still questioning and insistent ways.

HIV isn't working

Formulations of HIV citizenship in terms of economic contribution were a prominent focus in interview stories. Such stories positioned interviewees as exclusively and narrowly marketised subjects. Narrators were deserving, even existing, to the extent that they did paid work, rather than through social, political or human entitlements to citizenship or to subjectivity. At the same time, the narrators resisted this reduction of themselves, often by edging some other kind of work, or an explicit alternative to it, into the story. Many interviewees described the centrality of work, even work they did not value, within their lives. They particularly valued it if it was flexible, part-time and from home, especially when they were dealing with ongoing illness. A number of female and some male participants who were unemployed, like Gerry and Daniel, told life-affirming stories against the centrality of work, focused on family and friendship. However, many male and some female interviewees who were unemployed, like Olive, presented their lives in terms of the social and personal value of their voluntary 'work'. A few men, like Peter, whose interview traced in great detail how he had become shut out of his career, expressed sorrow and rage about being excluded from work.

The stories of migrant participants frequently, as in other research, were 'what-if' tales about wanting to work and to be included citizens. Penelope's story of her inability as an asylum seeker to gain voluntary work, to 'give back', is posed against the resources she has received as an HIV positive person, and contrasted to the absence of HIV resources in her home country. It presents her as exiled from citizenship by her inability to participate even in the voluntary sector, which, following Ong (2006), we could characterise as working at present partly against the discourses and practices of markets, but also increasingly as an unmarked, necessary, ameliorative, but market-mimetic and para-liberal 'exception' to neo-liberalism:

> **Penelope**: I don't want anything I just want to live a normal life and er, I'm not after benefits, where I come from, nobody gives you anything you have to work for everything /yeah/ you can go to the hospital if you don't have money they will not treat you so I really appreciate being in this country and um getting my treatment and accommodation you know in my country nobody will give you that and if I could I would really want to pay back you know, just do something just help somebody/ of course of course sure/yeah like a/like a support worker or a/Yeah help somebody, an elderly lady, somebody, I want to pay back and do something but it's not easy because there a lot of um, I dunno if I should say it nasty, nasty criminals you know who are after something who are not really willing to help, I don't want, I don't want any payment I just want to help somebody you know because to be where I am now if I was in my country I would of been dead...yes, I don't know what else to do, you know who to turn to, can't do anything can't plan can't do nothing just doing the same thing every day, go out come back sit watch TV go to bed wake up same thing.

Penelope's story has HIV as its starting point, but it concerns the marketised exclusion of non-citizens, rather than only HIV positive people. For Penelope, these two exclusions are lived with together. Her narrated experiences of HIV stigma intensify the social exclusion of the asylum seeker. A narrative approach allows us to see how each narrative strand potentiates the other. Reading this story against the dominant narrative of the naturalised and marketised HIV citizen also allows us to see how Penelope, like other interviewees, must put herself into the position of that citizen, and must set herself against those who break with it, such as the 'nasty criminals'.

More ability to negotiate a kind of para-liberal place from 'outside' of employment appeared in participants' narratives when they had more resources, as with Olive, who had citizenship status, or Gerry, who was both a citizen and someone with a history of knowing about and participating in HIV activism:

> **Gerry**: And as well, I had lately, been medically reassessed through benefits and, and quite, left a number of stresses um and again I don't know if I am about to be reassessed but when I do I am sure I

am going to be quite upset because I know who I am or ah, I mean I have read on the internet that there are charities that deal with that but again it's a little bit, that seems a little bit like, there's isn't a personal, someone to put inside, to put around, something to say 'don't worry', to be called for an interview with you...um it's almost that I feel like, I feel I am being told that I am out of life, because if you have a life then you don't need benefit and support, you can get up and work.

Gerry's narrative could be read as being about depression, illness and not working, rather than specifically about HIV. However, the particularities of 'living on' for a long time through the difficult history of the epidemic shape his narrative both of his current state and of what could be. The apparent 'incoherences' in the story, the stops and starts, operate to allow these different narrative trajectories a place, as well to express the problematic of finding a story that you can tell when it is also the story of how 'you are out of life' (Hyvarinen et al. 2010; Squire 2012, 2008, 2005). At the same time, Gerry's repeated articulation of his citizenly exclusion serves to put that exclusion in question.

Marketised exclusion

Exclusion from markets was described as restricting people's nutrition, transport, communication and leisure activities, to an extent that sometimes shut them out not just from the workforce but from almost all social interactions except those with their clinic. Such economic and consequently social sequestering of people living with HIV and ARVs regulates and punishes them as a subset of the poor (Piven and Cloward 1993; Wacquant 2009). It is of course not a process exclusive to people living with HIV; it happens much more generally to people living with severe or chronic illness. However, the sequestering performed by HIV's stigmatisation and the poor health often accompanying three-letter lives intensify this isolation. The result is that people living with HIV and ARVs are relegated to a deeply unnaturalisable but unremarked form of citizenship, outside the social order. It is almost as if contemporary marketisation results in HIV positive citizens not being citizens at all. As with the 'poor', a category which no longer seems to allow full citizenship within it, market thinking is pushing people living with HIV and perhaps those with other serious chronic illnesses to 'live on' a social borderline, where it is a struggle to keep on the vital side.

Quentin, for example, like many interviewees who were not working or who did not have family and friendship networks, described a life mapped out around clinic appointments and support group meetings, after which he went home once again to his isolated flat. This was the same kind of routine that Penelope described, even though, unlike her, Quentin had citizenship status and could and did intermittently work. Sean and Tyler, too, though they were not part of the earlier illness and treatment 'generations' who might seem most likely to become isolated, lived very largely within the confines of a small flat. They were 'shut away' by poor health and economic resources, with significant deficits also in their family and friendship resources. They presented themselves less as citizens living with HIV, more as non-citizens, pushed out of society by their HIV status. As Sean said:

> **Sean:** We don't feel we are living with HIV, well I don't, it's more like HIV is everything I am.

At the same time, both men spent large amounts of time engaging with processes operating outside this sequestered environment, which operated paradoxically to keep them there. These processes included clinic consultations, GP social worker appointments, sending emails and researching online. The processes preserved their physical and mental health, as well as the benefits they were entitled to and that would enable them to retain health. Yet they did this with, it seemed, the minimal aim of keeping them physically rather than socially alive. Sean and Tyler were thus imbricated in a mimetic welfare market within which they had to work for outcomes, and would lose out if they did not. This second marketisation operated practically, if not discursively, in concert with the first, managing these exceptional citizens that could not be brought into the neo-liberal economic or social project. It corralled Sean and Tyler into a socially excluded non-citizenly space, yet the men had to engage with the broader parameters of marketised citizenship all the time in order to ensure even that minimal space. Despite this doubled exclusion, Sean and Tyler told many counteracting stories of maintaining their own space, and criticising its boundaries.

Frequently, research participants who were living in a more socially included way, nevertheless seemed also to be living continuously with the possibility of exclusion. They told many stories about the present possibilities of reduced income, becoming unemployed, losing benefits. The what-if narratives of this liminal group about being made poor or otherwise excluded, index the borderline liveability of what is sometimes now called the precariat (Standing 2011). This term may gloss over some important differences between people living precarious economic lives, but it is useful, even across those differences, to describe the tightrope quality of some three-letter lives. Living in contemporary market conditions in the United Kingdom means that you are always living with the possibility of marketised exclusion. The resource strains imposed by HIV intensify this borderline experience. That polarising situation should not, though, lead us to conceptual simplism that misses out what people living with HIV and ARVs do within situations of potential exclusion to act against it.

Conclusion

The UK HIV situation could be read as a limit case for neo-liberalism because some of the neo-liberal options available may have fatal effects. These options include cheap medicines that are not the best for you, or that may produce other problems, or that interact badly; non-treatment, detention or expulsion of HIV positive migrants; and the cutting of psychosocial services around HIV lives, such as support groups, transport and training.

The recession and its marketised solutions are making counteracting narratives harder to produce. However, the material from the 2011 interviews indicates that people living with HIV and ARVs in the UK are producing numerous counteracting stories of resistance to and negotiation with the social and economic characteristics associated with neo-liberalism. These stories remake claims and reframe HIV activism, even though this is happening within a limited set of possible responses and effects.

The conceptual and practical limits of neo-liberalism suggest that we might do better to set it aside when describing what the contemporary situation looks like. Intense marketisation and living with the cuts, rather than neo-liberalism *per se*, characterise the UK epidemic situation. People excluded from HIV markets often have contracted, narrowed lives, like many others for whom recession constricts their experiences. In the case of HIV and, perhaps, other chronic conditions, citizens are being reduced by austerity policies to bodies kept more or less physically functioning and to subjectivities continually trying to keep on the living side of psychosocial as well as health borderlines. Activism in these circumstances can take the forms of constructing or reconstructing HIV collectivities, affirming HIV citizenship, asserting HIV subjectivity, or simply recording the processes that might make these conditions possible. 'Living on' activism could perhaps be as 'sly civility' (Bhabha 1994), a para-liberalism that does not confront the dominant forces around the epidemic head-on. Instead, it approaches them tangentially, sometimes undermining them. Instead of asking the socio-moral questions common in canonic self-narratives – 'what have you done?' and 'who are you?' – it responds to other questions: 'who might you have been?', 'what could be done?', and 'what might we say?'

It may be that these kinds of counteracting, 'living on' narratives, spoken and acted, are common in other borderline, resource-constrained situations at this conjuncture. For instance, they may appear around other health and disability issues, and around refugee and asylum contests. I cannot explore these 'translation' possibilities further here (Lincoln and Guba 1985). However, in the next chapter, I explore another translation possibility: of how similar moves might be said to be happening in the particular high-prevalence, medium-income context of HIV and ARVs in South Africa. That context demands, though, a distinct empirical and theoretical account.

9
Living with HIV: Three-letter Lives in South Africa

She had wondered earlier...where this thing could have come from. I wanted her to understand that there was no point, there could be no point in trying to dig out the roots. Sex and sex; love and sex; compassion, kindness, generosity and blood donations, the blood tests when the doctors tried to understand her earlier ailments, injections, needles...who could know where the roots lay?...We did not talk. We shed, shared tears. Platefuls of tears of love and sex...

Phaswane Mpe ('God doesn't smoke dagga', 2008: 187)

AIDS came with democracy. As we started our negotiations in 1990, the epidemic was seeping in and became a flood. By 1994...as we became a democracy nearly 20 years ago, 5 per cent national prevalence. And five years later, amongst young sexually active adults, an almost 20 per cent prevalence. Terrifying. And so [as] a defining feature we grappled with it...the Treatment Action Campaign, the street level activists, the township people and the unions and the churches took president Mbeki to court and won a court order saying that his policy on AIDS drugs was not reasonable, it was actually irrational. When we were told Africans can't take medications...told by our own black health minister, when were told that medical infrastructure will collapse...we've done it. And to me, as a very proud African and South African it means that we can do a lot of other things that we don't think we can do. And I think it's a good portent for a great future for our country.

Edwin Cameron (2013)

For {my family} to accept {my status}, I think it's because they
know that, maybe since things have been spoken about people
living with HIV killing themselves because of HIV. So I think
they saw me telling them that I am HIV positive, and I have
accepted that I am HIV, so I don't want anyone crying to me
because I am HIV positive, or someone avoiding me because I
am HIV positive. Because HIV is something that we are used to
now, it's like any other disease, it's like TB, all the diseases when
you take your medication you get well, so I never stressed about
that but my family was by my side.

                                      Nombulelo (South Africa, 2012)

Introduction

In summer 2012, I attend the International Congress of Psychology at the
Cape Town conference centre; the event overlaps with a South African
fashion exposition. Psychologists are, in the main, utilitarian dressers.
In the evening, though, this ferociously air-conditioned palace of glass
is taken over by the fashion crowd: immaculately coiffed, dressed to
impress, with dramatic shoes. Given the statistics, many of these South
Africans are likely to be living with HIV. But everyone looks healthy,
and the space is clearly hosting the upside of the country's record-
breaking Gini coefficient, the generally accepted measure of national
inequality. I have a meeting in the lobby with an acquaintance, a sometime worker in the HIV sector. Like most in that sector, my visitor could
be said to be a member of the South African 'precariat' (Standing 2011),
a group that in this country includes many with quite high levels of
social and cultural capital. Even for someone like my visitor, with high
school education and a good employment history, jobs are generally
short-term, with reduced benefits. This woman has just lost hers. Her
HIV treatment is assured and she receives a child support grant, but she
is too well to get a disability grant and the unemployment benefit for
which, like a small minority of South African workers, she is eligible,
will not last long (Bhorat et al. 2013). She does not have money for
minibus, taxis or trains, so her range of work-seeking opportunities is
limited. She takes a few photos of the beautiful people on her phone,
which she can still charge and which gives her free texts, before she
leaves.

Shortly after this encounter, I visit a support group I've worked with
before. My prior involvement with this group, among others, had led
to a book publication. It has been decided that the group's share of the

very modest royalties will be used to buy nutritious food to share out between all members. The group facilitator, a retired professional, has a car. She, I, and a couple of group members visit a cash and carry. We load up with sacks of beans, cornmeal, tinned fish, oil, and a few extras like cheap biscuits for the children. By the end, one of the group members is clearly fatigued by hefting large loads to the car; she sits out of the sun and rests. Around twenty core group members, contacted by a texting tree, and in some cases by neighbours from the group going round to their houses, arrive at the support group site. Food distribution is overseen with deep care and impartiality by a woman who has been in the group for over ten years. There is one extra packet of biscuits; these are distributed among the few children who've come along with their parents. Other parents grumble that their children have missed out on the extra biscuits, but there seems to be general satisfaction that things have been managed fairly.

Here, precarity is more extreme. In terms of social and cultural resources, the situation is similar to that described for people in higher-income countries living on the edge. Few group members have a formal employment history, though a couple have done small amounts of paid work with HIV organisations. Some group members are unwell enough to receive disability grants, despite being on ARVs; most get child support grants. None have the cultural capital of a finished high school education. Many have saleable skills such as sewing and cooking, but these are in abundance in the informal settlement where they live and they do not have ways to sell them elsewhere. The continuing social capital provided by the text tree, the middle-class facilitator, and the group itself, is, however, very helpful.

This chapter explores how HIV and ARVs are lived with in a country very different to the United Kingdom, as considered in Chapter 8: the high-prevalence, medium-income context of South Africa. The chapter considers how, in this context, HIV's naturalisation is both expressed and resisted in specific processes of medicalisation and demedicalisation, normalisation and denormalisation, marketisation and demarketisation, and 'being left behind'. In applying these considerations to an economic, social and cultural situation very different from that of the United Kingdom, the chapter will examine another field of particularities at work in three-letter lives, and will discern how processes may be held in common, differently articulated, or radically distinct.

In the United Kingdom, we have seen how the processes involved in 'living on' with HIV and ARVs are currently strongly shaped by market-oriented policies and austerity measures, common across the global north. At the same time, interviewee narratives analysed in Chapter 8 operated to counteract these dominant discourses and practices. They worked within the spaces and at the blurred borders that disturb the apparent homogeneity of 'neo-liberalism'. The research participants' narratives effected these disruptions and reformulations both by direct challenges, and by a kind of 'para-liberal' undermining of 'market' and 'austerity' discourses and practices.

In the case of South Africa, we might expect to see rather different particularities characterising lives lived with HIV and ARVs. For there, the resources available to address the epidemic are significantly fewer in people's everyday lives, the history of the epidemic has taken a unique form, and given the ubiquity of HIV, the whole country could be said to live a three-letter life. 'Living with' HIV is something that is in a broad sense common to almost all the population, since every family, every friendship group, and every workplace is affected. However, people 'live with' HIV differently, depending first of all upon HIV status, which continues to put an exceptional weight on people's lives that cannot, any more than in the United Kingdom, be fully normalised, that is treated as 'like' other kinds of physical, social and economic difficulties, and as a regular rather than exceptional part of human life.

In the quotation at the beginning of this chapter from a 2012 interview with Nombulelo, an HIV positive woman in her late 40s, Nombulelo asserts to her family that HIV is 'just like' other illnesses that can be treated, such as TB. ARVs have indeed turned HIV into a liveable condition in South Africa, as in the United Kingdom. Nombulelo's story of how her family thought things through after her diagnosis and how she explained things to them, would have been less likely to have been told in the first decade of the twenty-first century. Nevertheless, Nombulelo's insistence (here and in other places in the interview) on the simile, on how HIV is indeed '*just* like' (my emphasis) the other conditions, and her recounting of her and her family's response to earlier, suicidal responses, mark, by their very force, the difficulty, as in the United Kingdom, of making HIV liveable and normal. Nombulelo's account of HIV as something 'we are used to' is also ambiguous. It could, as here, be the grounds of acceptance and positive living. But in the context of high prevalence, with HIV affecting every family, 'something we are used to' sometimes grounds a story of a more fatalistic kind, in which HIV can be 'lived with' but nothing can be done about it. Such stories are less heard in the UK context, and perhaps would be less audible in well-resourced South African contexts, too (Zungu 2012).

Other particularities within the South African narratives I will be considering derive from patterns of past and present illness, whether ARVs are being taken and how they are working out, what kind of psychosocial support is available, and what the other difficulties and resources in people's lives are. Nombulelo marks the good socio-emotional resources she now has, contrasting them with back-stories of family rejection; but such stories are not all in the past.

The excerpt at the beginning of this chapter from a short story by Phaswane Mpe, which ends with the results of an HIV test, sketches some of the uncertain personal, medical and political histories that can swirl around an HIV diagnosis in the South African context. The 'platefuls of tears' shed between the young people trying to come to terms with the diagnosis might be served up anywhere. The current successes of medication may mitigate them for people diagnosed now, but they do not erase them. Moreover, the characters' narrative struggles to have things make sense are differently configured in this story than they would be for people living three-letter lives in other national contexts. They are inflected, for instance, by South Africa's history of neglecting or ignoring HIV, by years of deaths, silence, stigma and lack of treatment.

'Living with' HIV is always a matter of living with many other intersecting identities at the same time. In the South African context, as in many other low- and middle-income countries, resource limitations determine the narrative tracks of HIV positive lives, more strongly than in high-income countries like the United Kingdom (Brandt 2008; Long 2009). This limitation, rather than the history and invisible present of 'living on' that threads through the UK narratives, structured participants' accounts. Stories of contemporary three-letter lives in the UK trace, as we saw in the previous chapter, people's efforts to continue 'living on' the borderlines of markets and cuts, as well as of HIV's own difficulties. In contemporary South Africa, stories of living with HIV and ARVs are even less distinguishable from stories about resources. They are stories of 'living with' HIV and unemployment, poverty, food insecurity, ARV insecurity, other poverty-related health issues such as transport costs to clinics (Tuller et al. 2010), the expense of buying healthy food and personal hygiene items, health and social service deficits, and the particular issues facing, for instance, poor HIV positive women, or poor HIV positive youth, or older people, or non-South Africans living in South Africa, all at the same time.

A corollary of the complex intersectionality of 'living with' HIV in South Africa appears in recent changes in civil society. Here, community activism and policy engagements have shifted towards the mainstreaming of HIV within health and social policy, and the broadening of organisational remits from HIV towards health and social justice generally. For example, members of the Treatment Action Campaign and others have formed the Social Justice Coalition, campaigning on local issues such as xenophobia, crime, policing, gender-based violence, and infrastructure. Like Nathaniel, the young man whose move from HIV work into more general activism I described in Chapter 2, activists in this organisation who might previously have focused on HIV issues now view pressing community issues more broadly. Similarly, the influential AIDS Law Project has shifted to adopt a broader health remit, taking its new name, Section 27, from the section of the South African Constitution that guarantees health rights for all.

Nevertheless, many organisations retain their focus on HIV. The Treatment Action Campaign has taken on TB treatment, gender-based violence, xenophobia, pharmaceutical patent restrictions, and South Africa's new National Health Insurance scheme as current, closely HIV-related concerns. However, it continues to advocate for better HIV treatment options, and for more efficient HIV services, pressing for changes when there are problems with ARV supply in particular towns or provinces, for example (http://www.tac.org.za/). A smaller service organisation, the Etafeni Daycare Trust, operating in the Western Cape and Limpopo, has had a long-term mission to help children who have lost parents because of HIV, and to support those who care for HIV positive or HIV-affected children. Despite falling numbers of children orphaned through HIV, much-improved treatment for HIV positive children and carers, grant support for carers, and the pressing needs of other children in the community, the trust has maintained its original focus and continues to frame its work in terms of children's social and emotional development and community empowerment, as well as in terms of skills-building, employment and sustainability (http://www.etafeni.org/).

The following segment of the chapter describes some of the specific factors of the current South African epidemic that provide the context for 'living with' HIV.

Living with HIV in South Africa

All national epidemics have their own specificities, but the South African HIV epidemic has a highly particular trajectory and nature that is widely known. Currently, over 6 million South Africans are living with HIV, the highest number in any country. South Africa also has relatively good medical and social welfare provision for HIV positive people, including, since late 2012, universal access to ARVs (that is, 80% or more of people requiring them, according to the World Health Organisation's 2010 guidelines, are able to receive them, an increase of 75% over the past few years) and a disability grant available for those whose CD4+ T cell count falls below 200 T cells/mm^3, as well as for those in certain other HIV-related illness circumstances (Irin News 2012; UNAIDS 2012a). Life expectancy has risen by over three years since 2009, largely thanks to ARVs (Mayosi et al. 2012). The country has an effective hospital and clinic system and is able to treat effectively many difficult areas of HIV illness, with special expertise in working with children.

South Africa has also developed a slew of valuable public and voluntary sector programmes to support treatment, testing, education and care. For instance, its first community-linked treatment literacy and support programmes, in the Western Cape, have been models for ARV rollout in many low- and middle-income countries (World Health Organisation 2003). Its 'mothers to mothers' support programmes for women tested and treated during pregnancy to avoid vertical transmission have again been taken up in many other national contexts, particularly in sub-Saharan Africa (http://www.m2m.org/). Its cross-media and community education programmes, particularly *Soul City*, have been models for such programmes across Africa and beyond (Usdin 2009). Its HIV activism, drawing on the country's history of anti-apartheid struggle and lesbian and gay political organisation, as well as on developed-world AIDS activism of the 1980s and 1990s, has been powerfully effective in turning lives lived with HIV into lives lived with HIV and ARVs. It has become internationally influential for other similar NGOs as well as at larger policy levels, particularly through the Treatment Action Campaign and the AIDS Law Project (Mbali 2013; Robins 2009).

More recently, the country has had a series of health ministers knowledgeable about and committed to ending the epidemic. Its 2010 universal testing programme, normalising testing by encouraging everyone to test yearly and taking testing into everyday settings (SANAC Secretariat 2010), is something that is increasingly becoming part of testing policies in high-prevalence situations worldwide, for example, as we saw in the last chapter, for high-prevalence communities and neighbourhoods in the United Kingdom. In 2012, South Africa also restructured its National AIDS Council and launched a new National Strategic Plan for HIV/AIDS (Irin News 2012; Lancet 2012). In 2013, it committed to providing daily single-pill ARV medication, a regime that makes prescribing and distributing pills, as well as taking them, much easier (Irin News 2013).

As indicated by the quote at the beginning of this chapter, from Edwin Cameron, the judge who disclosed his HIV positive status to the nation in 1999, South Africa has taken an increasingly proactive and successful approach to this largest national epidemic, in very difficult circumstances (Cameron 2013).

The HIV epidemic's enormous scale in South Africa means that its naturalisation is in some ways inevitable, though in other ways it has had to be worked for. However, the serious popular, policy and political attention to it that is currently evident, still exists alongside a history that has included neglecting HIV, minimising it or silencing it through 'AIDS denialism' (Nattrass 2009). Many deaths have affected every family, in a non-normalisable way. Adequate medical treatment must still be worked for. Pharmaceutical supply chains often break. Patients may not, for this and other reasons such as high cost and poor availability of second- and third-line ARV regimes, receive the treatment that is best for them if their first-line ARVs fail. The health system is also working with many historical and current problems (Coovadia et al. 2009; Department of Health 2012; Irin News 2013; Treatment Action Campaign and Section 27 2013).

Today, steep and increasing resource inequalities (COSATU 2013) and severe resource shortages among people living three-letter lives in poverty mean that most such lives in South Africa are edged with want; HIV is lived with many resource constraints. Unemployment, at over 25%, and poverty are indeed the main concerns of people living with HIV and ARV treatment, and these factors have major effects on their treatment. Crime and violence, especially gender-based violence, are other large-impact issues (Cloete et al. 2010; Marais 2010). At the same time, social welfare payments are constrained and are being cut, both in response to the global fiscal crisis as it impacts South Africa, and in response to the increasing budget share that larger and larger numbers of people on ARVs take up. Psychosocial services are limited in extent, and the stigmatisation and 'othering' of people living with HIV, though attenuated, continue (Abrahams and Jewkes 2012; Petros et al. 2006; Zungu 2012). Public disclosure remains problematic, across the continent as well as in South Africa. As Cameron points out, 14 years after he disclosed his status, 'I'm still the only person in a public position, holding public office in the entire continent of Africa who has spoken out about myself' (Cameron 2013).

All these factors mean that people live with and talk about HIV and ARVs in South Africa with intensity, ubiquity, sadness and fatigue but also with a habitual, everyday quality of HIV knowledge and understanding, including about ARVs, their effects and the hopeful though still problematic future they can support. None of these elements could be said to characterise stories of HIV told in the United Kingdom, though for some groups, such as recent migrants from sub-Saharan Africa, gay men, current or former intravenous drug users, and haemophiliacs, the historical narrative of HIV's silencing may have some parallels.

The current HIV situation South Africa sees 6.4 million people living with HIV, an increase attributable to the success of ARV treatment (van der Linde 2013). The figures are skewed to make this a feminised epidemic. Prevalence is 23.3% among 15–49-year-old women, and 13.3% among men in the same age range. Women's greater physiological vulnerability is augmented in the South African case by economic need, the effects of other untreated sexually transmitted infections, the effects of gender-based violence and the age-based vulnerability of younger women who get married to older men with longer sexual histories. At the same time, numbers of new cases among young people generally, especially women, are falling, and young people here, as in a number of other sub-Saharan African countries, are reporting changes in their lives that protect them from HIV transmission, such as becoming sexually active later, having fewer partners, being circumcised (for men), and using condoms more. Similar changes have happened in all age groups, though less among adult men. Overall, incidence, the number of new cases, is now 50% of the 1999 figure. However, fewer people, especially in older age ranges, are using condoms than in earlier years, possibly a shift related to widespread ARV treatment's known transmission-reducing effects[1].

There are declining numbers of fatalities within the epidemic as ARVs become more widely used and are accessed earlier within people's lives with HIV. In 2011, 270,000 South Africans were reported as dying from HIV-related causes, a fall from around 350,000 in 2006. The percentage of people taking up treatment when they are already seriously ill has fallen. South Africa has also adopted World Health Organisation guidelines, prescribing ARVs when people's C4+ T cells reach 350/mm^3. By the end of 2011 the country was providing ARV coverage to 75% of people who needed them, up from 58% the previous year. By mid-2012, the level set by the Millennium Development Goals, 80% access, had been reached. South Africa's relatively good health infrastructure, along with effective strategies of devolving ARV prescription, evaluation and management to non-specialist settings, training health professionals in HIV and ARV issues, and making community-based support part of ARV programmes, has led to survival rates that are now 86% for people who have taken ARVs for a year, up 8% since 2010.

Since 2010, the country has been implementing a comprehensive universal testing programme, taking HIV tests into community settings such as taxi ranks, shopping malls, and train stations and promoting regular testing with immediate clinic referral and follow-up for those who test positive. The effectiveness of early treatment and of treatment as prevention have been argued strongly in relation to these policies. The arguments are often closely allied to cost-benefit analyses. In addition, the testing programme has enabled South Africa to progress much faster towards its Millennium Development Goal target and to normalise HIV testing and treatment, alongside HIV prevention, as part of lives 'lived with' HIV.

The rollout of treatment means that people living long-term on life-saving yet difficult and resource-intense ARV medications will constitute a large and increasing fraction of the population for some years. (Navario et al. 2010). The country's population also includes 460,000 children up to 14 living with HIV and 2.1 million AIDS orphans, whose lives 'with' HIV are presenting separate and new challenges of their own (Republic of South Africa 2012; UNAIDS 2011a; 2012a)[2].

It is clear that a great deal has changed quickly in South Africa in relation to HIV. Greatly improved treatment access, universal testing and lower levels of stigma were some of the reasons behind my return to research sites, largely NGOs and CBOs, visited first in 2001 and then again in 2003–4, in very different circumstances (Squire 2007). Another factor impelling my partly longitudinal revisiting of the earlier study was that the steeply increasing numbers of South Africans living long-term with HIV and ARVs might be experiencing some similar issues to those that have arisen since the late 1990s for people living three-letter lives in high-income countries such as the United Kingdom. My research participants from earlier interview years, particularly those who were already taking ARVs on trials or pilots in 2001, or who had started ARVs by 2003–4, had also by 2012 been living with HIV and ARVs for over a decade in some cases, much like many of the participants in my UK HIV support study. It would not be surprising in these circumstances to find some commonalities between UK and South African research participants' narratives of living with HIV and ARVs. In both cases, interviewees are having to address the positive, yet at the same time still problematic, 'borderline' aspects of living with HIV and ARVs today.

In South Africa too, as in the United Kingdom, the global financial crisis has generated economic recession. As a significant international trading partner, producer and consumer, the country has been harmed more than many others in sub-Saharan Africa by reductions in financial inflows (Arieff et al. 2010; Padayachee 2011). These issues, alongside the internal financial pressures caused by a growing public services budget, have led to restructuring and cuts in health and welfare services supporting HIV treatment, care and prevention. At the same time, the country has to address many wider and longstanding problems: a widening Gini coefficient, larger than anywhere in the world except perhaps Brazil; mass unemployment; service under-delivery; and slow infrastructural development and land reform. There are intense debates about nationalisation and the external control of assets. There is ongoing conflict between marketised or 'neoliberal' approaches, often associated with the previous Mbeki government and focused on Black Economic Empowerment for the few – people like the fashion entrepreneurs I described earlier – and a return to a development and social justice agenda, sometimes associated, particularly within HIV policy, with campaigns for initiatives such as food programmes or basic income and chronic illness grants (Nattrass 2004; Statistics South Africa 2013).

'Neoliberalism' does not adequately describe the complex and distinct history and contemporary ideologies or practices of South Africa, its history of anti-apartheid struggle, its transforming society and politics, and its emerging economy (Ferguson 2010). The new National Development Plan, strategising up to 2030, has however been criticised by the Congress of South African Trades Unions (COSATU) somewhat in these terms, as over-reliant on exports, the service sector and entrepreneurship; tolerant of continuing inequality; pro-deregulation, the financial sector and mining; reliant on the private sector to regenerate underdeveloped regions; weak on manufacturing, industry, agriculture and social investment (COSATU 2013). The proposed National Health Insurance scheme, now being piloted, also has what are often seen as neo-liberal features. It focuses on refinancing health services, moderates costs in the private sector and involves that sector with public provision (Republic of South Africa 2011). This is a structure that has not contained costs in other countries (Lister 2013). It also does not concentrate first, as many doctors think it should, on improving state sector provision (Baleta 2012; Good 2012). It is perhaps more useful to note, not that the scheme exhibits features often viewed as aspects of neo-liberalism, but that these particular features strongly shape the current context of the HIV epidemic, in the health and social welfare systems, and in people's everyday lives (Baker 2010).

The global economic crisis and South Africa's current attempts to address it alongside internal economic and political problems, have some quite specific implications for people living with HIV and ARVs.

The restrictions now applied to disability living allowance are, as in the United Kingdom, of particular significance. However, the absolute levels of need involved in the two countries have to be taken into account. They are of course much greater in South Africa, where for people with low incomes, food security – something widely found to impact HIV illness, the success of ARV treatment and HIV prevention – is at stake (Ivers et al. 2009; Tsai et al. 2012; Weiser et al. 2009; Weiser et al. 2007).

For unemployed HIV positive but healthy women with children, child support is often the only income source. Unemployed and healthy HIV positive men have no such income. Many HIV-affected low-income families, like low-income families generally, rely on older members' pensions. While informal economy participation often provides small amounts of income for such families, and such income has been relatively unaffected by fiscal crises and public spending curbs, it has not been able to expand to make up for cuts in those areas.

Even if paid work is available, it is not always suitable for or easily available to people with chronic ill health. In the absence of employment, the disability grant has been shown many times to be highly instrumental in enabling people to take and benefit from antiretrovirals, which are easier to take and work better if one can also eat. Food support for people who are healthy on ARVs but unemployed is only sporadically available through charities. Doctors, who have to recommend the grant, are faced with difficult decisions when a patient's physical health exceeds grant standards but may, in the absence of employment and in poor social conditions, deteriorate without the grant. The disability grant has major impacts on household wellbeing, too. Without it, people may refuse to access or regularly take ARVs if they are food poor. Some may attempt to negotiate the border of poor health requirements that allow them to claim the disability grant by skipping pills, especially when they are about to have blood tests. A few may obtain income by selling ARVs to people who cannot obtain them free at public clinics, such as migrants, or to people who use the drugs prophylactically or recreationally. Most people taking ARVs, however, carefully guard their health, even if that involves the exacerbated problems of losing their disability grant (Bloch 2010; de Paoli et al. 2012; Knight et al. 2013; Nattrass 2004; Phaswana-Mafuya et al. 2009; Thornton 2013).

Such financial pressures mean, for many people living with HIV and ARVs, that they are perpetually on the borders of poverty and hunger. They are not, like many UK interviewees, concerned first of all about having some disposable income for, for instance, pharmaceutical goods, healthier food, clothes, communications (phones especially), or bus and train fares. But of course these requirements for resources that are above the most basic survival level are also significant for people living three-letter lives in South Africa, as they are in the United Kingdom. People's survival as citizens depends on them.

Researching HIV support

The most recent round in my South African HIV support study, conducted in summer 2012, was of a smaller scale than the UK study. It involved 19 interviews with people living with HIV, including two HIV negative people working long-term in public welfare and statutory fields, who had been interviewed last in 2003–4, and two HIV positive people who had been interviewed in 2001 and in one case, also in 2003–4. There were thus 15 new research participants. There was also informal contact (not recorded) with three other interviewees from previous rounds, men, who could not participate because they had moved out of the research area. 17 women were interviewed, all defining themselves as black African, as well as two black African men. All HIV positive interviewees except two were taking antiretrovirals. Years of diagnosis ranged from 1999 to one participant diagnosed early in 2011. All the rest had been diagnosed before 2009, many in the early part of that decade. The participants thus tended not to be those recently diagnosed, those who had had no illness experience or those who were not taking ARVs.

Recruitment in 2001 included many participants with no ARV access, but also a large number of women diagnosed during pregnancy who were well, and who were accessed via specific prevention of mother–to-child transmission (PMTCT) groups for women taking ARV treatment perinatally and using formula milk rather than breast milk in order to prevent vertical transmission. (This guideline is no longer universally applied; in South Africa, as women are treated while breastfeeding; see World Health Organisation 2010c). The 2012 study did not recruit via PMTCT groups because testing has generalised, so that diagnosis is less concentrated around pregnancy for women and their male partners. For this reason, but also perhaps because recently diagnosed people living with HIV who are well may now find HIV a naturalised enough condition to render support groups unnecessary, the study does not include many participants who were recently diagnosed, not on ARVs and always healthy.

New participants were recruited via two community-based organisations previously involved in the research. In one case, this was a general HIV support group meeting weekly and occasionally hosting visiting speakers. The group has usually been, like many mixed-gender HIV support groups in the area, a mainly female group, but this tendency has increased; one out of the two men currently attending took part in the research, as did 6 out of the 18 women. During the 2001–4 interviews, out of 38 research participants, 8 were men, still a small fraction given the much more similar numbers of South African women and men living with HIV, but proportionally a larger group within the study than in this more recent interview round. It may be that as HIV issues become more naturalised within the South African context, men's use of mixed-gender psychosocial support services is decreasing, and that they are accessing aspects of them that they need through women family members and friends, as indeed they were already doing in 2001. Services directed specifically at men remain popular and are judged important by policymakers (see for instance Colvin and Robins 2009), but I did not recruit from such services since I had not done so in 2001.

The second group from which participants were recruited was a project directed at women living with HIV, which had income-generation as a major remit, and which had been involved with discussions but not recruitment during the prior research. This recruitment paralleled that from women-only PMTCT groups during earlier interviews. The income-generation group, though, served a function closer to the interests of the current study round because it supports long-term living with HIV and ARVs. Moreover, even by 2001 and especially 2003–4, many participants who were still healthy, or who aware of or taking ARVs, were discussing HIV in relation to income generation. How were they to live within a low-employment economy, given what would be ongoing health problems, even with successful ARV treatment, as well as stigmatisation? In the light of these speculations, starting a decade ago, it made sense to talk about living with HIV and ARVs with participants for whom income generation was a foregrounded issue.

The UK HIV support study interviews conducted in 2011 found that stories of 'living on' with HIV were also stories of living on the borderlines of economic viability, shadowed by recession and cuts. In conducting follow-up research in South Africa, it seemed likely that the global fiscal crisis might be affecting three-letter lives there, too. Recruiting from an HIV project that had income generation as a major part of its activities meant that characteristics of living with HIV alongside financial crisis were likely to be discernible.

A practical issue affecting recruitment was that of the interview fee, set at a research assistant hourly rate in South Africa, as in the United Kingdom. This fee was much more salient for many South African than for most UK interviewees. Indeed, research participation and assistantship are part of the income-generation possibilities open to people living with HIV in South Africa. Some income-generation programmes deliberately position themselves as providing interviewers, transcribers, translators or workshop facilitators or trainers. It could be argued that the income-generation project involved with this research was doing just this.

It is, of course, problematic that a study of this kind, originally intended to recruit sizeable numbers of men as well as women, ends up as a study almost entirely of South African women's three-letter lives. In what follows, I am acutely aware of this partiality, and how it describes and re-inscribes a specific pattern of engaged HIV citizenship that sometimes seems to be particularly associated with women (Squire 2007; Steinberg 2009). It is clear from research focused on men that living with HIV in contemporary South Africa generates some very different stories than the ones heard in this research (Colvin and Robins 2009; Zungu 2012).

Members of the support groups were of varying ages, and interview recruitment reflected this. Recruitment focused on groups where almost all members were black African, and in areas of high-unemployment and large percentages of informal housing with poor infrastructure. Predictably, then, all participants were black African and most were not in formal employment. Even activity in the informal economy was low-level.

Re-interviewed participants were relatively few; tracing and re-interviewing previous participants is harder in the South African than in the UK case, for a number of reasons. First, most participants live in informal settlements around Cape Town, where addresses can be imprecise and mobility is high. Second, participants living in peri-urban areas in South Africa often have strong family links to other areas in South Africa, to which they may return at times. Third, intranational movement for work purposes is common in South Africa; mechanisms for maintaining contact, such as address forwarding and retaining phone numbers, are variable. This was especially the case over the course of this study because in 2001–4, few participants had phones, though in 2012 most had some mobile phone access. Fourth, as ARV access widened during the 2000s, participants, especially those who had moved to Cape Town specifically to get HIV treatment for themselves or, during pregnancy, for their children, were freed to move away and take up treatment elsewhere. Lastly, as noted, the 2001 interviews included a large number of women who were in PMTCT programmes. These women were mostly well at the time of diagnosis; knowing and accepting their status, they were able to access ARVs in a timely way since around 2003. They were unlikely to be members of the groups from which I recruited.

In addition, the siting of the research in peri-urban areas of the Western Cape, particularly near Cape Town, strongly affects the findings. This area has service and infrastructure characteristics much better than that of many rural areas, and indeed of many other peri-urban areas in other regions of the province and other provinces. That is especially true in relation to HIV, since PMTCT and ARVs were both trialled early in Cape Town and were rolled out first in the Western Cape (Abdullah and Squire 2010).

The interviews were conducted at the support group, at the income-generation project and, for re-contacted participants, at their places of work or where they volunteered. Interviews were semi-structured and covered topics of medical, social, family, friendship, work, online and other media, and faith support. They ranged in time from 15 minutes to 2 hours. Constraints on interview time were much stronger in some South African than in UK cases, relating, in the case of support group interviewees, to the time the support group met. Some participants were time-constrained because of childcare and domestic duties, mainly cooking, and work in the informal economy, which could not be neglected without material recompense beyond what we were offering. Participants from the income-generation group could also not afford to take much time out of their working day. Interviewing at home might have avoided these constraints. However, difficulties around confidentiality and privacy associated with home-based interviewing meant that this route was not followed (although see Long [2009] and Brandt [2008] for alternative procedures).

At the income-generation group, some interviews were conducted in Xhosa and English, with translation provided by a friend chosen by the interviewee, since many in the group were willing to do this. At the support group, all participants spoke in English.

Interviews were narratively analysed, as described in the previous chapter.

In 2001, many personal narratives told by the South African research participants concerned diagnosis, and to a lesser extent getting treatment, By 2003–4, treatment stories were a much larger part of the material. By 2012, though, diagnosis and treatment stories were often told or revisited rather briefly. Instead, as the title of this chapter indicates, research participants produced a large number of stories which focused on how 'living with' HIV and ARVs was just one aspect of lives with many other problems.

People's stories about living with HIV have always intersected with stories about other difficult positions within their lives (Brandt 2008; Ciambrone 2001; Squire 2004). However, the South African participants' 2012 stories traced not just these borderlines between being HIV positive and on treatment, and other citizenly identities, but also the likely future borders of possibility in such lives. Most commonly, too, these borders were described narratively in terms of resources. The determining element in such resource stories might seem literally or metaphorically to be economic, but we can also and perhaps better understand them by reading their determination backwards, generating counteracting stories of social relief, action and fabrication. As the last chapter described, many of the UK research participants' narratives also took a counteracting form, operating within but also against a particular national context of 'living on' with HIV and the cuts in a context of marketisation. The counteracting narratives produced by South African participants had different features. They were also stories of searching out and making resources, but they were told within South Africa's particular epidemic context of having to 'live with' HIV, ARV treatment and many other difficult conditions all together.

HIV and resourcefulness

Chapter 7 discussed how not having resources consistently works against the naturalisation of HIV, and particularly its normalisation, in many epidemic contexts. Chapter 8 contained many examples of HIV-related and more general resource constraints inflecting the narratives of people 'living on' with HIV. This chapter analyses how narrators in the South African HIV support study evaluated resources, criticised their inadequacies and explored new ways of finding and building them, within their accounts of three-letter lives lived with and against naturalising processes of medicalisation, normalisation and marketisation. To begin this analysis, I want to consider the concept of 'resource' itself.

A resource is, most generally, a capacity, either economic, social, cultural or symbolic, which allows people to perform actions. I am going to use the concept to denote means that are discernible, from the research data, for participants to support their three-letter lives.

Resources are usually considered within larger theoretical frameworks, for instance, as aspects of social and other capitals. Campbell and colleagues (Campbell et al. 2007; Campbell et al. 2012), for example, have argued that people's competence in relation to HIV and ARVs depends strongly on service access and knowledge, but also on gathered resources that they frame as different kinds of social capital. Drawing on Putnam, they distinguish bonding social capital, that is, links between people who are similar, and bridging social capital, or links between people who are different. Both kinds of social capital can contribute strongly to competence, but bridging capital can perhaps more easily become a route to other resources. Some using this framework now expand this typology to include more explicitly 'vertical' links between people with different access to social power – for instance, Dageid and colleagues (2011), researching community care and support in relation to social capital in rural KwaZulu-Natal.

Campbell and colleagues' framing also draws on the broader ideas about capital of Bourdieu (1986), for whom the term applies to accumulations of sought-after, valued and productive resources. Bourdieu's additional forms of capital – social, cultural and symbolic – are interconnected and can be converted into each other and into economic capital. I do not use these concepts of social, cultural or symbolic capitals in relation to the material discussed here because they seem too strong for it. I did not obtain full information about South African or UK research participants' social, cultural and symbolic resources, or those resources' value, productivity or convertibility, and so a more legitimate approach here is to discuss resources as they appeared within participants' stories.

There are, moreover, many theoretical problems with the 'capitals' framework. It has been criticised for failing to address gender and ethnicity in its conceptualisation of capital's different forms. It is metaphorical, and it subordinates social cultural and symbolic capitals, conceptually, to economic capital. It reifies 'capitals' as fixed holdings in ways that concepts of resources do not. The divisions between forms of capital are uncertain and often difficult to operationalise when considering empirical material. In addition, after Bourdieu, suggested forms of 'capital' have multiplied to include human capital, emotional capital, relational capital, spatial capital, and many other forms, limited only, it seems, by the number of noun-derived adjectives in sociological English. The relation of social, cultural and symbolic capital, let alone these other capitals, to 'capital' in its initial economic definition is not easy to trace. The theorisation of capitals in the plural is also often said to fail to address the producers and owners of capitals and the conflicts between them and the state (Beasley-Murray 2000; Lehtonen 2004). And so in this chapter I am confining my discussion to *resources* of social, cultural, symbolic and economic kinds. However, I define the fields of the social, cultural, and symbolic much as does Bourdieu, as involving, respectively, horizontal and vertical social relationships, including friendships, acquaintanceships, group memberships and social networks; knowledge, skills, attitudes, beliefs and objects obtained from families and educational and other institutions; and honour, prestige, recognition and symbolic representation itself. This could perhaps be called a 'weak' or pragmatic social capital approach (Lehtonen 2004).

A resource is not just goods held; it allows people to do things. In this, it has some commonality with capability, a concept often invoked in development studies work, which I again want to leave aside in favour of resource.

A focus on capabilities addresses people's abilities to achieve certain kinds of functioning, rather than their reified capital or accumulations of resources (Seckinelgen 2012; Sen 1999). It pays attention, for instance, to emotional capabilities, of the kind emphasised by the UK study participants in their reframing of 'health as care' (Nussbaum 2000). As with capital, however, our data are not complete or extensive enough to allow for a full capabilities analysis. There are, too, considerable problems associated with this approach's assumptions about what is 'good' in life and how that can be measured, its lack of attention to entrenched political power or structural inequalities in contexts such as South Africa (Unterhalter 2003), and its problematic concepts of freedom and agency. In this chapter, I use the term 'resource' broadly to include 'capabilities', that is, abilities to function, as well as the resources supporting those abilities, without theoretically separating them.

'Resource' has some meanings more connected to process and motion than to holdings and capacities. In relation to the naturalisation and denaturalisation processes shaping HIV epidemics, these processual meanings can also be helpful to bear in mind. A particular resource can act to relieve existing conditions – from, for instance, an absence of other resources. In this case, 'resource' indicates how capacities can be mobilised or brought to bear, as a response to what already exists. Etymologically, 'resource' derives from words indicating relief and rising. It connotes development and improvement; it moves things forward; it indicates resource*fulness*. Some resources are able to fulfil requirements, some respond to marked absences, others allow further actions to be taken and change to happen, as Campbell and colleagues' (2007; 2009) and Dageid and colleagues' (2011) accounts of the potentiating powers of bonding, bridging and linking social capitals on HIV and ARV competencies and community responsiveness, indicate. Psychosocial aspects of living with HIV and ARVs are a strong focus of this book, posed as they often are against more simplistic aspects of the pandemic's naturalisation. The resources that support these aspects of three-letter lives are often capacities that allow actions and futures, as much as those that fulfil unmet needs. This chapter explores the resources associated with the particular narratives of 'living with' HIV and ARVs in contemporary South Africa. We could also relate these resources for 'living with' HIV and ARVs, to 'conviviality', a term for positive forms of social association that means, indeed, 'living with'. I am drawing here on Gilroy's theorisation of conviviality in postcolonial multicultural urban settings, where it results from 'the processes of cohabitation and interaction that have made multiculture an ordinary feature of social life in Britain's urban centres and in postcolonial cities elsewhere' (Gilroy 2004: xv). This concept has been deployed to understand everyday living in heterogeneous urban areas, in situations of boundary-crossing and boundary conflict (Karner and Parker 2011). It can also usefully be drawn on to make sense of the growing associations and the ongoing, always-renewed lines of division that characterise citizenship in a situation of 'living with' HIV, operating, as it does in South Africa, across HIV statuses, and across the intersectional patterns of HIV and other citizenships and identities.

Interactions across HIV statuses, and across HIV and other citizenships, have of course developed over a long time. People have been living together in this way in South Africa, in families, at work, across friendship networks, since the 1980s. However, HIV also created, or in some cases deepened, powerful physical, social and emotional splits within all these social groupings that eroded conviviality. Failures to 'live with' HIV in South Africa appear both in people who cannot contemplate it in themselves and among people who draw lines between themselves and the HIV positive, or specific groups of HIV positive people such as HIV positive women, HIV positive men, or HIV positive poor people. In a country where HIV diagnosis and illness were so widespread and for a long time so inextricably associated with terrible suffering and unavoidable death, and where HIV was often denied, minimised or attributed to moral failings, it is especially clear that othering, stigmatisation and isolation will still to some extent limit the ability of people of all statuses to 'live with' HIV, at the same time as such living with HIV becomes more and more a part of everyday activities, thoughts and feelings.

In what follows, I describe the particularities of South African research participants' narratives of their lives 'with' HIV and the resources that enable them to live convivially, in coalition and in solidarity with each other, with people of other HIV statuses, and with people living with other difficult conditions, as HIV citizens.

The medicalisation of HIV in South Africa

Universal access, local effects

HIV's naturalisation through medicalisation has, in South Africa, high levels of recent success. As mentioned earlier, over 80% of people who need ARVs can access them; 87% of pregnant HIV positive women also receive ARVs. (Republic of South Africa 2012). Treatment is also having powerful prevention effects and is raising life expectancy, in one study in KwaZulu-Natal by 11 years (Bor et al. 2013; Cohen et al. 2011; Tanser et al. 2013). At the same time, South African doctors and activists have often challenged developed-world and international NGO medical discourses and practices. Most recently, they have questioned WHO's new early-treatment guidelines' cost-effectiveness, their likely effects on HIV positive people's long-term health, and their potential to reduce transmission (Beaubien 2013; Geffen 2013). These arguments might be described as demedicalising; they assert medical treatment as a primary goal, but they focus on 'health for all', South Africa's constitutional guarantee to its citizens, rather than on medical progress as an end in itself. Such a framing of the medical field suggests that South Africans' medicalised HIV citizenship is, as in the United Kingdom, biopolitical from the ground up, not just the top down (Colvin and Robins 2009). This is especially the case because the history of HIV activism in South Africa, as in other middle- and low-income countries, has revolved very largely around campaigns for access to high-quality medical resources (Mbali 2013; Robins 2009). More broadly, too, a medically engaged HIV citizenship is claimed and acted on by people whose knowledge comes from community and media sources, as well as from activism (Abdullah and Squire 2010; Squire 2007).

It was perhaps to be expected that in this study, recruiting from support services rather than, for instance, clinics or the general community, there were few recently diagnosed or well HIV positive interviewees. (These are the people least likely to be in touch with HIV services other than clinics). The study's participants therefore told a preponderance of stories about South Africa's relatively recent, late-onset ARV treatment. Many interviewees' stories recounted the successes of medication against accounts of prior illness and often, the earlier unavailability of ARVs. All but two HIV positive interviewees were on ARVs, often with fairly recent starts, even if they had been diagnosed many years before – partly because of poor ARV access, but also because treatment at the 350 CD4+ T cell level had only recently been implemented. Their narratives were thus stories told in the long-wave aftershock of AIDS denialism and the treatment activist movement. They were replete with knowledge and strong appreciation of ARVs and their positive effects on living with HIV, as with Nicco's account, quoted at the beginning of Chapter 3. She recounts her medications; says, 'I like my status too much'; backtracks to her earlier difficulties in gaining acceptance; and ends with her commitment to contributing to education and change.

Nick, for instance, a man in his late 30s, diagnosed in 2009 but only recently started on ARVs, described his medical support as very good. In the questionnaire completed after the interview, he said that he had no HIV-related symptoms, although his tiredness during the support group meeting was noticeable and was remarked on by the group coordinator.

> **Nick:** I did go a lot of clinics, yes. I did got a lot of support in the clinic.
> **Interviewer:** Okay. So how long have you been using ARVs?
> **Nick:** I think it's two months now.
> **Interviewer:** You didn't have side effects?
> **Nick:** No, I didn't have side effects.

Nick also, like Nicco, positioned his medical success in relation to other kinds of engagement, in this case, the Treatment Action Campaign (TAC), with which he began the interview and which he returned to at later times, as indeed he had returned to the organisation itself:

> **Nick:** Because after I found out myself I'm HIV positive, I did go to TAC, so I've got a lot of friends there/Okay/Some of them close friends, they weren't affected, some of them they did get affected, so they did get a lot of support there.

As with Nick and Nicco, and as indeed with the UK interviewees, though in a more pronounced way, South African interviewees tended to locate medicalisation's successes within the frame either of local and national activisms which had significantly affected ARV provision or of their own education via radio, television, leaflets, and support group participation, that is, within the frame of local and national public health, HIV and ARV initiatives. Unlike in the United Kingdom, though, participants' stories might, as with Nick, ignore entirely some medical difficulties, such as fatigue and other side effects, as if they were not suitable or relevant to include. These are not, then, narratives of 'medicalisation' that can be read as wholly determined by medical discourses or practices, which would think those difficulties relevant. They have to be read, rather, inside their history of community engagement, like the convivial social resource of TAC that Nick describes here, but also the wider resources of the Western Cape's health and social services departments and media (especially radio), working across HIV statuses, across genders, possibly also in this case across language and national backgrounds. Such histories continue to be of considerable importance in campaigning for newer medications, expanded ranges of medications, and better medical supplies and services. Perhaps, too, it is not incidental that Nick, one of the few men in this mixed-gender support group, had a parallel history of involvement in TAC, an organisation with strong commitments to coalitional working and specifically, to addressing gendered aspects of the epidemic. He did not find working with the majority of women in the group difficult; he also had experience of politicised HIV support work, through TAC, that gave him a strong sense of what this more local support group could do.

The treatment, education and activist history of HIV's medicalisation in South Africa is also one within which side effects may not be registered or continuing symptoms may not be recognised as such, within the expressed trajectory towards treatment education and activism's successes. For Nick and others only recently using ARVs, this might especially be the case. However, many HIV positive people in South Africa, including some of the interviewees, have now lived over a decade with ARVs. For such people, HIV and ARVs have become twin aspects of their life paths. They are living three-letter lives in practice rather than in prospect. For these participants, the limits of medicalised addresses to HIV, outside of those addresses' connections to activist historical and present campaigns, were more strongly delineated in their narratives.

Medicalisation's problems

Many interviewees who defined themselves as symptom-free and who said early on in the interviews that they were having no problems with antiretrovirals later said, either spontaneously or in response to the reiteration of a simple question about how ARVs were going, that there were indeed problems. As in the UK interviews, allowing for long, unhurried and complex narrative co-construction in the interviews meant that later stories worked more explicitly to demedicalise contemporary three-letter lives. Depression, blood pressure, heart problems, other early ageing-related problems like arthritis and neuropathy were frequently noted later on, for example, as recalcitrant aspects of living with HIV. This disjunction within narratives was much more dramatic than in the

UK stories, largely because of the sometimes severe lack of treatment of these other problems. HIV-related problems such as shingles and some skin problems were indeed said at times to be untreatable. 'Fluctuating symptoms' such as fatigue and long-running flus were similarly storied as conditions to live with. Side effects were often narrated as 'going away', rather than actively being treated. The difficulties of treating side effects, and the limited possibilities for drug regime changes, were part of participants' stories to an extent only seen with older UK participants who had lived through precisely these limitations in earlier years of the epidemic.

Some participants criticised queuing structures and waiting times at clinics. More general criticisms of, for instance, waiting lists, or overall levels of drug provision, or medical professionals' attitudes, were rare. However, late on in interviews, participants sometimes came to criticise local, but not hospital, doctors, for not knowing enough about HIV and ARVs. HIV citizenship thus appears in these stories as a involving very different set of concrete medical requirements than in the UK case, over-lapping only in its resistance to the limited expertise of non-specialist doctors. Medicalised HIV citizenship is also not strongly marketised as in the United Kingdom, despite policy moves in that direction. It is connected much more to a broader narrative of health citizenship that is constitutionally guaranteed, which sets out principles of equitable and best-quality health care for all.

Nonkosi, for instance, a woman in her late 40s, was one of the few participants to mention spontaneously that she had had some trouble with ARVs. She had had to wait a considerable time to get help for ARV-related depression, something which UK interviewees like Jana (see previous chapter) explicitly critiqued. This was not, however, a resource lack that Nonkosi criticised. Indeed, it was only on inter-viewer follow-up that she told a full story about her difficulties with treatment. Then she told a demedicalising story about ARVs' difficul-ties and side effects as Quentin and many other UK interviewees did, although those interviewees tended to start such stories earlier and spontaneously:

Interviewer: What about you know you had some difficulties with your medicine and it took a long time with Efavirenz to stop it. Did you tell the hospital before that you were having problems with it?

Nonkosi: Yes I did I did, that's why they changed the tablets. But they didn't change the Efavirenz because of that they said they gave everybody, the people who was diagnosed with TB/I see/Yes, so they don't change any more the Efavirenz/So they changed some other things/Some other tablets, yes/Ah, and then you/ for 3TC which was damaging my liver.

Interviewer: Right, okay, and then only when you went back and you said you have this problem with your head.

Nonkosi: My head is nothing now. I've got nothing in my head...if I had my head comes again, {it would be} painful.

Interviewer: Really. And what about with the depression, how is that now?

Nonkosi: It took er three years to go away. Mhm.

Interviewer: And you had medication for that?

Nonkosi: No, I don't eat my depression medication now. But previously I was having those tablets.

Interviewer: Right. And do you think that was to do with, was it to do with the medications or was it to do with HIV or being on your own, or what do you think brought about the depression for you?

Nonkosi: The depression I think that it, it goes with those medication, it was the medication was too too heavy to go to this body, which this body was very sick.

This story also has to be read within the very distinct frame of the country's health and health services generally. The national frame can go relatively unmarked in the UK case, where treatment for, for instance, age-related cardiovascular conditions, can be assumed. In the South African narratives, however, it can be hard to distinguish under-treated HIV-related health problems from under-treated health problems generally. Even to describe cardiovascular problems that are age-related as intensified by HIV may be difficult, given the general under-treatment of such problems. The stories interviewees produce are indeed much more of 'living with' HIV, ARVs, and a raft of other problems of uncertain relationship to HIV, which are side-shadowed repeatedly in their narratives, rather than stories of 'living on' with HIV while other, related and non-related, but definitely treatable conditions, start to come into the picture, as in the UK case. Living with HIV and ARVs is thus not so much in these South African stories a matter of walking the borderline between HIV positive health and illness, but of living with HIV and ARVs alongside many other conditions that cross and recross that borderline.

It is also interesting to note that unlike many UK interviewees, Nonkosi is clear about the origins of her depression. She does not locate

it as a long-running aspect of individual personality, as some UK interviewees did, despite their having good knowledge of ARVs' potential
mental health side effects. Perhaps this radical refusal to take individual
responsibility for such a difficult-to-address aspect of Nonkosi's health is
also related to the legacy and ongoing of treatment literacy and activism
in the socio-medical context within which she lives. It indicates to us
again that HIV citizenship in its medical aspects, and health citizenship
generally, can mean very different things in distinct national contexts.
In the South African context, such citizenship may involve greater levels
of HIV knowledge and activism than in the UK context. It is indeed for
this reason that we can distinguish a different kind of demedicalising,
counteracting narrative in the South African than in the UK interviews:
surer of its medical expertise, less concerned with ambiguities, even
among interviewees with little direct access to expert HIV knowledge,
for instance through print or internet sources. This history and present
of activist but also community and media knowledge is a very important
resource, a kind of 'capital' that does not fit easily into either social or
cultural categories but lies across the borders of them. It is a resource
for 'living with' HIV at many levels: for individual participants, and for
their families, friends and neighbourhoods. It is also the resource that, at
the level of civil society could be said to have grounded the reformulation of the AIDS Law Project into the broader-remit Section 27 and the
development of the Social Justice Coalition.

As in the UK study, South African participants noted decreasing attention to psychosocial issues within their medical care, an aspect of cost-
conscious medicalisation which their stories explicitly counteracted.
Nonkosi, indeed, described the triaging-out, for people who are doing
well on ARVs, of psychosocial support services that take up too much
time:

> **Nonkosi:** Now I'm (stable)…as the time goes, they divide us. They
> said 'ok now you are not sick anymore so now you just take your
> pills {every three months} and go home'. So we haven't got that
> time to talk.

This was the only area of medical care where cost considerations were
clearly playing a role. However, constraints on medicalisation's successes
may have been under-represented in this interview material since the
research was performed within support groups. The research participants were well supported psychosocially by these services in relation to
their medical treatment, so they were unlikely to tell many stories about

the absence of treatment support. The groups frequently had treatment discussions and speakers on medical issues, for instance. Moreover, for many people living with HIV and ARVs, HIV knowledge and care is by this time spread across South African social contexts, generalising and informalising support, including support for medical aspects of living with HIV. One clear marker of this is the extent to which the women interviewed provided medical expertise for their male partners, many of whom were also HIV positive.

A final, counteracting narrative that operated rather clearly to mark the problems of HIV's medicalisation related three-letter lives to food. Many interviewees, in describing the success of ARVs for them, qualified their progress either by specifying the foods they must eat, or by noting their nutritional deficiencies. They told many 'what-if' stories of what had happened or could happen if ARVs and hunger coexisted. In these stories, the power of ARVs over bodies was vividly expressed, in a kind of counterpoint to the more medically enumerated side effects stories of current UK research participants. These stories of what even contemporary, relatively well-modulated ARVs do to bodies under the strain of poverty, already at the limits of wellness, recall stories from earlier in the UK epidemic, when people living with HIV had to manage their already-ill bodies' reactions to cruder medications. Morag's stories of her inability to manage the diarrhoea associated with ARVs (Chapter 7) without 'drug holidays' were examples. Nonkosi, emphasising how the medication is 'like a train, it hits you', embeds this description in a short story of her catch-22 situation: too ill to eat, but when hungry, too weak to benefit from the ARVs:

> **Nonkosi:** I was thin and always lying in the bed you see, I didn't want to eat anything. Then when I drink the medication, eish, I thought that the medication was going in my my blood, like, like, like a train, it hits you, (clap) you see, yeah. So that was my experience that I was taking it, I said 'No, it, I must first eat, then drink the medication'.
> **Interviewer:** Okay, otherwise it's very strong?
> **Nonkosi:** It's very strong, it's very very strong. Yeah I can say it. If you are drinking the medication at 8 o'clock you must first eat at 7 o'clock so that your body can have a food and then have those ARVs at 8 o'clock.

The failure to address these side effects via food security was suggested by a number of interviewees to produce ARV 'skipping', though this did not happen in their own lives. Only one interviewee, Siyanda, a woman in her 40s, told a habitual narrative, which I mentioned in Chapter 7, of her two HIV positive children's ARV skipping directly, out of shame, she said, for how lack of food made her a bad carer for her children:

> **Siyanda:** Sometimes they don't take ARVs before they go to school, because sometimes there's no food. Sometimes I'm feeling ashamed, I say, 'No, don't take ARVs', because stomach is empty.

To the extent that medicalisation processes operating within the South African epidemic do not consider food security, especially in situations where, as in these research environments, it is very unstable, they undermine their own successes. Interviewees' countervailing narratives of ARV problems pointed to this limitation. At the same time, because many interviewees were connected to support groups, and because the general South African context of HIV knowledge and action is shaped by histories of advocacy and activism, many medicalisation processes already have built into them resources of food support, by referrals to church groups, for instance, or via supplementary food programmes for children, or through grant support made available at the behest of doctors. The participants recruited from the income-generation project, for example, had access to transport to a free breakfast programme designed to address precisely the problem Siyanda encountered. The participants who attended the support group had occasional food support from a local church congregation. As with stories of medicalisation itself, research participants' narratives of medicalisation's problems thus traced those processes in a community-embedded way that went beyond medical boundaries and that were rooted in a sociality of health (Rabinow 2004).

Living healthily: counteracting medicalisation

Beyond their critical narratives counteracting the problems of HIV's medicalisation, the South African research participants also produced stories that counteracted medicalisation by a thoroughgoing reformulation of it, based in their own and other community-based ideas of healthy living. These stories related specific engagements with conventional medicine, for instance, questioning doctors, and having 'time' with doctors – aspects of HIV's contemporary medicalisation that were also foregrounded in UK interviewees' stories of holistic HIV care. In relation to ARVs specifically, and despite the examples in the previous chapter segment, such narratives were still mostly about 'living with' the positive realities of treatment expansion alongside their other pressing problems; continuing medical uncertainties were less troubling at present than in the United Kingdom. However, the growing lists of long-term side effects building up during the longer interviews, as they do during people's three-letter lives, suggest that this is becoming more of an issue.

The counteracting stories also mapped the terrain of healthy life beyond medication. Participants narrated how they implemented their own health rules, including good nutrition (fresh fruit and vegetables, no frying) reduced or no alcohol, and exercise, and these ways of living spread across families, becoming *de facto* grounds of health citizenship for everyone. Nonkosi, for example, described how this happened in her family. Without explicit discussion, new health practices derived from HIV knowledge were becoming part of regular domestic life:

> **Nonkosi:** I learn those things about food, I was eating junk food/ Okay, right/ was liking to eat just bread and meat, that's only. Then here they told us that we must eat veg and fruit. I start now a new life. Then I always eat at home, buying it/Okay/But the fresh food from the garden, not from those in the fridge, the mixed veg, I don't like it/So fresh veg/I like a fresh one.
>
> **Interviewer:** Okay. So did people say to you, 'Oh why are you changing your diet?' Does your family know you
>
> **Nonkosi:** No, they don't ask me. They don't ask me. I love cooking./ You do, okay./It's me who are cooking at home./Yes/They don't ask why now I changing what you are eating. Even with the eggs I didn't like to eat eggs, now I eat eggs.

Interviewees described using herbal medication for skin problems, as they have in many other studies. HIV was judged, like TB, not susceptible to herbal or spiritual medicine even by interviewees who use one or both in other circumstances, much less than in the 2001 interviews, when ARVs were a distant possibility for some interviewees and traditional medicines operated as what we might call 'pre-medicalised' ways of addressing the epidemic. Speaking out was identified as itself a means of producing health. Nonkosi, for instance, described how she had moved from not wanting to hear such speech, let alone produce it, since it was a secret cross to bear, to feeling relieved by it:

> **Nonkosi :** {Friends were} always talking about this sickness and I didn't want nobody to talk about it, I was very angry, even today,

to have friends, she told that 'No I'm HIV positive', 'It's a disgrace, why you talking like this?' I said to her, she said, 'No, they must know it, it's my sickness, how can I hide it. I say 'it's not sickness, you must know that the sickness that God gave you is your secret'. And then to know that you must talk, you see, so that it can come out, so now I experience those things/Okay. Is that how it feels to you? If you talk/If I talk, yes/You feel more healthy?/I feel comfortable.

Many participants reported healthy lifestyle elements as continuing, important accompaniments to ARVs, while prior to ARVs' accessibility, they had often been presented as the only solution (Squire 2007). These 'pre-medicalisation' approaches are still discussed in clinic support groups, perhaps to a greater extent than in the UK situation.

HIV citizenship in the medical field was, then, narrated as a matter for interviewees themselves and for others close to them, rather than for medical professionals. As we saw earlier, it was framed as operating within the fields of community advocacy and treatment activism, rather than medical efficacy. This may have happened partly because of the recruitment of relatively engaged research participants, via HIV-oriented projects; partly because of the history of South African HIV activism, operating directly for some participants like Nick, via their personal histories. The effects of this history have been strengthened by its transnational and international NGO links, tying it into much larger movements for HIV and health rights (Colvin and Robins 2009; Mbali 2013). More generally, many participants' resourceful relation to HIV's medicalisation seemed grounded not in activism but in HIV's widespread community and media presence which in this local context has, itself, a strong history (Abdullah and Squire 2010). (The situation may be different where activist NGOs such as TAC have played a more singular and less supported role, for instance, in parts of rural KwaZulu-Natal; Grønlie et al. 2011). National political discourse, within which health is a constitutional guarantee and the country's wider history of political activism have both contributed to these counteracting narratives of HIV within health citizenship (Nattrass 2009; Robins 2009). For the interviewees, all these constituted the assemblage of resources within which 'healthy living' with HIV could be narrated as a present phenomenon, a medical and psychosocial resource in itself, with a strong degree of autonomy from medicalised HIV discourses and practices. The conviviality of such healthy 'living with' HIV appeared in stories like Nombulelo's, about accepting HIV as an illness; in stories like Nick's and Nonkosi's, about the value and difficulties of treatment; and in Nonkosi's tales of eating good food and 'speaking out' about difficulties. These were stories told and in some cases, practices advised, for everyone, not just for people who were HIV positive. Through them, HIV citizenship becomes a resource for health citizenship generally.

HIV's normalisation

On the borders of the normal

It is commonly found that HIV's position in South Africa has shifted in a normalised direction (for instance, Abrahams and Jewkes 2012; Zuch and Lurie 2012). HIV is part of almost everyone's life; medical successes have made it a liveable condition; knowledge and treatment mean that stigmatisation is less. As in the United Kingdom, most stigmatisation involves gossiping, not overt stigmatisation or discrimination. However, these phenomena, fear of stigma and internalised stigma can lead to non-accessing of or withdrawing from support (Abrahams and Jewkes 2012).

The scale and visibility of HIV in South Africa means that by default it is part of everyday living and to some extent normalised, treated as a regular element in social discourses and practices. It is not, as in the United Kingdom, invisibilised. Much more than in the UK situation, stigma may be resisted by declaring that the condition is everywhere, and that at least the disclosing or disclosed HIV positive person knows their status and is doing the right things: getting ARVs, using condoms. Also unlike the United Kingdom, community support can often be accessed, and the law is invoked as a protection against discrimination rather than as a threat of criminalisation (Abrahams and Jewkes 2012).

However, the South African epidemic's visibility can grow into something that people who are not affected and even those who are affected by HIV pass over, so that HIV becomes hidden in plain sight. The gender-, class- and age-related discriminations associated with HIV positive status can also become part of the everyday landscape, with women and men becoming accustomed to concealing their status because of the threats to femininity and masculinity it poses; poor people being aware that their HIV status can be used further to abjectify them; and young people hiding their HIV positivity because of the continuing infantilisation it is perceived to bring (Abrahams and Jewkes 2012). Moreover, full public disclosure of your status, something that might be expected to characterise HIV's normalisation, is, Edwin Cameron recently pointed out, still relatively uncommon, especially among socially powerful and influential people:

> What we don't understand is internalised stigma.
> The person with HIV or at risk of it becomes self-condemnatory. It's very, very difficult to understand and to act upon. But I think the silence of our cabinet ministers, our national leaders, our presidents and prime ministers and kings – because there's widespread belief that some monarchs in Africa, in Southern Africa are living with HIV, are not on antiretrovirals. (Cameron 2013)

Normalisation was something that often appeared in my 2012 South African HIV support interviews as problematic as well as positive. It was a resource but sometimes a failure of resource, to the extent that HIV might turn into an unmarked condition whose mainstreaming erased the differences between it and other difficult conditions. A good example here is the story Sizeka, a woman in her mid-30s, told about her 'HIV Positive' T-shirt, and how she had negotiated from not wanting to wear it, through wearing it with others, to wearing it as a statement about HIV citizenship, independent of HIV status:

> **Sizeka:** Then we got the T-shirts from TAC that wrote 'HIV, HIV Positive'. And I didn't want to wear that T-shirt. I wear it when my friends wear that, they has their, their T-shirts/mhm/ but I had something, but er, when people read 'HIV' it's like, she says to me that I wrote big 'HIV', because there's HIV. I said, 'No, it's a T-shirt, as you can get a T-shirt that wrote it in Edgars {store}, so it's very (like) that.'/Just a T-shirt/ It's a T-shirt, not, but I used to wear that T-shirt and that T-shirt makes me strong. Because I had a way to, to answer when people are talking about this T-shirt, and I've got more T-shirt and I gave someone a T-shirt. I can give you if you need one. Doesn't mean you are HIV positive.

The 'HIV Positive' T-shirt, first popularised in South Africa by TAC, has a long history within the epidemic, with its 2002 adoption by Nelson Mandela a key moment in the broad public and political acceptance of the realities of the epidemic (Power 2003). In Sizeka's story, her use of the normalising 'HIV Positive' T-shirt allows her own speaking about HIV, which is both personally strengthening and socially educative, to happen in a safely non-disclosing way that at the same time limits the power of the apparently self-disclosing position from which she testifies (Squire 2007). In parallel, the normalisation performed by the T-shirt tells a higher-level social story: that we are all HIV citizens, that everyone needs to pay attention to HIV issues, that people of all HIV statuses are all humans who give and receive love and care, and that status cannot be distinguished from any stigmatising external marks. Yet the T-shirt also tells a more problematic story that undermines normalisation from within. For if these T-shirts are everywhere, worn by anyone, recast, perhaps, just as useful items of clothing, HIV's normalisation can erase three-letter lives, at the same time as seeming to affirm them.

In the 2012 interviews, participants did in fact tell many stories in which HIV was just a part of life, one of many other pressing issues such as worries about children, how to get a job, pursuing education, or, in two cases, past abuse experiences. As Siyanda put it, she 'feels free' with her HIV positive status, to not think about it, in order to think instead about her children and the future:

> **Siyanda:** Now I am, I am feeling free with my status because I don't want to always concentrate to, to my status/okay/It it comes, always, sometimes not always thinking about that, yes/Sure. Sure/ Yes/So you want to think about other things?/ Yes. Not about my status. Every time thinking about my status, I know my status but I am not always thinking about it because I am going be stressed if I just think about that./ Yes/I'm saying 'no, I will live longer'. Until my kids are old. /Because you are also/I have a hope, yes./ Yes/I have hope every time, yes.

If HIV's normalisation can invisibilise it for people who are not HIV positive, that normalisation can, for people who are HIV positive themselves, guarantee futures, as for Siyanda, and acceptance and strength, as for Sizeka. Few stories traced the ambivalent border between the particularities of HIV status and its normalisation, as in the UK interviews. Ongoing HIV-related health issues, for instance, were not cited 'against' HIV's normalisation, as in the UK. Perhaps this was because of widespread awareness of such issues, and of similar issues with other chronic illnesses, in a context of much lower resourcing of chronic illness treatment in general. Moreover, in South Africa after the long wait for effective medications for a fatal condition, and the wholesale 'othering' of millions of people on the basis of their positive status, a declaration of and an approach to HIV status as irrelevant to citizenship in the era of HIV and ARVs can operate as a political demand and even a political action. Once HIV's treatment has been addressed, the virus can be considered as both an issue for everyone, an everyday issue within convivial social lives, and as a side issue within individual lives, as Sizeka and Siyanda, respectively, declare. At the same time, HIV status still remains on the borders of the normal: not an internalised source of shame, but a stress and a secret, as these interviewees also tell us.

Family stories often described much more support than before because families were reported to be aware of the bad consequences of not supporting HIV positive members, and because HIV is now understood as ubiquitous and a treatable illness. Some of that support was very concrete, as in the United Kingdom, involving people who are not HIV positive taking active part in three-letter lives. Nonkosi's children help her take her medicine, for example, as in this habitual narrative of how they understand her status:

> **Nonkosi:** They know {my status}. It is when it is 8 o'clock they say 'mama, there is your water and the medication', I say 'ok'. So I drink it.
> **Interviewer:** So they're helpful?
> **Nonkosi:** They are helpful.

Normalisation also means separating from families and surrogate families with whom one is living because of HIV, and thereby becoming a proper adult. Several people wanted to move into their own places, something that they had not done earlier because of their illnesses, or illness-related lack of ability to work (Jury and Nattrass 2012). For young men, this has previously been reported as a reason to conceal their HIV status (Abrahams and Jewkes 2012). In this study, women also told stories of staying at home or with older friends or relatives because their status's associated illnesses or poverty meant they or others thought they could not manage independently.

Normalisation operates through media. South African broadcasters programme specific shows such as *Beat It!*, *Radio Zibonele* and *Soul City* which demonstrate, as one interviewee put it, 'different sides' to being HIV positive, normalising a range of different HIV experiences. Religious radio shows pray specifically for people living with HIV. Some interviewees were open about their HIV status with other HIV positive people at church; one had spoken to the whole congregation. Many more pastors and churches practice non-disclosing acceptance (Squire 2007). HIV is talked and prayed about, and members of the congregation get private solace from that, or at the most tell a few close church friends.

Boniswa, a woman in her late 30s, described how this worked as a kind of non-specific social inclusion:

> **Boniswa:** I do go to church, I am a believer. The church helps me.
> **Interviewer:** Do they talk openly about HIV at church or not?
> **Boniswa:** No I don't say that I have HIV at church.
> **Interviewer:** You're not {open}, no. But does the pastor say something about people, we must pray for people with HIV or
> **Boniswa:** Yes he does say, we must pray for people that have HIV, and I find comfort at that moment, but I do not say anything about being HIV positive.

There are limits to the value of such non-disclosing acceptance; it supports only a provisional conviviality. It is shadowed, as in the United Kingdom, by fear of stigma: fear that the pastor or other congregants will gossip, or blame. Nevertheless, among these interviewees, people told their pastor, individually, much more than they did before. And in family and friendship networks, religion may much more now drive normalisation than exclusion. HIV has become integrated into spiritual life and duty, not an excommunicated part of them: a big change. As Lusi, a woman in her mid-30s, narrated in dialogue with the interviewer, when asked how her family were treating her, their approach could be traced through their faith:

> **Lusi:** My family helps me a lot, by talking about it and by giving me strength that I am going to be okay and giving me hope.
> **Interviewer:** So how, why do you think your family reacted so well because some families don't react so well?
> **Lusi:** Most of my family they are religious, they are people that have Jesus, so they do understand a lot of things/ I see/They support me like this.

The many little failures of normalisation

Despite suggestions that stigma has reduced, there remained many narrated instances of stigmatisation and discrimination. In this study, interviewees did not talk about very severe stigmatisation, discrimination and violence, though such events happen. However, they did produce many small stories counteracting normalisation by pointing up moments of stigmatisation, problems of disclosure, and legacies of sadness and loss. Nicro, for example, despite her extremely positive account of her medication and HIV identity, went on, like many other interviewees, to describe 'a lot of challenges', ongoing, with family and friends. The narrative of least acceptance by family, social networks and community was produced by Nick, one of only two men then attending a 20-strong support group. Perhaps more-accepted men may access family support, of the kind women interviewees often described providing to partners, and therefore not take up voluntary-sector support:

> **Nick:** There is a problem, the problem is, in my community, there is no-one who can support me, even inside of my family you see. Sometimes if ever I'm eating, I've got my own dish, my own (spoon), because they don't know nothing about the HIV status...Yes. They think they are going to spread (with) all of us inside of the house, they feel so.

It remained difficult to tell parents, especially mothers, whose health causes worry. And the histories of deaths continue to hang over present realities: a non-normalisable grief sometimes amounting to melancholia, affecting people of all statuses, even when being HIV positive is accepted and understood. As Nonkosi put it, describing the path of loss in her family:

> **Nonkosi:** I didn't say {to my family} I am HIV positive, because I was having a brother who was HIV positive and I did saw him when he was sick and then he passed away in 2005. Then I didn't, didn't want to hurt my mother, then I said 'Eish, how can I told my mother?' Then I talked to my sister that the clinic doctor says to me I'm HIV positive. Then it's my sister who told my mother. It's not me. /Mhm/ Yes. And even the other sisters of me. Yes, they know that I'm HIV positive.
> **Interviewer:** And how were they? How did they respond?
> **Nonkosi:** No, they say that is not to, you mustn't I mustn't be worried because, the sickness is coming in the house, all the members of the house would have that sickness
> **Interviewer:** Yes, so everybody knows/Everybody knows/Yes. And your mum?
> **Nonkosi:** My mother passed away last year. All of them died. It's just, I must keep drinking my tablets and go to the hospital. Yes.

Here, normalisation means that HIV becomes accepted, but also that it could affect the whole family: 'all the members of the house would have that sickness... all of them died'. Nonkosi and similar others are just surviving, 'left behind' like many UK interviewees; but they are also committed to the futures they struggled for, guaranteed by ARVs. As Nonkosi affirms, 'I must keep drinking my tablets and going to the hospital. Yes'.

Normalisation meant that the two non-HIV positive interviewees had 'moved on' from HIV, seeing their future activism and caring as called forth by other requirements. Some younger HIV positive people were making the same decision. However, HIV fatigue tended not to be such an issue for the South African interviewees in this study as for interviewees as in the United Kingdom. The non-normalisable history of this enormous and at one point drastically under-recognised, under-resourced epidemic kept them involved, as a long-term worker in the sector, Yoliswa, clarified:

> **Yoliswa:** For now, I really do not think my involvement will ever drop, neither my interest and passion. Kaloku {Because} remember, we have different reasons why we got involved in the 1st place. In my case, and that of others, I think it is understandable that HIV has become part of us as it has robbed of one thing or another. HIV took my baby, and that will always be part of me, and that's the deal! Sometimes I even feel I am not involved enough. (Email follow-up to interview)

Such stories were not just counteractions to normalisation. They also started to spell out a specific narrative of HIV's contemporary place, both regularised and particular, within South Africa.

The specific normalisations of HIV

The particular forms of HIV's condition-specific, country-specific normalisation were charted in interviewee stories that counteracted a more generalised normalisation. Instead, these stories traced a process of HIV normalisation that ended up strongly focused on HIV-literate small socialities, a micro-social world of HIV citizenship. This social resource was storied, from many different sides, as highly valuable. 'Health' is often currently framed in African HIV epidemics as a matter of individual responsibility (Cornwall et al. 2011; Hickel 2012). However, as in the UK context, but more generally here, South African interviewees' stories consistently turned individual responsibility for living well with HIV into something socially negotiated, a collective 'response-ibility', as Dageid and colleagues have described it (2011)[3].

Unlike in earlier years, when many interviewees only mentioned their 'new' HIV positive friends, now there was a much more mixed picture. For some, only family and not friends could be trusted, or friends were of mixed value. For others, all friends were supportive. However, few described friendships as completely undifferentiated across HIV statuses. Most found particular value with other HIV-affected friends. Nolundi, for example, had accepting but uncomprehending HIV negative friends. She 'lived with' HIV-affected people in a closer association. This assertion of the role of HIV experience in generating a particular kind of HIV citizenship appeared in UK interviews too. However, it did not constitute a parallel 'normal', as in South Africa:

> **Nolundi:** They {friends}are still not understanding it {HIV}...But what there is one thing that I can say, after I had been diagnosed, and I have also accepted. There was happiness to stay with people living with HIV, talking the same talk, I was not longer happy staying with people who are not HIV positive.

Husbands and boyfriends were also narrated by the women interviewees as often very supportive. Some participants reported past partners as negative but these are not usually current experiences. Boniswa's boyfriend, for example, like Nonkosi's children, in the previous chapter segment, was closely connected to her HIV normalisation, a part of it, despite his negative status:

> **Boniswa:** I am happy that my boyfriend knows about my status, when it's time for me to the clinic, he sometimes reminds me that 'Do not forget to go to the clinic'. And when, if he is at work he calls me at nine to remind me to take my pills. He reminds me.

Relationships are thus HIV-normalised here. Partners who understand HIV, and who will not cause trouble to an HIV positive person (by, for instance, violence, drug use, drinking or malicious talk), were wanted by the participants. HIV status and sero-sorting were not described as prominent issues in this high-prevalence context, though many interviewees told stories of their strategies of early disclosure in relationships.

HIV normalisation also happens through HIV support groups, which become major friendship networks in themselves, even surrogate families. One research participant, the youngest, had been abused by her family and husband, and had been helped by the support group and its wider friendship network not just to come to terms with HIV and

ARVs, but materially and socially. The group had aided her with housing when she left her husband, and with encouragement to act as other young women do in the township and wear fashionable clothes, rather than the conservative dresses her husband had favoured. In the interview, this young woman, speaking mostly in Xhosa, gave some of her most troubling stories to the older woman friend who was translating, trusting them to her, explicitly instructing her, 'you tell it'.

More casually, members gossip when they meet at the local supermarket, like 'sisters', whatever their other differences. And senior support group members, like older sisters, volunteered for our research first. This kind of particularised HIV collectivity also characterises neighbourhoods. Nomonde, though not trained as a counsellor, still gave regular advice and support to friends around her who were hesitant to approach clinics or support groups. In this way, she sustained an informal support network similar to those operated by Olive and Queenie in previous chapters. However, as in the United Kingdom, in resource-constrained circumstances such social capacities have limited potential unless they can reach outside themselves. Several interviewees described wanting to leave the support group or project buildings, leave the township even, see normal things, go to the seaside, but with each other, in an HIV-accepting context:

> **Nonkosi:** All my friends here {support group}/yes/ I love them all. Yes/Yes/...But we need to go out {of the project}, so we can freshen our minds.

Such 'what-if' stories were shadowed by constraints on cash in both HIV-centred and other contexts. Siyanda, for instance, was planning to use the interview fee to buy fruit for her own and other children at a church-organised outing. Her normalised citizenship thus derived at least partly from the marketisation of her participation. As with Gerry, who described a similar HIV-centred normalcy in the previous chapter, a strong HIV sociality is part of the resources on which participants built another resource: the capacity to 'live with' the condition. However, in this case, they had to build resources to 'live with' HIV alongside poverty, from conditions of poverty.

This HIV sociality can also encompass, in the South African case, 'living with' national difference, most obviously in the case of anti-xenophobic attacks during 2008, within the townships where we later carried out this research. In 2008, TAC and other civil society organisations provided humanitarian relief, sanctuary and protection for non-South Africans under attack. This kind of intersectional action, based on the parallels of HIV discrimination and xenophobia, was not fore-grounded in participant interviews, but it was part of the broader under-standing of the conditions of living with HIV and ARVs that led some interviewees from previous rounds to become involved with broader forms of community action.

Support groups are too spread out to constitute a full alternative friendship network, especially given that travel is expensive. Maybe this *lack* of familial closeness is also part of their particular, 'HIV normal', appeal. One interviewee, Rosy, pointed out that it is good to talk with people who do not know you, are not your friends. This might be espe-cially the case where, as for her, other issues such as abuse have come up in their lives now that HIV has been to some extent addressed. Again HIV's normalisation is limited when, as is often the case, there are other issues tied to it. It can be an illness tied to histories of subjection, for instance, via abuse or gender-based violence, and to other illnesses, as well as to poverty.

'Younger' HIV generations are not much represented in this sample. Perhaps this is they have experienced more community and family normalisation, because older generations are more affected psychoso-cially by HIV's fatal history, and because of recent drops in diagnoses among younger people. At any rate, normalisation is not operating for this younger generation through the groups where I recruited. However, HIV normalisation also affects the younger generations' ways of under-standing HIV. They are specially educated, as Nolundi indicates, when they live within families affected by HIV:

> **Nolundi:** These children I don't know if maybe they do not accept or what is happening or maybe they don't understand even though they could see people who are sick and seeing them dying some of them, they still do not want to use a condom, that is when they are being irresponsible even though they see that HIV is spreading, they just being irresponsible
> **Interviewer:** So is this what you talk to your children?
> **Nolundi:** Yes I teach them.

In the South African interviewees' stories, then, a developing convivi-ality around HIV made itself felt, in stories of HIV-aware and supportive families, friends, partners and children, despite many instances of incomprehension, stigma and discrimination also being reported. Such conviviality can be an extremely powerful resource. It seems much more difficult to find or develop in the low-prevalence, low-HIV-literacy, high-austerity context of the UK epidemic. However, it contains within itself also the difficulties of HIV's normalisation, which divide some kinds of 'living with' HIV from others. Such difficulties include losses that constitute what Yoliswa described as 'what has been robbed from us'; what people, even your own children, as Nolundi emphasises, still do not want to know; the resource deficits with which Siyanda struggles; the 'platefuls' of tears, love, sex and uncertainty that Mpe describes at the beginning of this chapter; and Nombulelo's family's acceptance of HIV, hanging with some fragility between affirmation and fatalism. All these must also be 'lived with', and acknowledging them, at least, can be counted as a resource.

As with narratives counteracting medicalisation, stories of complex, HIV-normal socialities depend on resources if they are to develop and be effective: on the ability to communicate, to move from place to place, to be able, like Siyanda, to bring something appropriate to social interactions. How do such resources relate to South Africa's marketisation? Is that process at odds with both this coalitional HIV normality, and with the citizenly health expertise that also, I have argued, characterises many South African participants' accounts of their three-letter lives?

Marketisation, demarketisation, and not having resources

Market failures and resource shortages: 'I need support'

South Africa's HIV epidemic is a massive financial burden for the country, especially as its own health department is being pushed to cover more of the costs. Historically, the unaffordability of ARV provision was often used to argue against treatment rollout in the country (Boulle et al. 2010). Today, UNAIDS (2011a) describes all the efforts made in this country context and within an 'era of financial austerity' – to provide integrated one-a-day pills, for instance – as 'investment' as well as a quality of life improvement for patients. The country negotiates hard with its 21% share of the global ARV market for discount deals. But supporting at least 3 million people on ARVs by 2015, however cost-effective the solutions developed, is not easy to achieve within a marketised framework. External funding and pharmaceutical company discounts will be required for the foreseeable future, with attendant budget and supply uncertainties. NGOs and health departments have, indeed, been dealing with budget reductions since 2009.

What suffers in such circumstances, as in the United Kingdom, tends to be psychosocial services and non-essential support such as additional medical services and food aid. It is clear that food security plays a large part in medium- and low-income countries in the success or otherwise of ARV treatment (Campbell et al. 2012; Ivers et al. 2009; Tsai et al. 2012; Weiser et al. 2009; Weiser et al. 2007). Cash availability has additional major impact on for instance transport to clinics (Tuller et al. 2010). Cash subsidies have also been used as a means of reducing HIV risk among young people (UNAIDS 2012a). Moreover, many policy initiatives, such as UNAIDS's commitment to keeping HIV positive mothers alive (UNAIDS 2011c), as well as non-HIV-specific Millennium Development Goals 4 and 5, concerned with reducing child mortality and improving maternal health, mean that market-focused approaches must be mitigated in low- and middle-income countries with social welfare. These contradictions are approached more directly by many HIV doctors, NGOs and activists within South Africa, who consider cost arguments not from a profit or investment perspective, but rather because they take seriously the constitutional promise of 'health for all' and the country's commitment to a sustainable social justice-oriented economy (see for instance Beaubien 2013; Geffen 2013). Such approaches (though they are themselves sometimes criticised by those politically opposed to them as 'neo-liberal') are more directly undermining of marketisation than the para-liberal approaches considered in the previous chapter, because they present more defined policy alternatives.

How do policy contests around marketisation affect people living with HIV and ARVs in South Africa? In my interviews, some participants, like Yoliswa (see Chapter 7), pulled international limits to funding into their narratives, or tracked national service cuts and the local effects of global recession. However, day-to-day experiences of 'living with' HIV, ARVs and poverty were a far more common thread in their storying of markets.

Resource constraints have already appeared as powerful features of South African participants' three-letter lives in this chapter. Such constraints did not, though, shape the participants' narratives of themselves as HIV citizens as ubiquitously as in the UK interviews. Narratives of extreme resource lack, of attempting or planning economic participation through work, and of needing public or voluntary services when work was not available or when poor health precluded it, were very common. However, they were articulated intersectionally with 'living with' HIV, alongside other issues such as unemployment, undereducation, poverty, and gender, relationship and parenting concerns.

The participants were also much more markedly aware of the failures of markets than UK interviewees. They described living with these failures daily, via, for instance, high local unemployment, coupled with the pervasive encouragement and requirement to do paid work.

Given such clearly articulated contradictions, it would be very hard to describe the South African interviewees' stories as in any simple sense neo-liberal, even when those stories used vocabularies of hard work, individual responsibility and self-determination. For this reason, I am describing all the narratives described in this chapter segment as counteracting narratives, which acknowledge while also working against HIV's marketisation.

In framing this counteraction, research participants positioned themselves as resourceful, bringing existing resources to bear to counteract resource deficits, and using resources to move their lives forward, at the same time as they described their lack of required resources. They storied themselves as entrepreneurs who were nevertheless well aware of the context-limited grounds and attainments of their entrepreneurship. They articulated forms of socially resourceful HIV citizenship in ways that recalled the stories of many UK research participants, but with a stronger recent history within HIV and other activisms.

Resource worries were very frequently of a basic kind, about food and funerals, or cash to send your child to school:

> **Nombulelo:** I have a child at home who goes to school, so I have that problem that will make me get up at home (cries)/Sorry./Since I am not working, you see, I need support, when my child for {is at} school I think, 'When she comes back what is she going to eat?' Sometimes I don't even have the money for school transport, and again when I am dead who is going to bury me, with what? Those are the things I think about.

In some ways, resource deficits did not need to be storied within the interviews, even to an outsider interviewer like me. For a start, the participants were living in obviously low-income, low-employment situations, with manifest threats to their health and other resources, and in a national climate of welfare cuts. Participants were, indeed, largely recruited through an income-generation project widely known, like other similar projects, to be struggling to provide adequate work, or a support group whose food support provision was, again as with other such groups, precarious.

'Support', the topic of the study, means practical as well as psychosocial support, both when used in South African English, as an English term within Xhosa, and when translated into the lexically closest two words. So the study itself foregrounded resources of all kinds in the South African context. In the UK context, 'support' was understood almost entirely psychosocially, although here too the word can indicate practical assistance. In South Africa ten years ago, 'support', whatever its linguistic context, was understood to mean medical and psychosocial but also practical help. In 2012, though, it was taken by interviewees, when they referred to the present and future, primarily as referring to material support for everyday lives.

Work and citizenship: ' I want to work'

Getting work was a major theme of the 2001 stories. In 2012, it was even more than before a priority for interviewees, particularly since their HIV needs were less immediate and intense and they were planning lengthy, healthy lives with ARV treatment. Boniswa provided a typical future-story of how she would like to live through work:

> **Boniswa:** I want work, like working with my hands, to do things with my hands, things that are going to make me to have money and sewing. Those are the things I want in my life ... I want to work for myself.

This entrepreneurial approach to living with HIV and markets was very common. Several interviewees, for instance, wanted a sewing machine or hairdressing materials to work at home, or wanted more resources to expand existing small businesses within the informal economy. The absence of such resources, and of opportunities for paid employment, did not generate stories of political and psychosocial dispossession, as with UK participants. Rather, these absences produced stories of unmet personal and familial requirements for living and of shame, like that of Siyanda, faced with children she could not feed, limiting their own and her HIV citizenship.

As stories like Boniswa's of small-scale, 'work for myself' initiatives might suggest, interviewees' tales of what work might be done were foreshadowing stories, strongly grounded in present resources. They did not imagine towards large-scale social mobility. Like Boniswa, interviewees recognised the resources they already had and liked – 'working with my hands' – or more generally in the case of the income-generation project, the craft skills they had acquired there, and made those resources determinants of the story. Many had voluntary experience also of working as counsellors or home carers. The contemporary HIV market in South Africa, contracting in the wake of successful treatment, normalisation and destigmatisation, and financial cuts, means that these skills were less likely to be woven into stories of a remunerated future than in the past, or than in the contemporary United Kingdom. As skills of which the country has an abundance, they can rarely provide economic capital, although they are powerful social and cultural resources.

Participants' stories of their employment and education plans in 2001 tended to cover a broader span, perhaps related to the country's larger possibilities at the time, a growth-oriented global economy, and the narrators' deeply embattled situations within the epidemic, in response to which they constructed powerful projections of an ideal future. The newer participants in this interview round were all from low-income backgrounds, which might be argued to constrain their narratives of life progression. However, such constraint did not characterise the earlier interviews with people living in similar poverty. Nor did it appear in re-interviews this time around with middle-income participants from the earlier rounds, in which those participants, like the others, generated stories of economic participation that built in a careful and step-wise manner on their past and present work.

Small-scale entrepreneurship stories like those of Boniswa and many other interviewees are not just tales of the beginning or lowest, small-scale, informal, insecure level of marketised societies. As narrated here, this was affirmed as work for yourself, under your own control. It was not part of larger structures, which might seem in South Africa, both historically and in the present, unreliable and unaccountable to individual employees and to society. Moreover, while interviewees' focus on entrepreneurship might read as parking responsibility for happy three-letter lives on individuals, their stories were about improving things for their children, families and communities, rather than about individualised success. Providing for children, needy siblings, or ageing, ill parents, were the expressed goals of productive employment.

As in the UK material, therefore, though in a very different national political context, interviewees narrated and sometimes in so doing, planned their attempts to create resources for themselves, their children and community. In this case, unlike in the United Kingdom, participants' accounts were of the building of economic as well as social HIV citizenship. They found ways to 'live with' HIV and low resources, rooting out what resources they had, building on them, and searching for new ones. In these narrated strategies, HIV was also a much less determining part of the context of work and productivity than in the United Kingdom, intersecting with, for instance, education and employment histories and opportunities, and restrictions around gender, age, and access to capital and means of production.

Health markets and social welfare

As Ong (2006) notes, marketised societies operating under the rubric of the 'neo-liberal' must of necessity also work with non-marketised social arrangements that maintain the lives of citizens and non-citizens who fall outside market logic. The South African interviews provided a number of stories of health and social services operating according to market constraints, in rationing professional time, for instance, and in cutting the availability of free medications beyond those directly required to deal with HIV illness and such medications' own most severe side effects. For example, interviewees said that medicated cream for eczema, which some reported as an ARV side effect, now had to be bought; only a moisturising cream was provided free. Social grants, particularly the disability grant, were narrated as moving towards stricter criteria, were being time-managed, and depended more strongly on doctor discretion for their continuation. Yet participants provided many counteracting narratives of managing health and grant income at the same time. These stories criticised the arbitrariness, unfairness, and long-term uneconomic nature of such short-term savings; often they also involved negotiations with and between doctors.

It was reported, for instance by Siyanda, that some people did not take ARVs at times in order to maintain the grant. She herself had thought of this action, but she, like other study participants, did not report pursuing it. Given these participants' involvement in highly HIV-literate groups of HIV citizens, they are perhaps some of the least likely to adopt it:

> **Siyanda:** I only get only six months {disability grant}. By the time I was taking ARVs./I see/Then I lost it. I didn't go back and do it again, I say, 'No, the grant is not important more than my health. I don't want go back and start it again, again'.
> **Interviewer:** No. Do you think some people want the grant more than their health?
> **Siyanda:** Mhm, some people. Some people they default with ARVs because they want CD4 count to drop.
> **Interviewer:** Yes. Do you think many people do that?
> **Siyanda:** I don't encourage that.
> **Interviewer:** No. Do you think many people do that?
> **Siyanda:** Yes, some. They do it.

This is an obvious example, as Siyanda knew, of people already living in poverty compromising health resources for monetary ones which could provide, for instance, food and children's education. HIV can propel people into poverty and food insecurity, and it appears an 'austerity' welfare policy can do the same, with health the only resource that can be traded for nutrition and cash.

People apparently more resource-secure, trying to move into a more middle-class life, are also affected by loss of grant support. Nonkosi, living in a family with some earned income and using part of her disability grant to buy a fridge by instalments, lost her disability grant, failed the payments, and told the company to take the fridge back. That fridge guaranteed fresh and nutritious food, which could be bought in reasonable quantities and therefore more cheaply for a large household. Economically, participants in such situations lived with HIV precariously (Standing 2011), despite their relatively good educational and other social and cultural resources. As with people living in poverty, their economic position was always on the point of determining their health. The struggled-for value of social and cultural resources within a convivial HIV citizenship, of Nonkosi's wide-reaching HIV-aware friendship network, for instance, were always on the brink of being broken up and lost because of economic failure. Such things as reduced ability to pay for transport, which allows connections to be made and kept with different support groups and with central training facilities, would have diminished Nonkosi's social resources. Sometimes such losses can be recouped by accessing other resources, for instance, by relying more on free phone texts or making walking part of one's health regime. Face-to-face meetings provide a different kind of support though, and poor health may mean that long walks are not the best fitness exercise.

On the other hand, people already living in poverty, like Siyanda, cannot contribute economically towards developing their social and cultural resources in the first place, and have less existing resources with which to be resourceful. They always need transport in order to contribute to collective life outside their neighbourhood. They often cannot afford to spend money on healthy rather than caloric food. They may not be able to meet basic nutritional needs, let alone the food needs exacted by ARVs, without a grant. In such situations, a sympathetic doctor who approves the disability grant, a church group that provides regular transport to activities and occasional food parcels, friends from the support group who come by with food they have cooked, or help from partners or family members are essential, convivial aspects of living with HIV and ARVs. These non-market resources are the ubiquitous, often-unremarked companions of the market economy, keeping people alive.

Living with the market economy

In Chapter 3, Yoliswa saved for the end of her story of 'living with' HIV and ARVs, her concerns about global financial uncertainties in relation to donor drug supply. Most of the participants in the 2012 study articulated such concerns more locally. Loss of capital flows meant that the middle- and high-income church supporters of food aid to the support group from which many participants came were donating less. Participants from that group noted the now-sporadic nature of this help. Participants from the income-generation group narrated the recent abolition of a regular stipend; price undercutting; fewer orders than before; and loss of full-time paid staff. The regional, national and international markets into which their work was tied, were suffering. Local markets were in a different position: the trickle-down of fiscal crisis and austerity was not affecting the informal economy as much. Interviewees with small businesses of their own, selling food, sewing or hairdressing, said that little had changed for them, economically.

Although in South African HIV policy, successful ARV treatment is described as allowing full-time employment, people living with HIV and ARVs experience particular difficulties in integrating themselves into market economies. Especially in a high-unemployment economy, uncertain and weaker health disadvantages a person. Such health can itself be worsened by the demands of full-time work. There are related difficulties in attending school, and in getting money to go back to and finish school. Also, as in the United Kingdom, HIV can cause a problematic employment break. Several interviewees who were longer-diagnosed told stories about being excluded from work because employers want younger people, not people who, because of illness, have not worked or developed their skills for a long time. The exclusions that keep people living with HIV and ARVs from 'normal' lives, that is, lives with paid work, are ineluctably tied to such employment markets.

Occasionally, market discourse inflected participant narratives in a usefully analytic way, as other work on neo-liberalism's effects within low- and middle-income countries has found (Ong 2006). Some interviewees, for instance, told critical stories of NGOs protecting their resources, like computers, minibuses and trainings, rather than making them available for general up-skilling of their clients that would let them become more knowledgeable, more competitive and more integrated into the economy. While such broad availability might not have been practical, or even part of the NGOs' remits, such critical 'market' narratives pointed to issues of transparency and accountability that are important for NGOs' functioning.

More often, though, cracks in neo-liberal approaches appeared within the interviews, particularly in participants' counteracting stories about 'living with' HIV and ARVs in ways that cannot make market sense. As described already in this chapter, some stories about 'living with' HIV and ARVs alongside poverty were simply about keeping oneself and others alive. Even within policy discourse, such stories can only secondarily be parsed as 'investments' in potential workers and parents of future contributors to the economy. Their primary storied meaning is of human suffering and collective human responsibility.

In participants' counteracting narratives, the lived contradictions to neo-liberalism were strongly developed, and mostly lacked the qualifying self-descriptions as marketised subjects that were present in the UK material. These narratives paid attention to the marketised frame of HIV lives, but argued, implicitly or explicitly, for more than the provision of just enough resources to sustain people for future work. Nonkosi, for example, dismissed the current occasional work-day activities of the income-generation group in a compact one-sentence story.

Nonkosi: We just work, eat and go home.

Instead of regular hours of work for a regular stipend, small amounts of product were now just occasionally required. Training and other work-based activities had ceased, though a meal was still provided for the workers by donor money.

Similarly, Nombulelo described the eking out of orders and money at a level that had little to do with more general citizenly resource requirements:

Nombulelo: What is happening here, as we are sewing, we receive a small amount of money {for small orders} and it's not enough because we do not have work that give us support. We get work when there is an order, that is how we get money, you see what we need is that we get the support {stipend}. You stay the whole month without any food, you stay here for the whole month working here and get no money.

Participants' stories did not present the income-generation group itself as implementing marketised policies The stories did, however, often evaluate the group's contemporary difficulties by explicating how it was no longer possible for the group to obtain funding without showing that its work made economic sense, in terms of human 'investment', if not profit from goods. Participants were aware that the profit and even the investment requirement were almost impossible to meet within the flat-lining economic present. Their narratives thus constituted a highly analytic account of the limits of marketised policies in high-unemployment, low-income contexts, where citizens must negotiate the boundaries of health and illness as well as poverty. Once again, HIV citizenship was offering resources of cultural and political knowledge that could have important and more general benefits.

Participants' demarketising narratives referenced a wide range of existing resources, such as skills, contacts, time and motivation to work. Even though the narratives arose from the specificities of living with HIV and ARVs, they applied to people who were not HIV positive or HIV-affected; they described an HIV-inflected citizenship. And they had, as their hoped-for ends, a local conviviality of community-owned and controlled forms of work within which HIV statuses, while recognised, were lived with alongside other social conjunctions.

Conclusion

Contemporary narratives of living with HIV and ARVs in South Africa demonstrated the strong national particularities of the pandemic. In many ways, these narratives were distinct from those that appeared within the accounts of people living with HIV in the UK, even though they operated with similar processes of naturalisation and denaturalisation. This chapter's analysis of the South African narratives might, though, have some translatable applicability to other high-prevalence, low-resourced national, local and community situations, where ARVs are accessible and stigmatisation is reducing, though still marked.

The chapter's 'living with' title refers to the ways in which the inter-sectionalities of HIV citizenship with health in general, poverty, education and gender were consistently articulated in the participants' stories. These 'living with' stories thus had a narrative form different from the ambiguous 'living on' stories of the previous chapter. The South African stories were characterised more by the blurring of borders than by their negotiation.

Participants' narratives of medical discourses and practices performed these discourses and practices, even more than in the UK study, as owned and implemented by the narrators, via activist but also community knowledges. These stories were consistently shaped by resource constraints, particularly around food. Participants also articulated an HIV-inflected 'normality', a convivial HIV citizenship much more intersectionally 'lived with' than in the UK study stories, but again, constrained by resources. Finally, in narrating the marketised contexts of current three-letter lives, the South African interviewees once more spoke from positions defined multiply by HIV and other conditions. They did so in more explicitly critical voices, with a fuller articulation of alternatives, than in the UK study. Perhaps this difference could be ascribed to the country's own specific political history, perhaps also to HIV's higher prevalence and people's relatively greater openness about it in South Africa.

Throughout the stories, interviewees narrated and performed resourcefulness: both a critical awareness of resource constraints, and an ongoing attention to existing and possible resources. Participants' resource mobilisations rested on the convivialities of community, neighbourhood, and family engagements, as much as on activist histories (Abdullah and Squire 2010; Mbali 2013; Squire 2007). But such mobilisations could not meet the requirements of everyday life, intensified by HIV life. More than some policy narratives, participant stories were clear about such limits.

10
Hopeful Futures, Inertial Histories and the Complex Present

Optimism and momentum has been building around the real possibility that an AIDS-free generation is imminent. Public enthusiasm is fuelled by news about the rapid scale-up of antiretroviral therapy, evidence that HIV treatment can prevent new infections, and expanded coverage of programmes to prevent mother-to-child transmission of HIV. Yet, the most recent estimates of HIV prevalence and incidence and of AIDS-related mortality released by UNAIDS... make it clear that AIDS is not over... while much progress has been made in treatment and prevention, the persistent and substantial global burden associated with HIV and AIDS compels us to do more – and do better – to achieve the AIDS-free generation the world is waiting for.

Sidibé et al. (2012)

Rebecca: You know, now back home... the people that grew up together, their friends, they don't just ask 'where is', uh-uh!

Susan: Generations have been wiped out.

Rebecca: They have gone! They have gone. My brother told me, the people have died.

Susan: Generations have really been wiped out.

Rebecca: It's only the older people remaining, with young people.

Susan: Yeah, the young people. As long as they are negative, because if they are positive, they are bound to die at some point.

Rebecca and Susan, UK (2011)

For two of my UK interviews, I travel to the outer reaches of South London, to a small block of flats where the borough council houses asylum-seekers. The flats are a long bus ride away from the train station and the central shopping area. Rebecca has offered to host myself and Susan, a friend of hers, for the afternoon. Both will do interviews. Before Susan arrives, Rebecca describes her ARV treatment, still only moderately successful – her CD4+ T cell count remains under 500, five years after she started – and her difficult citizenship status. Eleven years after arriving in the UK and seven years after her first asylum application, she is still awaiting a decision from the Home Office on whether she can stay in the UK. She talks briefly of her children in her country of origin and, upset, switches topic to her own current situation. The council provides her housing and a pre-paid £40-a-week card to pay for food, clothes, other personal necessities and transport. To welcome myself and her friend, she offers water, fruit juice, and a bowl of fresh fruit, all kept in a pristine refrigerator. In severely constrained economic circumstances, she makes a priority of good nutrition to support her still-precarious health. This happens at the direct expense of travel outside her area, for instance, to centralised HIV NGOs that provide trainings and legal advice. As happens at our meeting, Rebecca also often contributes food resources to her convivial relations with HIV positive friends like Susan, to other non-HIV-affected friends living in the flats, and even to one-time visitors like me. This hospitable sharing supports the HIV-inflected social citizenship that, in the absence of other forms of citizenship, sustains her.

How much is held in common and how much is different across Rebecca's situation, and South African lives lived with HIV and ARVs? During my research in South Africa, I spend time with the support group from which I have recruited new participants, and with their facilitator. From these visits, as well as the interviews, a complex picture emerges of health, feelings and resources within group members' three-letter lives. Most members live in a rapidly growing, very poor, under-serviced and crime-troubled informal settlement that spreads out around the group meeting place. It can take members over an hour to get to the group. Many members are too resource-constrained to take advantage of other resources that could help them. For instance, their homes are dispersed and far from large shops. They are cash-strapped for transport, with no transport of their own. Though their treatment is successful on physiological measures, in most cases much more than Rebecca's, they also live with significant levels of HIV- and ARV-related symptoms and other illnesses. Almost all members are women, with large responsibilities for domestic work. These factors make it hard for the group members to make and keep clinic appointments, to attend support groups beyond a short walk away, to network with HIV positive friends, or to look for work. They would find it very difficult to bulk-buy food collectively in the way I described a group doing in Chapter 9.

Often, too, home circumstances make resourceful everyday living with HIV and ARVs problematic. If group members have HIV positive children and no food in the morning, then theoretically they could take advantage of organisations offering such children free pre-school breakfasts and transport to them, in order to support their children's treatment regimes. However, their parents often wake up fatigued and in ill health, needing to wash, clean and get the children ready for school in a one-room wood or metal home with very little infrastructure (no running water or electricity and poor sanitation, for instance). Most live some distance from places where free transport to the breakfast facility is available. They may also not want to be seen using services – such as free meals and a special minibus – that might reveal their child's HIV positivity, however open they are about their own status. In such conditions, the human resources required to pursue food security may be too great to allow it.

Since treatment adherence is key to healthy three-letter lives, the sustainability of survival itself, let alone more general positive aspects of living with HIV, is in doubt here, especially for children living with HIV. This may also be true for adults, who sometimes similarly skip medications when they do not have food, who may also do this at times to get or preserve a grant, and who are distanced in many ways from medical and psychosocial support.

Some group members are discouraged. They describe, for example, the fruitlessness of looking for work, the impossibility of caring properly for their children. At the same time, all the members I talk to describe and evidence, in the activities of their lives, intense and ongoing efforts at resourcefulness. They keep their main clinic appointments and search out better doctors and medications if they think their health needs them. They are assiduous in building their social and cultural resources: they tend to their neighbourhood friendship networks, particularly with other HIV positive people; they chat to nurses and doctors; they visit support groups all over, sometimes walking long distances; they take up volunteer or other work in NGOs and CBOs whenever it is offered and accessible, as with my research; they establish friendships with people in such organisations. But it would be unrealistic to expect the powerful social and cultural convivialities of HIV and ARV lives that these members develop to translate into economic self-sufficiency in the conditions of still-problematic health and economic and other material resource scarcity in which they live.

This book has tried to show the importance of particularity, rather than exceptionality, within specific HIV contexts, especially within the two distinct national epidemics in the United Kingdom and South Africa. I have tried to demonstrate this particularity against the background of many commonalities in contemporary three-letter lives. Such lives are characterised by earlier treatment and increasing treatment success; lowered levels of stigmatisation and discrimination in some national and local contexts; the strong abilities of HIV positive citizens to find and build resources for their lives; and policy discourses and practices that have the 'end of AIDS' in sight. These are important, progressive and hopeful commonalities, as Sidibé and colleagues (2012) acknowledge at the beginning of this chapter. As those writers emphasises, though, the HIV pandemic continues to present large problems of higher and sustainable funding, targeted prevention, treatment and care integration, political mobilisation, and community education. Today, people living with HIV and ARVs experience the failures to deliver those policies and services, and the complexities that both cause and result from those failures. They live with the instabilities and limitations of treatment; powerful constraints on resources; and difficult, and often neglected psychosocial aspects of 'living on' and 'living with' HIV and ARVs, when the condition becomes an acknowledged or invisible part of everyday life, while at the same time still carrying with it the abjection of long-term illness and social difference or exclusion.

For instance, in both national situations, the treatment possibility era can make it difficult to address ongoing health difficulties. Nevertheless, these difficulties are prevalent, and will escalate as more people take ARVs for longer. In the South African case especially, medical resource constraints intensify such problems. Despite reduced stigma in high-prevalence contexts such as South Africa, there exists, even there, the possibility of a kind of second-class 'HIV' citizenship, which women seem more able to turn around by their imbrication in social resources that span family and community, church, clinic and support groups. In countries like the United Kingdom, HIV's invisibilisation remains relatively unchallenged. Rebecca and Susan, the two friends in the story that begins this chapter, do not have local HIV positive or HIV aware friends. They must travel long distances to see each other, and the main support group they both used to frequent has closed. At the same time, HIV can turn citizenship itself into something new in high-prevalence contexts, rewriting popular stories of health and resources in ways that counteract dominant, marketised narratives, as can be seen from the story of the South African support group at the beginning of this chapter. Socially and culturally, it is harder for this to happen in low-prevalence contexts like the United Kingdom where narratives of HIV citizenship are hardly spoken. The resurgent HIV activism of ACT UP in the United States is one example of an attempt to counteract such silence. The micro-social convivialities constructed by texting, phoning and where possible, visits, by some of my UK research participants, like Olive and Queenie, across networks of migrant and asylum-seeker women living with HIV, are others. In South Africa, as the story of the group at the beginning of this chapter also suggests, such resources must be seen, despite their effectiveness, in the context of drastic shortages in economic resources. Within the United Kingdom, too, HIV positive people who are not working are living in economic circumstances that severely limit their three-letter lives, especially if, like Rebecca, they are asylum-seekers.

The book has attempted to explicate the particularities of HIV by tracing the contemporary processes through which HIV is becoming a naturalised part of health and social citizenship. The ambiguities of naturalisation, that is, the operation and the simultaneous undoing of medicalisation, normalisation, and marketisation, work differently in various national environments. In the United Kingdom, a kind of para-liberalism characterises people's counteracting narratives. It negotiates the borderlines of naturalisation processes, mapping out ways in which people 'live on' long-term with HIV. In the South African context, narratives are more occupied with tracing processes of 'living with' HIV across different HIV statuses and alongside many other difficult conditions. Here, counteracting narratives are less tied to market logics, more connected to recent HIV and other activist traditions. They are more occupied with the building of economic and social resources. They are also able to draw on a developing, cross-status sociality that is inflected by the country's recent HIV history, that foregrounds HIV knowledge, acceptance and campaigning.

In both national contexts, however, there are many elements of experience on the edges even of these counteracting narratives. Being 'left behind' by situations of uncertain knowledge, inadequate resources and failures to understand HIV's abjections and ineluctability persist in both epidemic contexts. It appears in what the South African support group members show about their ongoing health difficulties in their fatigue and the time it takes them to walk short distances; what Rebecca cannot say about the children she cannot see; how Rebecca and Susan live with an inertial history of HIV suffering and death that until relatively recently characterised most epidemics in the world and that can bring a degree of fatalism with it. 'Generations have been wiped out!' Rebecca says, and, 'They have gone!' Susan affirms, later extending this future to all the young people who are HIV positive, too.

The book has quoted extensively from the stories told by research participants living with HIV and ARVs in the United Kingdom and South Africa, in order to trace the complexities of three-letter lives as people express and develop them across multiple narrative threads. Sometimes such narratives are spoken as highly personal stories, opaque even to the teller, sometimes as social narratives, 'stories of us'. The participants produced many stories that explicitly and implicitly criticised and presented alternatives to discourses and practices of HIV's naturalisation. It was important to recognise such elements of their narratives, without over-romanticising them or treating them as substitutes for other, larger-scale forms of politics. For such stories are the grounds of HIV citizenship. They give narrators and their audiences accounts of the HIV world that entangle and extend the simpler stories of HIV politics and policy. They are stories that present micro-theories of epidemics' particularities and that, in the process, open up the possible futures of three-letter lives.

Notes

2 From HIV's Exceptionalism to HIV's Particularity

1. Here and in all interview excerpts, round brackets indicate paralinguistic elements like laughs, substitutions for purposes of anonymity, words that are not entirely audible, or transcription gaps. Curly brackets indicate insertions to improve sense.
2. Some term this position normalisation; I have reserved that term for social rather than biosocial regularisations of HIV, since naturalisation refers especially to the making-natural, making part of the biological world, of phenomena. For further discussion of naturalisation and normalisation, see Chapters 3 and 5.
3. See the *Lancet* July 2012 special issue on HIV and men who have sex with men.
4. Derrida gives exceptionality a double character, both part of and radically dissociated from the norm. I am naming the aspect of it that involves partial assimilation, particularity.

3 Being Naturalised

1. Chapters 3–7 draw on and expand arguments first sketched in Squire (2010).
2. This term has been taken from a song within Roger Bourland's song cycle, *Hidden Legacies*, discussed further in Chapter 7.

5 A Long-term Condition: HIV's Normalisation

1. This portion of Mhiki's interview was cited also in Squire (2007), in a different context.

6 Investing in the Pandemic: The Marketised HIV Citizen

1. This interview was also used, within a different interpretive framework, in Squire (2007).

7 Being Left Behind

1. Some of this portion of Mhiki's interview has been analysed in a different context in Squire (2007).
2. This material has been analysed with a different emphasis in Squire (2007).
3. Thanks to Dr. Lillian Cingo for this insight.

8 Living on: Three-letter Lives in the United Kingdom

1. Most of this information is taken from the Health Protection Agency's reports (Health Protection Agency 2011a; 2012).
2. Previous interview rounds were done in 1993, 1994, 1997 and 2001–2, and have involved 70 interviewees in total (see Squire 1998; 2004; 2006 for further procedural details). Interviews were preceded by me giving participants details about the research, though these had already been received in some cases, and asking them to sign a consent form. All these documents could be discussed orally, particularly helpful in cases where English was not participants' first language. After interviews, participants were asked to provide some optional data on age, ethnicity, sexuality, employment, study or profession, dates of diagnosis and of becoming HIV positive, and treatment experience. I made field notes about aspects of the research such as where it was conducted, and general nonverbal aspects of the interview, that do not appear within the transcripts.

9 Living with HIV: Three-letter Lives in South Africa

1. Most recent figures come from Republic of South Africa (2012) and van der Linde (2013).
2. The account in the paragraphs above is drawn from all three of these references.
3. See also Colvin and Robins (2009) on men's negotiations of responsibilised masculinities in a close-by study area, and Campbell and colleagues' (2012) account of collective responsibility for support in rural Zimbabwe.

References

AbdoolKarim, Q., AbdoolKarim, S., Frohlich, J., Grobler, A., Baxter, C., Mansoor, L., et al. (2010) Effectiveness and safety of tenofovir gel, an antiretroviral microbicide, for the prevention of HIV infection in women. *Science* 329: 1168–74.

Abdullah, F., and Squire, C. (2010) Technologies of treatment: Scaling up ART in the Western Cape, South Africa. In *HIV technologies in international perspective*, edited by M. Davis and C. Squire. London: Palgrave Macmillan.

Abrahams, N., and Jewkes, R. (2012) Managing and resisting stigma: A qualitative study among people living with HIV in South Africa. *Journal of the International AIDS Society* 15, article 17330. http://www.jiasociety.org/index.php/jias/article/view/17330. Accessed 20 July 2013.

ACT UP NY. (2013) LGBT NY mayoral forum, ACT UP NY Announce, April 1. http://justiceunity.com/cgi-bin/dada/mail.cgi/list/actupnyann/. Accessed 20 June 2013.

Althusser, L. (1998) *Reading Capital*. London: Verso.

Arieff, A., Weiss, M., and Jones, V. (2010) The global economic crisis: Impact on sub-Saharan Africa and global policy responses. Washington, D.C.: Congressional Research Service. April 6. http://www.fas.org/sgp/crs/row/R40778.pdf. Accessed 20 July 2013.

Babb, D., Pemba, L., Seatlanyane, P., Charalambous, S., Churchyard, G., and Grant, A. (2007) Use of traditional medicine by HIV-infected individuals in South Africa in the era of antiretroviral therapy. *Psychology, Health and Medicine* 12: 314–20.

Bad Object Choices (1991) *How do I look?* San Francisco, CA: Bay Press.

Baeten, J., Donnell, D., Ndase, P., Mugo, R., Campbell, J., Wangisi, J., et al. (2012) Antiretroviral prophylaxis for HIV prevention in heterosexual men and women. *New England Journal of Medicine* 367, 5: 399–410. August 2.

Baker, P. (2010) From apartheid to neoliberalism: Health equity in post-apartheid South Africa. *International Journal of Health Services* 40, 1: 79–95.

Baleta, A. (2012) South Africa rolls out pilot health insurance scheme. *The Lancet* 379, 9822: 1185. 31 March. http://www.thelancet.com/journals/lancet/article/PIIS0140-6736%2812%2960495-4/fulltext. Accessed 20 July 2012.

Bamberg, M., and Andrews, M. (2004) *Considering counter-narratives*. Amsterdam: John Benjamins.

Barnett, C., Cloke, P., Clarke, N., and Malpass, A. (2008) The elusive subjects of neoliberalism. *Cultural Studies* 2, 5: 624–53.

Barnett, A., and Whiteside, A. (2006) *AIDS in the twenty-first century*. London: Palgrave Macmillan.

Baubock, R. (2008) Stakeholder citizenship: An idea whose time has come? In *Delivering citizenship: The Transatlantic Council on Migration*, edited by Berlsmann Stiftung, European Policy Centre, Migration Policy Institute. Gütersloh, Germany: Verlag Bertelsmann Stiftung. pp. 31–48.

Bayer, R. (1999) Clinical progress and the future of HIV exceptionalism. *Archives of Internal Medicine* 159, 10: 1042–8. May 24.

Beasley-Murray, J. (2000) Value and capital in Bourdieu and Marx. In *Pierre Bourdieu: Fieldwork in culture*, edited by Brown, N., and Szeman, I. Lanham, MD: Rowman and Littlefield. pp. 100–19.

Beaubien, J. (2013) South Africa weighs starting HIV drug treatment sooner. *Shots, Health News from NPR*. July 16. http://www.npr.org/blogs/health/2013/07/16/202381945/south-africa-weighs-starting-hiv-drug-treatment-sooner. Accessed 20 July 2013.

Bernays, S., and Rhodes, T. (2009) Experiencing uncertain HIV treatment delivery in a transitional setting: A qualitative study. *AIDS Care* 21, 3: 315–21.

Bernays, S., Rhodes, T., and Prodanovic, V. (2007) *HIV Treatment Access, Delivery and Uncertainty: A Qualitative Study in Serbia and in Montenegro*. Belgrade: United Nations Development Programme.

Bertagnolio, S., Parkin, N., and Jordan, M. (2012) HIV drug resistance surveillance in low- and middle-income countries: 2004 to 2010. *Journal of the International AIDS Society* 11: 15, Supplement 4.

Bhabha, H. (1994) *The Location of Culture*. London: Routledge.

Bhabha, H. (2011) *Our Neighbours, Ourselves*. Berlin: Walter de Gruyter.

Bloch, A. (2010) The right to rights? Undocumented migrants from Zimbabwe living in South Africa. *Sociology* 44, 2 (April): 233–50.

Bogart, L., Wagner, G., Galvan, F., and Banks, D. (2010) Conspiracy beliefs about HIV are related to antiretroviral treatment nonadherence among African American men with HIV. *Journal of Acquired Immune Deficiency Syndrome* 53, 5: 648–55.

Bogere, H. (2009) AIDS crisis: patients turned away as drugs dry up. *Observer* (Uganda). July 5. http://www.observer.ug/index.php?option=com_content&task=view&id=4133&Itemid=59. Accessed 20 July 2013.

Bor, J., Herbst, A., Newell, M-L., and Bärnighausen, T. (2013) Increases in adult life expectancy in rural South Africa: Valuing the scale-up of HIV treatment. *Science* 339, 6122: 961–5.

Bhorat, H., Goga, S., and Tseng, D. (2013) *Unemployment Insurance in South Africa*. Washington, DC: Brookings Institution. April. http://www.brookings.edu/~/media/Research/Files/Papers/2013/04/04_unemployment_insurance_south_africa.pdf. Accessed 20 July 2013.

Borzekowski, D. (2011) Successfully reaching the youth of Nairobi: Evaluating the Project Ignite campaign. *Journal of Adolescent Health* 48, 2, Supplement S46–7.

Bosniak, L. (2006) *The Citizen and the Alien: Dilemmas of Contemporary Membership*. Princeton, NJ: Princeton University Press.

Boulle, A., Hilderbrand, K., Menten, J., Coetzee, D., Ford, M., Mathys, F., et al. (2008) Exploring HIV risk perception and behaviour in the context of antiretroviral treatment: Results from a township household survey. *AIDS Care* 20, 7: 771–81.

Bourdieu, P. (1977 [1972]) *Outline of a Theory of Practice*. Cambridge: Cambridge University Press.

Bourdieu, P. (1986) The forms of capital. In *Handbook of Theory and Research for the Sociology of Education*, edited by Richardson, J. Westport, CT: Greenwood.

Bourdieu, P. (1998) *Acts of Resistance*. London: Polity Press.

Bourland, R. (2006) 'Left behind' by John Hall and Roger Bourland. http://roger-bourland.com/2006/02/18/left-behind-by-john-hall-and-roger-bourland/. February 18. Accessed 20 June 2013.

Bourland, R., and Hall, J. (1992) *Hidden Legacies*. Los Angeles: Gay Men's Chorus of Los Angeles.

Bower, M., Powles, T., Newsom-Davis, T., Thirlwell, C., Stebbing, J., Mandalia, S., et al. (2004) HIV-associated anal cancer: Has highly active anti-retroviral therapy reduced the incidence or improved the outcome? *Journal of Acquired Immune Deficiency Syndrome* 37, 5: 1563–5.

Brandt, R. (2008) Is it all chaos, loss and disruption? The narratives of poor, HIV-infected South African women. Cape Town: Centre for Social Science Research. CSSR Working Paper 224. http://www.cssr.uct.ac.za/sites/cssr.uct. ac.za/files/pubs/WP224.pdf. Accessed 20 June 13.

British HIV Association and Expert Advisory Group on AIDS (2013) *Position Statement on the Use of Antiretroviral Therapy to Reduce HIV Transmission*. London: BHIVA and EAGA. January.https://www.gov.uk/government/uploads/system/ uploads/attachment_data/file/213284/BHIVA-EAGA-Position-statement- on-the-use-of-antiretroviral-therapy-to-reduce-HIV-transmission-final.pdf. Accessed 20 July 2013.

Bunton, R., Burrows, J., and Nettleton, S. (1995) *The Sociology of Health Promotion*. London: Routledge.

Bury, M. (1982) Chronic illness as biographical disruption. *Sociology of Health and Illness* 4, 2: 167–82.

Butler, J. (2005) *Giving an Account of Oneself*. Fordham, NY: Fordham University Press.

Cameron, E., Mathers, J., and Parry, J. (2008) Health and well being: Questioning the use of health concepts in public health policy and practice. *Critical Public Health* 16, 4: 347–54.

Campbell, C. (2003) *Letting Them Die? Why African AIDS Prevention Programmes Often Fail*. Bloomington: Indiana University Press.

Campbell, C., Nair, Y., Maimane, S., and Gibbs, A. (2009) Strengthening community responses to AIDS: Possibilities and challenges. In *HIV/AIDS in South Africa: 25 Years on*, edited by P. Rohleder, L. Swartz, S. Kalichman, and L. Simbayi. New York: Springer.

Campbell, C., Nair, Y., Maimane, S., and Sibiya, Z. (2007) Building contexts that support effective community responses to HIV/AIDS. *American Journal of Community Psychology* 39, 3–4: 347–63.

Campbell, C., Skovdal, M., Mupambireyi, Z., Madanhire, C., Nyamukapa, C., and Gregson, S. (2012) Building adherence-competent communities: Factors promoting children's adherence to antiretroviral HIV/AIDS treatment in rural Zimbabwe. *Health and Place* 18, 2: 123–31. March.

Carlisle, S., and Hanlon, P. (2008) 'Well-being' as a focus for public health? A critique and defence. *Critical Public Health* 18, 3: 263–70.

Carr, R., and Gramling, L. (2004) Stigma: A health barrier for women with HIV/ AIDS. *Journal of the Association of Nurses in AIDS Care* 15, 5: 30–9.

Carricaburu, D., and Pierret, J. (1995) From biographical disruption to biographical reinforcement: The case of HIV-positive men. *Sociology of Health and Illness* 17, 1: 65–88.

Centers for Disease Control. (2013) Study finds first evidence that PrEP can reduce HIV risk among people who inject drugs. Atlanta, GA: Centers for Disease Control. http://www.cdc.gov/nchhstp/newsroom/2013/PrEP-Study- Press-Release.html. Accessed 20 June 2013.

Ciambrone, D. (2001) Illness and other assaults on self: The relative impacts of HIV/AIDS on women's lives. *Sociology of Health and Illness* 23: 517–40.

Cloete, A., Strebel, A., Simbayi, L., van Wyck, B., Henda, N., and Nqeketa, A. (2010) Challenges faced by people living with HIV/AIDS in Cape Town, South Africa. *AIDS Research and Treatment* 2010, Article ID 420270, 8 pages, doi:10.1155/2010/420270. Accessed 20 July 2013.

Cohen, M., Chen, Y., McCauley, M., Gamble, T., Hossenipour, M., Kumarasamy, N., et al. (2011) Prevention of HIV-1 infection with early antiretroviral therapy. *New England Journal of Medicine* 36: 493–505.

Cohen, M., McCauley, M., and Gamble, T. (2012) HIV as prevention and HPTN 052. *Current Opinion in HIV/AIDS* 7, 2: 99–105.

Colvin, C., and Robins, S. (2009) Positive men in hard, neoliberal times: Engendering health citizenship in South Africa. In *Gender and HIV/AIDS:Critical Perspectives from the Developing World*, edited by J. Boestan, and N. Poku. London: Ashgate.

Conceicao, P., and Bandura, R. (2008) Measuring subjective wellbeing: A summary review of the literature. UNDP Working Paper, May.

Coovadia, H., Jewkes, R., Barron, P., Sanders, D., and McIntyre, D. (2009) The health and health system in South Africa: Historical roots of public health challenges. *Lancet* 374, 9692, 817–34. 5 September. http://www.thelancet.com/journals/lancet/article/PIIS0140-6736%2809%2960951-X/. Accessed 20 July 2013.

Cornwall, A., Robins, S., and Von Lieres, B. (2011) States of citizenship: Contexts and cultures of public engagement and citizen action. IDS Working Paper 363. Brighton, Sussex: IDS. http://www.drc-citizenship.org/system/assets/1052734719/original/1052734719-cornwall_etal.2010-states.pdf. Accessed 20 July 2013.

COSATU (2013) Summary of critique of the National Development Plan, March 2013 (draft). Johannesburg: COSATU. http://www.cosatu.org.za/docs/discussion/2013/NDPcritiquesummary.pdf. Accessed 20 July 2013.

Crenshaw, K. (2003) Traffic at the crossroads: Multiple oppressions. In *Sisterhood is Forever: The Women's Anthology for a New Millennium*, edited by R. Morgan. New York: Washington Square Press.

Crimp, D. (2002) *Melancholia and Moralism: Essays on AIDS and Queer Politics*. Cambridge, MA: MIT Press.

Crossley, M. (2000) *Introducing Narrative Psychology: Self, Trauma and the Construction of Meaning*. Buckinghamshire, UK: Open University Press.

Dageid, W., Sliep, Y., Akintola, O., and Duckert, F. (2011) *Response-ability in the Era of AIDS*. Bloemfontein: Sun Media.

Dangerfield, A. (2011) Doctors criticise London HIV drug cost-cutting deal. BBC News London, November 1. http://www.bbc.co.uk/news/uk-england-london-15525537. Accessed 20 June 2013.

Dangerfield, A. (2012) Faith leaders across England in 'HIV healing' claims. BBC News London, September 24. http://www.bbc.co.uk/news/uk-england-london-19656649. Accessed 20 June 2013.

Daniel, L., and Squire, C. (2010) Experiences of living with HIV. In *HIV in South Africa 25 Years on*, edited by P. Rohleder, L. Swartz, and S. Kalichman. New York: Springer.

Davis, M. (2009) *Sex, Technology and Public Health*. Houndmills, UK: Palgrave Macmillan.

Davis, M., and Squire, C. (2010) HIV technologies. In *HIV Technologies in International Perspective*, edited by M. Davis, and C. Squire. London: Palgrave Macmillan.

De Waal, A. (2006) *AIDS and Power: Why There Is No Political Crisis – Yet*. New York: Zed Books.

Denning, P., and DiNenno, E. (2010) Communities in crisis: Is there a generalised HIV epidemic in impoverished urban areas of the United States? International AIDS Conference, Vienna, July. http://www.cdc.gov/hiv/risk/other/poverty. html.Accessed 10 August 2010.

Department of Health (2013) The South African antiretroviral treatment guidelines. Pretoria: Department of Health. March 24. http://www.doh.gov.za/docs/ policy/2013/ART_Treatment_Guidelines_Final_25March2013.pdf. Accessed 20 July 2013.

Derrida, J. (1979) Living on: Borderlines. In *Deconstruction and Criticism*, edited by H. Bloom. New York: Seabury Press.

Derrida, J. (2002) Forces of law. In *Acts of Religion*, edited by Anidjar, G. London: Routledge.

Doctors Without Borders (2010) The lives of survival migrants and refugees in South Africa. Geneva: Doctors Without Borders. http://www.doctorswithoutborders.org/publications/article.cfm?id=4465&cat=briefing-documents. Accessed 20 June 2013.

Donnell, D., Baeten, J., Kiarie, J., Thomas, K., Stevens, W., Cohen, C., et al. (2010) Heterosexual HIV-1 transmission after initiation of antiretroviral therapy: A prospective cohort analysis. *The Lancet* 375, 9731: 2092–8.

Doyal, L., and Anderson, J. (2005) 'My fear is to fall in love again': How HIV positive African women survive in London. *Social Science and Medicine* 60, 8: 1729–38.

Doyal, L., and Doyal, L. (2013) *Living with HIV and Dying with AIDS*. London: Ashgate.

Elliott, J. (2013) Suffering agency: Imagining neoliberal personhood in North America and Britain. *Social Text* 31, 2: 83–101.

Elsey, H., Tolhurst, R., and Theobald, S. (2005) Mainstreaming HIV/AIDS in development sectors: Have we learnt the lessons from gender mainstreaming? *AIDS Care* 17, 8: 988–98.

England, R. (2008) The writing is on the wall for UNAIDS. *British Medical Journal* 336, 7652 (May 10): 1072.

Epstein, H. (2006) *The Invisible Cure*. New York: Farrar, Straus and Giroux.

Epstein, S. (1996) *Impure Science: AIDS, Activism and the Politics of Knowledge*. Los Angeles: University of California Press.

Esin, C., and Squire, C. (2013)Visual autobiographies in East London. *FQS* 14, 1.http://www.qualitative-research.net/index.php/fqs/article/view/1971. Accessed 20 June 2013.

Fahlgren, S., and Sawyer, L. (2011) The power of positioning: On the normalisation of gender, race/ethnicity, nation and class positions in a Swedish social work textbook. *Gender and Education* 23, 5: 535–48

Fang, C.-T., Hsu, H.-M., Twu, S.-J., Chen, M.-Y., Chang, Y.-Y., Hwang, J.-S., et al. (2004) Decreased HIV transmission after a policy of providing free access to highly active antiretroviral therapy in Taiwan. *The Journal of Infectious Diseases* 190: 879–85.

Farmer, P. (2001) *Infections and Inequalities*. Los Angeles: University of California Press.

Fassin, D. (2007) *When Bodies Remember*. Berkeley: University of California Press.

Fine, M., and Harris, A. (2001) *Under the Covers: Theorising the Politics of Counter Stories*. London: Lawrence and Wishart.

Flowers, P., and Davis, M. (2012) Obstinate essentialism: Identity transformations among gay men living with HIV. *Psychology and Sexuality Online*, Epub ahead of print 18 May 2012. DOI: 10.1080/19419899.2012.679364.

Flowers, P., Davis, M., Hart, G., Imrie, J., Rosengarten, M., and Frankis, J. (2006) Diagnosis and stigma and identity amongst HIV positive Black Africans living in the UK. *Psychology and Health* 21, 1: 109–22.

Food and Drug Administration (2012) FDA approves first drug for reducing the risk of sexually acquired HIV infection. Silver Spring, MD: US Food and Drug Administration. http://www.fda.gov/NewsEvents/Newsroom/PressAnnouncements/ucm312210.htm. Accessed 20 June 2013.

Foucault, M. (1988 [1964]) *Discipline and Punish*. New York: Vintage.

Foucault, M. (1991) Governmentality. In *The Foucault Effect: Studies in Governmentality*, edited by G. Burchill, C. Gordon, and P. Miller. Chicago: University of Chicago Press.

Foucault, M. (2000) *Power*. London: Penguin Books.

Frank, A. (1997) *The wounded Storyteller*. Chicago, IL: University of Chicago Press.

Frosh, S., and Baraitzer, L. (2008) Psychoanalysis and psychosocial studies. *Psychoanalysis, Culture and Society* 13: 346–65.

Geertz, C. (1973) *The Interpretation of Cultures*. New York: Basic Books.

Geffen, N. (2013) World Health Organisation guidelines should not change the CD4 count threshold for antiretroviral therapy initiation. *South African Journal of HIV Medicine*, Forum, 14, 1: 6–7.

Germond, P., and Cochrane, J. (2010) Healthworlds: Conceptualising landscapes of health and healing. *Sociology* 44, 2 (April): 307–24.

Gill, R., and Scharff, C. (2011) *New Femininities: Postfeminism, Neoliberalism and Subjectivity*. London: Palgrave Macmillan.

Gilroy, P. (2004) *Postcolonial Melancholia*. New York: Columbia University Press.

Global Fund (2010) Donors meet to assess Global Fund support needs. http://www.theglobalfund.org/en/mediacenter/newsreleases/2010-03-24_Donors_meet_to_assess_Global_Fund_resource_needs/, 24 March. Accessed 10 August 2013.

Good, A. (2012) Doctors glum over SA health plan. *Mail and Guardian* 23 November. http://mg.co.za/article/2012-11-23-doctors-glum-over-sa-health-plan. Accessed 20 July 2013.

Government of the District of Columbia (2010) Annual Report HIV/AIDS, Hepatitis, STD and TB (HAHSTA). Washington, DC: Government of the District of Columbia. http://doh.dc.gov/sites/default/files/dc/sites/doh/publication/attachments/HAHSTA_ANNUAL_REPOR_2011.pdf. Accessed 20 June 2013.

Granich, R., Gilks, C., Dye, C., De Cock, K., and Williams, B. (2009) Universal voluntary HIV testing with immediate antiretroviral therapy as a strategy for elimination of HIV transmission: A mathematical model. *Lancet* 373, 9657 (January 3): 48–57.

Grant, R., Lama, I., Anderson, P., McMahan, V., Liu, A., Vargas, L., et al. (2010) Preexposure chemoprophylaxis for HIV prevention in men who have sex with men. *New England Journal of Medicine* 363, 27: 2587–99.

Green, C. (2009) *The End of Stigma?* London: Routledge.

Grønlie, A., Nesje, K., and Dageid, W. (2011) Improving the response-ability of people living with HIV/AIDS: Individual and group factors. In *Response-ability in the Era of AIDS*, edited by W. Dageid, Y. Sliep, O. Akintola, and F. Duckert. Bloemfontein: Sun Media.

Hall, S. (1990) Cultural identity and diaspora. In *Identity: Community, Culture, Difference*, edited by J. Rutherford. London: Lawrence and Wishart.

Harvey, D. (2005) *A Brief History of Neoliberalism*. Oxford: Oxford University Press.

Havlir, D., and Beyrer, C. (2012) The beginning of the end of AIDS? *New England Journal of Medicine* 367 (August 23): 685–7.

Hayek, F. (2011 [1960]) *The Constitution of Liberty*. Chicago: Chicago University Press.

Haynes, B., Gilbert, P., McElrath, J., Zolla-Pazner, S., Tomaras, G., Alam, M., et al. (2012) Immune-correlates analysis of an HIV-1 vaccine effectivity trial. *New England Journal of Medicine* 366: 1275–86.

Health Protection Agency (2011a) HIV in the United Kingdom. London: Health Protection Agency.http://www.hpa.org.uk/webc/HPAwebFile/HPAweb_C/1317131685847. Accessed 20 June 2013.

Health Protection Agency (2011b) Areas where wider HIV testing policies should be considered. London: Health Protection Agency. http://www.hpa.org.uk/webc/HPAwebFile/HPAweb_C/1221722386448. Accessed 20 June 2013.

Health Protection Agency (2012) HIV in the United Kingdom: 2012 report. London: Health Protection Agency. http://www.hpa.org.uk/webc/hpawebfile/hpaweb_c/1317137200016.Accessed 20 June 2013.

Hecht, R., Bollinger, L., Stover, J., McGreevey, W., Muhib, F., Madavo, C., et al. (2009) Critical choices in financing the response to the global HIV/AIDS pandemic. *Health Affairs* 28, 6: 1591–605.

Henrich, T., Sciaranghella, G, Li, J., Gallien, S., Ho, V., LaCasce, A., et al. (2012) Long-term reduction in peripheral blood HIV-1 reservoirs following reduced-intensity conditioning allogeneic stem cell transplantation in two HIV-positive individuals. XIX International AIDS Conference, Washington, July 22–7.http://pag.aids2012.org/Abstracts.aspx?AID=6016. Accessed 20 June 2013

Herman, D. (2013) Approaches to narrative world making. In *Doing Narrative Research, Edition 2*, edited by M. Andrews, C.Squire and M.Tamboukou. London: Sage.

Herek, G. (2002) Thinking about AIDS and stigma: A psychologist's perspective. *Journal of Law, Medicine, and Ethics* 30: 594–607.

Hickel, J. (2012) Neoliberal plague: The political economy of HIV transmission in Swaziland. *Journal of Southern African Studies* 38, 3: 513–29.

Higgins, J., Hoffman, S., and Dworkin, S. (2010) Women's vulnerability to HIV/AIDS. *American Journal of Public Health* 100, 3 (March): 435–45.

House of Lords (2011) No vaccine, no cure. London: House of Lords. http://www.publications.parliament.uk/pa/ld201012/ldselect/ldaids/188/188.pdf. Accessed 20 July 2013.

Hutter, G., Nowak, D., Mossner, M., Ganepola, S., Mussig, A., Allers, K., et al. (2009) Long-term control of HIV by CCR5 Delta32/Delta32 stem-cell transplantation. *New England Journal of Medicine* 360 (February 12): 692–8.

Hyvarinen, M., Hyden, L.-C., Saarenheimo, M., and Tamboukou, M. (2010) *Beyond Narrative Coherence*. Amsterdam: John Benjamins.

ILO/WHO (2005) Joint ILO/WHO guidelines on post-exposure prophylaxis (PEP) to prevent HIV infection. http://www.who.int/hiv/pub/guidelines/PEP/en/. Accessed 30 May 2010.

Innes, E. (2013) HIV 'cure'may be possible for some patients diagnosed within ten weeks of infection. March 15. http://www.dailymail.co.uk/health/article-2293789/HIV-cure-possible-patients-diagnosed-weeks-infection.html. Accessed 20 June 2013.

International Association of Providers of AIDS Care (2012) Controlling the epidemic with antiretrovirals: HIV treatment as prevention and pre-exposure prophylaxis: Consensus statement. IAPAC. http://www.iapac.org/tasp_prep/assets/TPSIon12_consensus.pdf. Accessed 20 July 2013.

Irin News (2012) South Africa: Revamped AIDS council makes its debut. New York: UN Office for the Coordination of Humanitarian Affairs. http://www.irinnews.org/report/96492/south-africa-revamped-aids-council-makes-its-debut. Accessed 20 June 2013.

Irin News (2013) Shortages of new one-a-day ARV pills in South Africa. 13 April. http://www.irinnews.org/report/97880/shortages-of-new-one-a-day-arv-pills-in-south-africa. Accessed 20 July 2013.

Ivers, L., Cullen, K., Freedberg, K., Block, S., Coates, S., and Webb, P. (2009) HIV/AIDS, under-nutrition, and food insecurity. *Clinical Infectious Diseases* 49, 7: 1096–102.

Jain, V., and Deeks, S. (2010) When to start antiretroviral therapy. *Current HIV/AIDS Reports* 7, 2: 60–8.

Jessop, B. (2002) Liberalism, neoliberalism and urban governance. *Antipode* 34, 3: 452–72.

Joffe, H. (2006) Anxiety, mass crisis and 'The Other'. In *Public Emotions,* edited by P. 6, S. Radstone, C. Squire, and A. Treacher. London: Palgrave Macmillan.

Josephs, J., Fleishman, J., Gaist, P., and Gebo, K. (2007) Use of complementary and alternative medicines among a multistate, multisite cohort of people living with HIV/AIDS. *HIV Medicine* 8, 5 (August): 300–5.

Jury, C., and Nattrass, N. (2012) Parental presence and the impact of antiretroviral treatment in Khayelitsha, South Africa. Cape Town: Centre for Social Science Research. CSSR Working Paper 318. http://www.cssr.uct.ac.za/pub/wp/318. Accessed 20 July 2013.

Kalichman, S. (2009) *Denying AIDS: Conspiracy Theories, Pseudoscience and Human Tragedy*. New York: Springer.

Karner, C., and Parker, D. (2011) Conviviality and conflict: pluralism, resilience and hope in inner-city Birmingham. *Journal of Ethnic and Migration Studies* 37, 3: 355–72.

Kielman, K., and Cataldo, F. (2009) Tracking the rise of the 'expert patient' in evolving paradigms of HIV Care. *AIDS Care* 22, 1: 21–8.

Killian, S., Suliman, S., Fakier, F., and Seedat, S. (2007) Rape survivors and the provision of HIV post-exposure prophylaxis. *South African Medical Journal* 97 (November), 8: 585–6.

Kippax, S. (2012) Effective HIV prevention: The indispensable role of social science. *Journal of the International AIDS Society* 15: 17357–65.

Kitahata, M., Gange, S., Abraham, A., Merriman, B., Saag, M., Justice, A., et al. (2009) Effect of early versus deferred antiretroviral therapy for HIV on survival. *New England Journal of Medicine* 36, 18: 1815–26.

Kleinman, A. (1988) *The Illness Narratives*. New York: Basic Books.

Knight, L., Hosegood, V., and Timaeus, I. (2013) The South African disability grant: Influence on HIV treatment outcomes and household well-being in KawZulu-Natal. *Development South Africa* 30, 1: 135–47.

Konings, E., Ambaw, Y., Dilley, K., Gichangi, P., Arega, T., and Crandall, B. (2012) Implications of adopting new WHO guidelines for antiretroviral therapy initiation in Ethiopia. *Bulletin of the World Health Organization* 90: 659–63.

Krentz, H., and Gill, M. (2013) The effect of churn on 'Community Viral Load' (CVL) in a well defined regional population. *Journal of Acquired Immune Deficiency Syndrome*, early online edition. DOI: 10.1097/QAI.0b013e31829cef18. 2013.

Kymlicka, W. (2003) New forms of citizenship. In *The Art of the State: Governance in a World Without Frontiers,* edited by T. J. Courchesne and D. J. Savoie. Montreal: IRPP (Institute for Research in Public Policy), pp. 265–310.

Lamontagne, E., Haacker, M., Ventelou, B., and Greener, R. (2010) Macroeconomic impact of HIV: The need for better modelling. *Current Opinion in HIV and AIDS* 5, 3 (May): 249–54.

Lana, O. (2009) From risk to reason: Understanding young people's perception of HIV risk in South Africa. PhD thesis, University of York.

Lancet (2011) Treatment as prevention for HIV 11: 651. http://download. thelancet.com/pdfs/journals/laninf/PIIS1473309911702195.pdf. Accessed 20 July 2013.

Lancet (2012) South Africa's AIDS response: The next five years. Editorial. 379, 9824: 1365. 14 April. http://www.thelancet.com/journals/lancet/article/ PIIS0140-6736(12)60578-9/fulltext. Accessed 20 July 2013.

Langlois-Klassen, D., Kipp, W., Jhangri, G., and Rubaale, T. (2007) Use of traditional herbal medicine by AIDS patients in Kabarole district, western Uganda. *American Journal of Tropical Medicine and Hygiene* 77, 4 (October): 757–63.

Larkin, P. (1964) *The Whitsun Weddings*. London: Faber and Faber.

Latour, B. (2004) *The Politics of Nature*. Cambridge, MA: Harvard University Press.

Lazzarini, Z., Galletly, C., Mykhalovskiy, E., Harsono, D., O'Keefe, E., Singer, M., et al. (2013) Criminalisation of HIV transmission and exposure: research and policy agenda. *American Journal of Public Health* 103, 8: 1350–3.

Lehtonen, M. (2004) The environmental–social interface of sustainable development: capabilities, social capital, institutions, *Ecological Economics*, 49: 199–214.

Lincoln, Y., and Guba, E. (1985) *Naturalistic Inquiry*. Newbury Park, CA: Sage Publications.

van der Linde, I. (2013) Plenary session 3, 20 June 2013 – HIV/AIDS in South Africa: At last the glass is half-full. Cape Town: Human Sciences Research Council. http://www.hsrc.ac.za/en/media-briefs/hiv-aids-stis-and-tb/plenary-session-3-20-june-2013-hiv-aids-in-south-africa-at-last-the-glass-is-half-full. Accessed 20 July 2013.

Lister, J. (2013) *Health Policy Reform: Global Health versus Private Profit*. London: Libri Books.

Lodi, S., Phillips, A., Touloumi, G., Geskus, R., Meyer, L., Thiébault, R., et al. (2011) Time from human immunodeficiency virus seroconversion to reaching

CD4+ cell count threshold <200, <350, and <500 cells/mm³: Assessment of need following changes in treatment guidelines. *Clinical Infectious Diseases* 53: 817–25.

Logie, C., and Gadalla, T. (2009) Meta-analysis of health and demographic correlates of stigma towards people living with HIV. *AIDS Care* 21, 6: 742–53.

Long, C. (2009) *Contradicting Maternity: HIV Positive Motherhood in South Africa.* Johannesburg: Wits University Press.

Maane, E. (2009) *Umzala.* Cape Town: Openly Positive Trust.

MacArthur, R., and DuPont, L. (2012) Etiology and pharmacologic management of noninfectious diarrhea in HIV-infected individuals in the highly active antiretroviral therapy era. *Clinical Infectious Disease* 55, 6: 860–7.

MacIntyre, A. (1984) *After Virtue.* Bloomington, IN: Indiana University Press.

Madge, S., Matthews, P., Singh, S., and Theobald, N. (2011) *HIV in Primary Care, Edition 2.* London: Medical Foundation for AIDS and Sexual Health. http://www.medfash.org.uk/uploads/files/p17abjng1g9t9193h1rsl75uuk53.pdf. Accessed 10 August 2013.

Malawi Government (2012) 2012 global AIDS response progress report. http://www.unaids.org/en/dataanalysis/knowyourresponse/countryprogressreports/2012countries/ce_MW_Narrative_Report[1].pdf. Accessed 20 June 2013.

Marais, H. (2010) *South Africa Pushed to the Limit: The Political Economy of Change.* Cape Town: UCT Press.

Mars-Jones, A. (1992) *Monopolies of Loss.* London: Faber and Faber.

Mayosi, B., Lawn, J., van Niekerk, A., Bradshaw, D., Abdool Karim, S., Coovadia, A., et al. (2012) Health in South Africa: Changes and challenges since 2009. *The Lancet* 380, 9858 (8 December): 2029–43. http://www.thelancet.com/journals/lancet/article/PIIS0140-6736(12)61814-5/fulltext. Accessed 20 July 2012.

Mbali, M. (2005) The Treatment Action Campaign and the history of rights based patient-driven HIV/AIDS activism in South Africa. *Centre for Civil Society Research Report* 29: 1–23.

Mbali, M. (2013) *South African AIDS Activism and Global Health Politics.* London: Palgrave Macmillan.

McAdams, D. (2006) *The Redemptive Self.* New York: OUP USA.

McGregor, L. (2007) *Khabzela.* Johannesburg: Jacana Media.

Médecins Sans Frontières (2009) Challenges: second-class AIDS treatment. http://utw.msfaccess.org/background/challenges. Accessed 30 May 2010.

Médecins Sans Frontières (2011) Activity report. Geneva: MédecinsSansFrontières. http://www.msf.org.uk/sites/uk/files/MSF_Activity_Report_2011_lowres_201208200807.pdf. Accessed 30 June 2013.

Men, C., Messen, B., and van Pelt, M. (2012) I wish I had AIDS: A qualitative study on access to health care services for HIV/AIDS and diabetic patients in Cambodia. *Health, Culture and Society* 1, 2: http://www.who.int/alliance-hpsr/alliancehpsr_iwishihadaids.pdf. Accessed 20 June 2013.

Mendel, G. (2009) Through positive eyes. http://throughpositiveeyes.org/mexico-city/alejandro. Accessed 20 June 2013.

Milan, F., Arnsten, J., Klein, R., Schoenbaum, E., Moskaleva, C., Buono, D., et al. (2008) Use of complementary and alternative medicine in inner-city persons with or at risk for HIV infection. *AIDS Patient Care and STDs* 22, 10 (October): 811–16.

Mishler, E. (1986) *Research Interviewing: Context and Narrative.* Cambridge, MA: Harvard University Press.

Mlambo, M., and Peltzer, K. (2011) HIV sero-status disclosure and sexual behaviour among HIV positive patients who are on antiretroviral treatment (ART) in Mpumalanga, South Africa. *Journal of Human Ecology* 35, 1: 29–41.

Modood, T., Triandafyllidou, A., and Zapata-Barrero, R. (2006) *Multiculturalism, Muslims and Citizenship: A European Approach.* London: Routledge.

MMWR (2011) Vital signs: HIV prevention through care and treatment – United States. *MMWR* 60, 47 (December 2): 1618–23. http://www.cdc.gov/mmwr/preview/mmwrhtml/mm6047a4.htm. Accessed 20 June 2013.

Monk, D. (2009) Reckless trials? The criminalisation of the sexual transmission of HIV. *Radical Philosophy* 156, (July-August): 2–6.

Moore, O. (1996) *PWA: Looking AIDS in the Face.* London: Picador.

Morgan, J., and the Bambanani Women's Group (2004) *Long Life.* Cape Town: Double Storey.

Morin, S., Yamey, G., and Rutherford, G. (2012) HIV pre-exposure prophylaxis. *British Medical Journal* 345 e5412 (13 August).

Mouffe, C. (2006) *On the Political.* London: Routledge.

Mpe, P. (2008) *Brooding Clouds.* Durban: University of KwaZulu-Natal Press.

Mykhalovskiy, E., and Rosengarten, M. (2009) HIV/AIDS in its third decade: Renewed critique in social and cultural analysis. *Social Theory and Health* 7, 3: 187–95.

Naidu, T. (2012) Home-based care volunteer identity and participation in HIV/AIDS care and support in rural KwaZulu-Natal, South Africa. PhD thesis, University of KwaZulu-Natal.

National AIDS Trust (2011a) The impact of social care support for people living with HIV. London: National AIDS Trust. http://www.nat.org.uk/Media%20library/Files/Policy/2011/Social%20Care%20Survey%20June%202011%20FINAL.pdf. Accessed 20 June 2013.

National AIDS Trust (2011b) Fluctuating symptoms of HIV. August. London: National AIDS Trust. http://www.nat.org.uk/media/Files/Policy/August_2011_Fluctuating_symptoms_of_HIV.pdf. Accessed 20 June 2013.

Nattrass, N. (2004) Trading-off income and health: AIDS and the disability grant in South Africa. CSSR Working Paper 82. Cape Town: Centre for Social Science Research, University of Cape Town. http://www.cssr.uct.ac.za/sites/cssr.uct.ac.za/files/pubs/wp82.pdf. Accessed 20 July 2013.

Nattrass, N. (2012) *The AIDS Conspiracy: Science Fights Back.* New York: Columbia University Press.

Navario, P., Bekker, L.-G., Blecher, M., Darkoh, E., Hecht, R., McIntyre, J., et al. (2012) Special report on the state of HIV/AIDS in South Africa. *Global HealthMagazine.* http://www.cssr.uct.ac.za/sites/cssr.uct.ac.za/files/pubs/South%20Africa%20HIV%20strategy%20GHMag.pdf. Accessed 20 July 2013.

Nguyen, V.-K. (2011) *The Republic of Therapy.* Chapel Hill, NC: Duke University Press.

Nguyen, V.-K., Bajos, N., Dubois-Arber, F., O'Malley, J., and Pirkle, C. (2011) Remedicalizing an epidemic: From HIV treatment as prevention to HIV treatment is prevention. *AIDS* 23, 5: 291–3.

Niehaus, I., and Jonsson, G. (2005) Dr. Wouter Basson, Americans and wild beasts: Men's conspiracy theories of HIV/AIDS in the South African lowveld. *Medical Anthropology* 24, 2: 179–208.

Nigatu, T. (2012) Integration of HIV and noncommunicable diseases in health care delivery in low- and middle-income countries. *Prevention of Chronic Disease*

9: 110331. http://www.cdc.gov/pcd/issues/2012/11_0331.htm. Accessed 10 August 2013.

Noah, T. (2012) Health care as consumption. *New Republic* March 30. http://www.newrepublic.com/blog/timothy-noah/102221/health-care-consumption. Accessed 20 June 2013.

Nussbaum, M. (2000) *Women and Human Development: The Capabilities Approach.* Cambridge: Cambridge University Press.

Odets, W. (1995) *In the Shadow of the Epidemic.* London: Cassell.

Ong, A. (2006) *Neoliberalism as Exception.* Chapel Hill, NC: Duke University Press.

Ooms, G., Hill, P., Hammonds, R.,Leemput, L. van, Assefa, Y., Katabaro, M., and Damme, W. van (2010) Applying the principles of AIDS 'exceptionality' to global health. *Global Health Governance* 4, 1: 1–9.

Padian, N., MacCoy, S., Balker, C., and Wasserheit, J. (2010) Weighing the gold in the gold standard: Challenges in HIV prevention research. *AIDS* 24, 5: 621–5.

Parker, R., and Aggleton, P. (2003) HIV and AIDS-related stigma and discrimination: A conceptual framework and implications for action. *Social Science and Medicine* 57, 1: 13–24.

de Paoli, M., Mills, E., and Grønningsaeter, A. (2012) The ARV rollout and the disability grant: A South African dilemma? *Journal of the International AIDS Society* 15, 6: doi: 10.1186/1758-2652-15-6

Patayachee, V. (2011) Global economic recession: Effects and implications for South Africa at a time of political challenges. LSE International Development 20th anniversary conference: Responding to the crisis in international development. http://www.lse.ac.uk/internationalDevelopment/20thAnniversaryConference/ImpactoftheGlobalFC.pdf. Accessed 20 July 2013.

Pateman, C. (1989) *The Disorder of Women: Democracy, Feminism and Political Theory.* Cambridge: Polity Press.

Patton, C. (1991) *Inventing AIDS.* London: Routledge.

Perrin, B., and Nirje, B. (1985) Setting the record straight. *Australia and New Zealand Journal of Developmental Disabilities* 11, 2: 69–72.

Persaud, D., Gay, H., Ziemniak, C., Chen, Y., Piatak, M., and Chun, T-W. (2013) Functional HIV cure after very early ART of an infected infant.20th Conference of retroviruses and opportunistic infections. Atlanta, Georgia, March.Paper.

Persson, A. (2012) Non-infectious corporealities: Tensions in the biomedical era of 'HIV normalisation.' *Sociology of Health and Illness* Early view. http://onlinelibrary.wiley.com/doi/10.1111/1467-9566.12023/abstract. Accessed 20 June 2013.

Petros, G., Airhihenbuwa, C., Simbayi, L., Ramlagan, S., and Brown, B. (2006) HIV/AIDS and 'othering' in South Africa: The blame goes on. *Culture, Health and Sexuality* 8, 1: 67–77.

Phaswana-Mafuya, N., Peltzer, K., and Petros, G. (2009) Disability grant for people living with HIV/AIDS in the Eastern Cape of South Africa. *Social Work in Health Care* 48, 5: 533–50.

Pinfold, V. (2000) 'Building up safe havens… all around the world': Users' experiences of living in the community with mental health problems. *Health and Place* 6, 3: 201–12.

Piot, P. (2006) AIDS: From crisis management to sustained strategic response. *Lancet* 368: 526–30.

Piot, P., Kazatchkine, M., Dybul, M., and Lob-Levyt, J. (2009) AIDS: Lessons learnt and myths dispelled. *Lancet* 374, 9685 (March 20): 260–3.

Piven, E., and Cloward, R. (1993) *Regulating the Poor*. New York: Vintage.

Plummer, K. (1995) *Telling Sexual Stories*. London: Routledge.

Plummer, K. (2001) *Documents of Life 2*. London: Sage.

Poku, N., Whiteside, A., and Sandkjaer, B. (2007) *AIDS and Governance*. Aldershot, Hampshire: Ashgate.

Polletta, F. (2006) *It was Like a Fever*. Chicago: Chicago University Press.

Portelli, A. (2010) *They Say in Harlan County*. Oxford: Oxford University Press.

Power, L., Bell, M., and Freemantle, I. (2010) A national study of ageing and HIV (50 Plus). London: Joseph Rowntree Foundation. http://www.tht.org.uk/~/media/Files/Publications/Policy/50-plus-final-report.ashx. Accessed 20 June 2013.

Power, S. (2003) The AIDS rebel. *New Yorker* May 19, 54–67.

Prince, R., Denis, P., and van Dijk, R. (2009) Introduction to special issue on engaging Christianities, negotiating AIDS, health and social relations in east and southern Africa. *Africa Today* 56, 1: v–xviii.

Quine, W. (1969) *Ontological Relativity and Other Essays*. New York: Columbia University Press.

Rabinow, P. (2004) Assembling ethics in an ecology of ignorance. First Conference on Synthetic Biology, MIT, 10–12 June. http://openwetware.org/images/7/7a/SB1.0_Rabinow.pdf. Accessed 10 August 2013.

Rachlis, B., Sodhi, S., Burcial, B., Orbinski, J., Cheng, A., and Cole, D. (2013) A taxonomy for community-based care programs focused on HIV/AIDS prevention, treatment and care in resource-poor settings. *Global Health Action* 6, 10: http://www.ncbi.nlm.nih.gov/pmc/articles/PMC3629264/. Accessed 20 July 2013.

Rao, D., Kekwaletswe, T., Hosek, S., Martinez, J., and Rodriguez, F. (2007) Stigma and social barriers to medication adherence with urban youth living with HIV. *AIDS Care* 19, 1: 28–33.

Republic of South Africa (2011) National Health Insurance in South Africa policy paper. 5 August. http://www.hst.org.za/sites/default/files/2bcce61d2d1b8d972af41ab0e2c8a4ab.pdf. Accessed 20 July 2013.

Republic of South Africa (2012) Global AIDS response progress report. Pretoria: Republic of South Africa. http://www.unaids.org/en/dataanalysis/knowyourresponse/countryprogressreports/2012countries/ce_ZA_Narrative_Report.pdf. Accessed 20 July 2013.

Republic of Uganda (2012) Global AIDS response progress report. Kampala: Uganda AIDS Commission. http://www.unaids.org/en/dataanalysis/knowyourresponse/countryprogressreports/2012countries/ce_UG_Narrative_Report[1].pdf. Accessed 20 June 2013.

Rerks-Ngarm, S., Pitisuttithum, P., Nitayaphan, S., Kaewkungwal, J., Chiu, J., Paris, R., et al. (2009) Vaccination with ALVAC and AIDSVAX to prevent HIV-1 infection in Thailand. *New England Journal of Medicine* 361: 2209–20.

Riessman, C. (2008) *Narrative Methods for the Human Sciences*. Thousand Oaks, CA: Sage.

Robins, S. (2009) *From Revolution to Rights in South Africa*. Durban: University of KwaZulu-Natal Press.

Robinson, C. (1993) Managing life with a chronic condition: The story of normalisation. *Qualitative Health Research* 3, 1: 6–28.

Rodlach, A. (2006) *Witches, Westerners and HIV: AIDS and Cultures of Blame in Africa.* Walnut Creek, CA: Left Coast Press.

Rose, N. (2007) *The Politics of Life Itself: Biomedicine, Power and Subjectivity in the Twenty-first Century.* Princeton, NJ: Princeton University Press.

Rosengarten, M. (2009) *HIV Interventions: Biomedicine and the Traffic between Information and Flesh.* Seattle, WA: Samuel and Althea Stroum Press.

Rosengarten, M., and Michaels, M. (2010) HIV: Pre-exposure prophylaxis or PrEP and the complexities of biomedical prevention. In *HIV Technologies in International Perspective,* edited by M. Davis, and C. Squire. London: Palgrave Macmillan.

Roura, M., Busza, J., Wringe, A., Mbata, D., Urassa, M., and Zaba, B. (2009) Barriers to sustaining antiretroviral treatment in Kisesa, Tanzania: A follow-up study to understand attrition from the antiretroviral program. *AIDS Patient Care and STDs* 23, 3 (March): 203–10.

Russell, S. (2010) City endorses new policy for treatment of H.I.V. *New York Times,* 2 April. http://www.nytimes.com/2010/04/04/us/04sftreatment.html. Accessed 10 August 2010.

Ryan, M.-L. (2004) *Narrative Across Media.* Lincoln, NE: University of Nebraska Press.

Saez-Cirion, A., Bacchus, C., Hocqueloux, L., Avettant-Fenoel, V., Girault, I., Lecuroux, C., et al. (2013) Post-treatment HIV-1 controllers with a long-term virological remission after the interruption of early initiated antiretroviral therapy ANRS VISCONTI study. PloS http://www.plospathogens.org/article/info%3Adoi%2F10.1371%2Fjournal.ppat.1003211. Accessed 20 June 2013.

SANAC (South African National AIDS Council) Secretariat. (2010) The national HIV counselling and testing campaign strategy. Cape Town: SANAC. http://www.westerncape.gov.za/other/2010/6/hct_campaign_strategy_2_3_10_final.pdf. Accessed 20 July 2013.

Sanders, D., Stern, R., Struthers, P., Ngulube, T., and Onya, H. (2008) What is needed for health promotion in Africa: Band aid, live aid or real change? *Critical Public Health* 18, 4: 509–19.

Scott, J. (1991) The evidence of experience. *Critical Inquiry* 17, 4 (Summer): 773–97.

Seckinelgen, H. (2012) The global governance of success in HIV/AIDS policy: Emergencyaction, everyday lives and Sen's capabilities. *Health and Place* 13. 3: 453–60.

Semple, I. (2013) US doctors cure child born with HIV. *Guardian,* March 4. http://www.guardian.co.uk/society/2013/mar/03/us-doctors-cure-child-born-hiv/. Accessed 20 June 2013.

Sen. A. (1999) *Commodities and Capabilities.* Oxford: Oxford University Press.

Shachar, A. (2009) *The Birthright Lottery: Citizenship and Global Inequality.* Cambridge, MA, and London: Harvard University Press.

Sidibé, M., Piot, P., and Dybul, M. (2012) AIDS is not over. *Lancet* 380, 9859: 2058–60.

Sirkeci, I., Cohen, J., and Ratha, D. (2012) *Migration and Remittances during the Global Financial Crisis and Beyond.* Washington, DC: World Bank.

Sloan, J. (2012) 'You can see your face in my floor': Examining the function of cleanliness in an adult male prison. *Howard Journal of Criminal Justice* 51, 4: 400–10.

Smith, J., and Whiteside, A. (2010) The history of AIDS exceptionalism. *Journal of the International AIDS Society* 13: 47. http://www.biomedcentral.com/1758-2652/content/13/1/47. Accessed 20 June 2013.

Sontag, S. (1988) *AIDS and its Metaphors*. London: Penguin.

Sools, A. (2012) 'To see a world in a grain of sand': Towards future-oriented what-if analysis in narrative research. *Narrative Works* 2, 1: 83–105.

Soul City (2008) The OneLove campaign in South Africa: What has been achieved so far? http://www.soulcity.org.za/research/evaluations/campaigns/onelove-evaluation/onelove%20interim%20eval%20Report-final%20incl%20cover.pdf/view. Accessed 10 August 2013.

Squire, C. (1999) 'Neighbors who might become friends': Selves, genres and citizenship in stories of HIV. *The Sociological Quarterly* 40, 11 (February): 109–37.

Squire, C. (2003) Can an HIV positive woman find true love? Romance in the stories of women living with HIV. *Feminism and Psychology* 13, 1: 73–100.

Squire, C. (2005) Reading narratives. *Group Analysis* 38, 1: 91–107.

Squire, C. (2006) Feeling entitled: HIV, entitlement feelings and citizenship. In *Public Emotions*, edited by P. 6, S. Radstone, C. Squire, and A. Treacher. London: Palgrave Macmillan.

Squire, C. (2007) *HIV in South Africa*. London: Routledge.

Squire, C. (2008) From experience-centred to culturally-oriented narrative research. In *Doing Narrative Research*, edited by M. Andrews, C. Squire, and M. Tamboukou. London: Sage.

Squire, C. (2010) Being naturalized, being left behind: The HIV citizen in the era of treatment possibility. *Critical Public Health* 10, 4: 401–27.

Squire, C. (2012) What is narrative? National Centre for Research Methods Working Paper. http://eprints.ncrm.ac.uk/3065/. Accessed 20 June 2013.

Squire, C. (2013) Narratives, connections and social change. *Narrative Inquiry* 22, 1: 50–68.

Squire, C., Esin, C., and Burman, C. (2013) 'You are here': visual autobiographies, cultural-spatial positioning, and resources for urban living. *Sociological Research Online* 18, 3, (August 31). http://www.socresonline.org.uk/18/3/1.html. Accessed 25 June 2013.

Statistics South Africa (2013) Quarterly labour force summary. 6 May. Pretoria: Statistics South Africa. http://www.statssa.gov.za/publications/P0211/P02111stQuarter2013.pdf. Accessed 20 July 2013.

Steinberg, J. (2008) *Three Letter Plague*. London: Vintage.

Stenner, P., and Taylor, D. (2008) Psychosocial welfare: Reflections on an emerging field. *Critical Social Policy* 23, 4: 415–37.

Stich, S. (1993) Naturalizing epistemology: Quine, Simon and the prospects for pragmatism.In *Philosophy and cognitive science*, edited by C. Hookway, and D. Peterson. Cambridge: Cambridge University Press.

Supreme Court of Canada (2012) R. v. Mabior. October 5. http://www.aidslaw.ca/EN/lawyers-kit/documents/6a_Mabior2012SCC-EN.pdf. Accessed 20 June 2013.

Tanser, F., Bärnighausen, T., Grapsa, E., Zaidi, J., and Newell, M. (2013) High coverage of ART associated with decline in risk of HIV acquisition in rural KwaZulu-Natal, South Africa. *Science* 339, 6122: 966–71.

Terrence Higgins Trust (2013) Statement.*Guardian*, March 4. http://www.guardian.co.uk/science/blog/2013/mar/04/doctors-cure-child-born-with-hiv. Accessed 20 June 2013.

Thigpen, M., Kebaabetswe, P., Smith, D., Rose, C., Segolodi, T., Henderson, F., et al. (2012) Antiretroviral preexposure prophylaxis for heterosexual HIV transmission in Botswana. *New England Journal of Medicine* 367, 5 (August 2): 423–34.

Thomas, S., and Crause, Q. (1991) The Tuskegee syphilis study, 1932 to 1972: Implications for HIV education and AIDS risk education programs in the black community. *Public Health Then and Now* 18, 11: 1498–505.

Thomson, E., Fidler, S., Ayers, M., McDonald, S., and Foster, S. (2013) Applicability of stable patient HIV service provision for young adults. *HIV Medicine* 14: 12.

Thornton, S. (2013) South African patients forced to choose between death or a disability grant. *Huffington Post*, 12 March. http://www.huffingtonpost.com/2013/03/12/south-african-hiv_n_2862800.html. Accessed 20 July 2013.

Tilly, C. (2002) *Stories, Identities and Political Change.* Oxford: Rowman and Littlefield. Online edition.

Treatment Action Campaign and Section 27 (2013) Monitoring our health: An analysis of the breakdown of health care services in selected Gauteng facilities. Cape Town and Johannesburg: Treatment Action Campaign and Section 27. http://www.tac.org.za/sites/default/files/campaigns/%3Cem%3EEdit%20Campaign%3C/em%3E%20HEALTH%20SYSTEMS%20STRENGTHENING%20FOR%20QUALITY%20HIV%20AND%20TB%20TREATMENT/file-uploads/Monitoring-Our-Health-March-2013.pdf. Accessed 20 June 2013.

Treichler, P. (1999) *How to Have Theory in an Epidemic: Cultural Chronicles of AIDS.* Durham, NC: Duke University Press.

Tsai, A., Bangsberg, D., Frongillo, E., Hunt, P., Muzoora, C., Martin, J., and Weiser, S. (2012) Food insecurity, depression and the modifying role of social support among people living with HIV/AIDS in rural Uganda. *Social Science and Medicine* 74, 12(June): 2012–19.

Tuller, D., Bangsberg, D., Sekungu, J., Ware, M., Emenonyu, N., and Weiser, S. (2010) Transportation costs impede sustained adherence and access to HAART in a clinic population in southwestern Uganda: A qualitative study. *AIDS and Behavior* 14, 4: 778–84.

Uganda Radio Network (2012) Panic in Gulu as ARVs are sold in drug shops. 2 October. http://ugandaradionetwork.com/a/story.php?s=46049. Accessed 20 June 2013.

UNAIDS (2009a) *Towards Universal Access: Scaling up Priority HIV/AIDS Interventions in the Health Sector.* Geneva: UNAIDS. http://data.unaids.org/pub/Report/2009/20090930_tuapr_2009_en.pdf. Accessed 10 August 2013.

UNAIDS (2009b) Governments and civil society expand access to HIV testing and counselling. http://www.unaids.org/en/resources/presscentre/featurestories/2009/september/20090930whotc/. Accessed 10 August 2013.

UNAIDS (2009c) Impact of the global financial and economic crisis on the AIDS response. 25th Meeting of the UNAIDS Programme. 8–10 December. http://www.unaids.org/en/media/unaids/contentassets/dataimport/pub/informationnote/2009/20091030_impact_economic_crisis_on_hiv_final_en.pdf. Accessed 10 August 2013.

UNAIDS (2010a) *The Treatment 2.0 Framework for Action.* http://data.unaids.org/pub/Outlook/2010/20100713_outlook_treatment2_0_en.pdf. Accessed 10 August 2010.

UNAIDS (2010b) *Getting to Zero*. Geneva: UNAIDS. http://www.unaids.org/en/ media/unaids/contentassets/documents/unaidspublication/2010/jc2034_ unaids_strategy_en.pdf. Accessed 2 May 2013.

UNAIDS (2011a) *Report on the Global AIDS Epidemic*. Geneva: UNAIDS. http://www.unaids.org/en/media/unaids/contentassets/documents/ unaidspublication/2011/JC2216_WorldAIDSday_report_2011_en.pdf. Accessed 22 September 2012.

UNAIDS (2011b) *Chronic Care of HIV and Non-communicable Diseases: How to Leverage the HIV Experience*. UNAIDS report. Geneva: UNAIDS. http://www.unaids.org/en/ media/unaids/contentassets/documents/unaidspublication/2011/20110526_ JC2145_Chronic_care_of_HIV.pdf. Accessed 5 December 2011.

UNAIDS (2011c) *Countdown to Zero: Global Plan Towards the Elimination of New HIV Infections among Children by 2015 and Keeping their Mothers Alive*. Geneva: UNAIDS. http://www.unaids.org/en/media/unaids/contentassets/documents/ unaidspublication/2011/20110609_jc2137_global-plan-elimination-hiv-children_en.pdf.

UNAIDS (2012a) *UNAIDS World AIDS Day Report*. Geneva: UNAIDS. http://www. unaids.org/en/media/unaids/contentassets/documents/epidemiology/2012/ gr2012/JC2434_WorldAIDSday_results_en.pdf. Accessed 20 June 2013.

UNAIDS (2012b) 30th meeting of the UNAIDS Programme Coordinating Board. Report by the PCB NGO representative. Geneva: UNAIDS.

Unterhalter, E. (2003) The capabilities approach and gendered education. *Theory and Research in Education* 1, 1: 7–22.

Usdin, S. (2009) Interview with Shereen Usdin. *World Health Organisation Bulletin*. http://www.who.int/bulletin/volumes/87/8/09-050809/en/index.html. Accessed

Van Damme, L., Corneli, A., Ahmed, K., Agot, K., Lombaard, J., Kapiga, S., et al. (2012) Preexposure prophylaxis for HIV infection among African women. *New England Journal of Medicine* 339, 6122: 966–71.

Van Damme, W., Kober, K., and Laga, M. (2006) The real challenges for scaling up ART in sub-Saharan Africa. *AIDS* 20: 653–6.

Veenstra, N., Whiteside, A., Lalloo, D., and Gibbs, A. (2010) Unplanned antiretroviral treatment interruptions in southern Africa: How should we be managing these? *Globalisation and Health* 6, 4. http://www.globalizationandhealth.com/ content/6/1/4. Accessed 20 May 2010.

Wacquant, L. (2009) *Punishing the Poor: The Neoliberal Government of Social Insecurity*. Durham, NC: Duke University Press.

Wada, N., Jacobson, L., Cohen, M., French, A., Phair, J., and Muñoz, A. (2013) Cause-specific life expectancies after 35 years of age for Human Immunodeficiency Syndrome-infected and Human Immunodeficiency Syndrome-negative individuals followed simultaneously in long-term cohort studies, 1984–2008. *American Journal of Epidemiology* 177, 2: 116–25.

Walkerdine, V., and Jiminez, L. (2012) *Gender, Work and Community after De-industrialisation*. London: Palgrave.

Wallerstein, I. (1995) *After Liberalism*. New York: New Press.

Walmsley, J. (2001) Normalisation, emancipator research and inclusive research in learning disability. *Disability and Society* 16, 2: 187–205.

Watney, S. (2000) *Imagine Hope: AIDS and Gay Identity*. London: Routledge.

Watt, M., Maman, S., Jacobson, M., Laiser, J., and John, M.(2009) Missed opportunities for religious organisations to support people living with HIV/AIDS: Findings from Tanzania. *AIDS Patient Care and STDs* 23, 5: 389–94.

Weait, M. (2007) *Intimacy and Responsibility: The Criminalisation of HIV Transmission*. London: Routledge-Cavendish.

Weiser, S., Fernandes, K., Brandson, E., Lima, V., Anema, A., Bangsberg, D., et al. (2009) The association between food insecurity and mortality among HIV-infected individuals on HAART. *Journal of Acquired Immune Deficiency Syndrome* 52, 3(November 1): 342–9.

Weiser, S., Leiter, K., Bangsberg, D., Butler, L., Percy-de Korte, F., Hlanze, Z., et al. (2007) Food insufficiency is associated with high-risk sexual behavior among women in Botswana and Swaziland. *PLoS Med* 4: e260. doi:10.1371/journal. pmed.0040260.

Western Cape Government (2012) Social relief of distress programme. http://www. westerncape.gov.za/eng/directories/services/11586/. Accessed 20 June 2013.

Wills, J., and Douglas, J. (2008) Health promotion: Still going strong? *Critical Public Health* 18, 4: 431–4.

Winskell, K., Hill, E., and Obyerodhyambo, O. (2011) Comparing HIV-related symbolic stigma in six African countries: Social representations in young people's narratives. *Social Science and Medicine* 73, 8: 1257–65.

World Bank (2009) *Averting a Human Crisis during the Global Downturn*. Washington, DC: World Bank.

World Health Organisation (2003) *Antiretroviral Therapy in Primary Health Care: Experience of the Khayelitsha Programme in South Africa*. Geneva: WHO. http:// www.who.int/hiv/amds/case8.pdf. Accessed 20 July 2013.

World Health Organisation (2005) *National Policy on Traditional Medicine and Regulation of Herbal Medicines*. Geneva: World Health Organisation.

World Health Organisation (2006) *HIV/AIDS in Europe: Moving from Death Sentence to Chronic Disease Management*. Geneva: WHO. http://www.who.int/hiv/pub/ idu/hiv_europe.pdf. Accessed 20 June 2013.

World Health Organisation (2009) *Rapid Advice: Antiretroviral Therapy for HIV Infection in Adults and Adolescents*. Geneva: WHO. http://www.who.int/hiv/ pub/arv/advice/en/index.html. Accessed 30 May 2010.

World Health Organisation (2010a) *Mental Health and Psychosocial Support in Humanitarian Emergencies*. Geneva: WHO. http://www.who.int/mental_health/ emergencies/what_humanitarian_health_actors_should_know.pdf. Accessed 20 June 2013.

World Health Organisation (2010b) *Antiretroviral Therapy for HIV Infection in Adults and Adolescents: Recommendations for a Public Health Approach*. Geneva: WHO, HIV/AIDS Programme.

World Health Organisation (2010c) *Guidelines on HIV and Infant Feeding*. Geneva: WHO. http://www.who.int/maternal_child_adolescent/documents/ 9789241599535/en/.

World Health Organisation (2011) *Global Health Sector Strategy on HIV/AIDS 2011–2015*. Geneva: WHO. http://whqlibdoc.who.int/publications/2011/ 9789241501651_eng.pdf. Accessed 20 June 2013.

World Health Organisation (2012) *Global Monitoring Framework and Strategy for the Global Plan Towards the Elimination of New HIV Infections among Children by*

2015 and Keeping Their Mothers Alive (EMTCT). Geneva: WHO. http://apps.who.
int/iris/bitstream/10665/75341/1/9789241504270_eng.pdf. Accessed 20 June
2103.

World Health Organisation (2013) *WHO Issues New HIV Recommendations Calling
for Earlier Treatment*. Geneva: WHO. June 30. http://www.unaids.org/en/media/
unaids/contentassets/documents/unaidspublication/2013/20130630_treat-
ment_report_en.pdf. Accessed 30 June 2013.

World Health Organisation (not dated) *HIV/AIDS: Psychosocial Support*. Geneva:
WHO. http://www.who.int/hiv/topics/psychosocial/support/en/. Accessed 20
June 2013.

World Health Organisation/International Labour Organisation (2007) *Joint ILO/
WHO Guidelines on Post-exposure Prophylaxis (PEP) to Prevent HIV Infection*. http://
www.who.int/hiv/pub/guidelines/PEP/en/. Accessed 30 May 2010.

World Health Organisation/UNAIDS/UNICEF (2011) *Global HIV/AIDS Response:
Epidemic Update and Health Sector Progress Towards Universal Access 2011*. Geneva:
WHO.

World Health Organisation/UNAIDS/UNICEF (2013) *Global Update on HIV
Treatment 2013*. Geneva: WHO. http://www.unaids.org/en/media/unaids/
contentassets/documents/unaidspublication/2013/20130630_treatment_
report_en.pdf. Accessed 30 June 2013.

Young, I. (1989) Polity and group difference: A critique of the ideal of universal
citizenship. *Ethics* 99: 250–74.

Yuval-Davis, N. (2006) Intersectionality and feminist politics. *European Journal of
Women's Studies*, special issue on intersectionality, 13, 3: 193–209.

Zablotska, I., Prestage, G., De Wit, J., Grulich, A., Mao, L., and Holt, M. (2012) The
informal use of anti-retrovirals for preexposure prophylaxis among gay men in
Australia. *Journal of Acquired Immune Deficiency Syndrome* 62, 3: 334–8.

Zuch, M., and Lurie, M. (2012) 'A virus and nothing else': The effect of ART on
HIV-related stigma in rural South Africa. *AIDS Behaviour* 16, 3: 564–70.

Zungu, N. (2012) Social representations of AIDS and narratives of risk among
Xhosa men. PhD thesis, University of Cape Town.

Index